DISASTER VICTIMS' CARE IN HOSPITALS

DISASTER VICTIMS' CARE IN HOSPITALS

DISASTER VICTIMS' CARE IN HOSPITALS

(Encyclopaedia of Hospital Management—10)

DR. S.L. GOEL

Professor of Public Administration (Retd.),
Panjab University, Chandigarh
Editor, Indian Journal of Public Administration, IIPA, New Delhi
Former Member, UGC, Former Member Distance Education Council
Former Member All India Board of Management, AICTE
Member, Executive Council, IIPA, New Delhi.
Former Vice-President, IIPA, New Delhi.
Emeritus Fellow, University Grants Commission
Former Director, State Bank of India (Local Board) Chandigarh
Former Director, National Horticulture Board, Ministry of Agriculture,
Government of India, New Delhi.

and

DR. R. KUMAR

MBBS, MS, Ex. PGI
President, Chandigarh Ophthalmological Society, 2000-01,
Columnist on Health Education and Management,
Advisor on Health Care and Medical Tourism,
Member Tourism Advisory Forum,
Chandigarh Administration, Chandigarh

DEEP & DEEP PUBLICATIONS PVT. LTD.

F-159, Rajouri Garden, New Delhi-110027

DISASTER VICTIMS' CARE IN HOSPITALS
(Encyclopaedia of Hospital Management—10)

ISBN 978-81-8450-225-1

Typeset by S.S. COMPOSERS
3190, Mohindra Park, Shakur Basti, Delhi-110034.

Printed in India at MAYUR ENTERPRISES
WZ Plot No. 3, Gujjar Market, Tihar Village, New Delhi-110018.

Published by DEEP & DEEP PUBLICATIONS PVT. LTD.
F-159, Rajouri Garden, New Delhi-110027.
Phones: 25435369, 25440916
E-mail: ddpbooks@yahoo.co.in • ddpubs@gmail.com
Showroom:
2/13, Ansari Road, Daryaganj, New Delhi-110002 • Telefax: 23245122

Contents

Contents

Preface

In disasters, people lose loved ones, relatives and friends, and they lose property, above all, in psychological terms, they lose faith. It may involve a flood, torrential rain or tidal wave. Others include earthquakes, volcanic eruptions, lava, firestorms, lightening strikes, tornadoes, typhoons, cyclones, hurricanes, or some other desolation. Man-made disasters include attacks by atomic bombs, chemical warfare, terrorist attacks and so forth. One is usually terrified in a catastrophe situation, as the life seems in jeopardy. When the disaster strikes, power goes out, all modes of communication becomes inoperable, lifts stop functioning, drinking water becomes contaminated, normal modes of transportation suddenly becomes impossible, and casualties start coming in groups that is not the time for planning but that is the time of acting. This fact makes it imperative for community disaster preparedness and particularly health care system with its critical component "the hospital" which are to be prepared consistently to mobilize all their facilities for maximum use. To create a medical community, which is adequately knowledgeable about the disasters, natural or otherwise, it is likely to face and the safe ways of surviving community affected. The ultimate aim of disaster management plan is to save as many lives as possible by providing best possible medical care under those circumstances. The use of satellite, computers, electronics, better communication facilities are going to make significant difference in disaster management. The data processing and computers are providing a useful tool in decision-making in disaster.

Declaration of disaster depends on gravity or magnitude of situation, number of victims involved, time factor, i.e. Suddenness of an event, availability of medical care in terms of space, equipments, medical and paramedical staff, medicines and other basic human needs, i.e. food, shelter and clothing, weather conditions in the locality of incident, etc. Thus, enhancing human sufferings and create human needs that the victims cannot alleviate without assistance.

The aims and objectives after the victims are shifted to a hospital—

- To ensure immediate medical intervention in life threatening situation.
- To expedite the care of patients through an accurate initial assessment of urgency.

- To ensure that patients are prioritized for treatment in accordance with the severity of their medical condition.
- To reduce the morbidity associated with medical conditions through early intervention.
- To assist patient requiring treatment in another hospital, department, or community health services.
- To improve public relations by communicating accurate information to friends and relatives who accompany patients.
- Sorting of dead from injured.
- Fixing of identity is a great challenge for Forensic Expert and in almost all cases autopsy is to be performed as unknown, unclaimed dead bodies.
- Postmortem examination of all the casualties is must to confirm the cause of death.
- Fixing Identity and confirmation of event by preservation and collection of evidences for Forensic Examination (DNA Evidence, Blood Grouping, etc.).
- Almost all wounded patients need Casualty Services.
- For Postmortem Examination, Demarcation of additional staff and space and rapid disposal of cases is the need of hour in cases of Mass Casualties.
- For creating Temporary Mortuary, use of tents, folding tables and adequate quantity of equipments may be needed.
- Mobile Vans may be used for 'On the Site Postmortem Examination'.
- Facility of 'Cold Storage Cabinets' or arrangement of Ice Cubes (blocks) for keeping the dead bodies till waiting for relatives or final disposition of dead bodies may be available.
- Provision for adequate water supply, arrangement of lights must be ensured before performing 'On the Site Postmortem Examination'.
- Another important point needs emphasis here is to ask for adequate security arrangements to avoid 'Secondary Disaster' due to Law and Order problems.
- Removing traffic jams or road blocks so that clear passage may be available for relief vehicles, ambulance, and fire brigade vehicles, etc.
- Prevention of any untoward effects like break down of electric, water, and gas supply.
- To assist Fireman in obtaining adequate water for Fire Fighting.
- Rescue operations particularly of removing victims from under debris, etc.
- Prevention of 'Secondary Disaster': 'Disaster Over Disaster' due to law and order problems during treatment, like public outrage, conflicts between hospital staff and attendants of patient's or so called self-made local leaders, creating strike like situation.

The Disaster Management mechanism is needed to take care of the following:

A. Saving human life and providing medical help to the victims.
B. Controlling/preventing further damage to the property.
C. Restoring normal living conditions in the affected area.

The hospitals have to be in a state of preparedness for dealing with a disaster situation, since there is no time to be lost. The resources have to be optimally mobilized and utilized since the demands outweigh the supply. (See Appendix at the end of the Book.)

It is hoped that this book on "Disaster Victims' Care in Hospitals" would make a modest contribution to the knowledge and existing literature on this expanding field. Besides, this would help the academicians, national health officials, public health administrations, medical research workers and the policy-makers and planners in the proper understanding of health care delivery system. We will consider our labour well rewarded if the findings of the study are translated to provide decent health care to the millions of people living in rural areas, urban slums and tribal areas. Comments and suggestions from the readers would always be welcome.

The authors have dealt the aspects of hospital management for disaster casualties in the following chapters.

1. Introduction to Disaster Management; Hospitals' Role
2. First Receivers of Disaster Victims in Hospitals
3. Triage in Mass Casualty Disasters
4. Role of Appropriate Medical Leadership and Technology during Disaster
5. Preparedness and Emergency Communication Systems
6. Management of Blast and Burn Injuries during Disaster
7. International Agencies in Relief of Natural Disasters
8. Lapses in Health Care of Disaster Victims
9. Weapons of Mass Destruction and Hospital Preparedness

Appendix 1: Incident Command System (ICS)

Chandigarh

S.L. GOEL
R. KUMAR

1

Introduction to Disaster Management: Hospitals' Role

The period of 1970 alone accounted for deaths of over 1 million persons and destruction of property over 46 billion dollars by Cyclones, Hurricanes, Tornados, Earthquakes, Floods and other disasters (UNDRO, 1979). In Past Century more than 10 million people died due to Floods, Earthquakes and Tropical Storms (United Nation, 1983). Disasters strike with sudden violence, snuffing out lives, mutilating bodies, and setting families apart. It seems to have a peculiar ferocity in terms of suddenness and violence, and kindle powerful emotions such as anger and despair. 'This will never happen again', is the wish that everybody will like to cherish. To believe that the current disaster is the last is a dangerous fallacy, because it leaves us unprepared in planning the management of victims and also preparing hospitals to manage future victims of disasters. Sitting at home witnessing natural disasters such as the Bhuj Earthquake or attack by terrorists on Taj Hotel Mumbai through the eye of the television camera, there may be little sense of reality. When a disaster strikes the feeling of the onlookers or TV watchers is that 'It won't happen to us, it always happens to someone else.' The fact is that we are living in the thick of disasters, which can happen everyday and everywhere. The bus and rail accidents, community and class clashes, riots, political rivalry based attacks esp. during the elections and many others. The Nuclear Bomb was dropped in Hiroshima and Nagasaki in 1945, since then the threat of Nuclear War is ever increasing (Mass Casualties Management, 1983). Increasing Nuclear Power Plants the world over inevitably carry the risk of accidents like manifested in the Three Mile Island and Chernobyl. One of the worst Industrial Disasters in the World "Bhopal Gas Tragedy" occurred in the Night of 3rd-4th December, 1984 which killed 2500 victims and led to hospitalization of 17,500 victims, besides, incapacitating thousands. Many deaths, morbidity and suffering of thousands could have been saved in Bhopal with proper disaster management. The 'Chemical Disaster Prevention Day' being observed all over India on 4th December every year is a grim reminder of the worst recorded accident in the history of Chemical Industry.

What can happen?

In disasters, people lose loved ones, relatives and friends, and they lose property, above all, in psychological terms, they lose faith. It may involve a flood, torrential rain or tidal wave. Others include earthquakes, volcanic eruptions, lava, firestorms, lightning strikes, tornadoes, typhoons, cyclones, hurricanes, or some other desolation. Man-made disasters include attacks by atomic bombs, chemical warfare, terrorist attacks and so forth. One is usually terrified in a catastrophe situation, as the life seems in jeopardy.

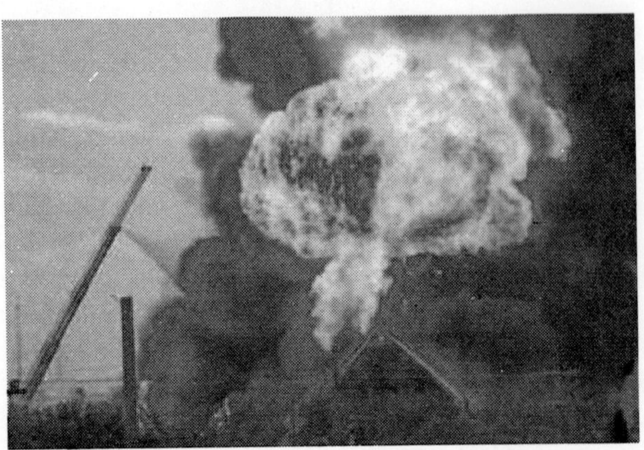

When the disaster strikes, power goes out, all modes of communication becomes inoperable, lifts stop functioning, drinking water becomes contaminated, normal modes of transportation suddenly becomes impossible, and casualties start coming in groups that is not the time for planning but that is the time of acting. This fact makes it imperative for community disaster preparedness and particularly health care system with its critical component "the hospital" which are to be prepared consistently to mobilize all their facilities for maximum use. To create a medical community, which is adequately knowledgeable about the disasters, natural or otherwise, it is likely to face and the safe ways of surviving community affected. The ultimate aim of disaster management plan is to save as many lives as possible by providing best possible medical care under those circumstances. The use of satellite, computers, electronics, better communication facilities are going to make significant difference in disaster management. The data processing and computers are providing a useful tool in decision-making in disaster.

There is a need for change of strategy from 'post-disaster reactive approach' to 'pre-disaster pro-active approach' to reduce the damage, losses to the property, and human sufferings along with prevention of human lives on one hand and reduce the cost of relief, rehabilitation and reconstruction on the other hand. The aim of disaster management is basically the prevention and minimization of death, disability, sufferings and losses. Disaster management means a planned and systemic approach towards understanding and solving problems in the wake of disasters.

Definition

The Oxford Dictionary describes disaster as "A sudden Calamitous event bringing great damage, loss or destruction". WHO Definition: "A situation, which implies unforeseen serious and immediate threat to public health". Colin Grant's Definition: "Catastrophe causing injury or illness simultaneously to at least thirty people who will require hospital emergency treatment" (Colin Grant's, 1973). Rutherford's Definition: "An emergency of such magnitude as to require extraordinary mobilization of medical services" (Rutherford, 1974). Jenkins's Definition: "Disaster needs declaration when immediate patient load in the emergency medical services system is greater than normal, operator can care for" (Jenkins, 1978).

It entails Unforeseen, Serious and Immediate threat to Public Health, i.e. Suddenness in terms of time; and a state of Emergency; Calamity, Catastrophe, Misadventure, Tragedy, Epidemic, Cataclysm, etc.; where number of casualties far exceeds medical facilities in normal situation that disrupts the normal routine of life, i.e. Magnitude in terms of severity of damage or deaths. In other words declaration of disaster depends on gravity or magnitude of situation, number of victims involved, time factor, i.e. Suddenness of an event, availability of medical care in terms of space, equipments, medical and paramedical staff, medicines and other basic human needs, i.e. food, shelter and clothing, weather conditions in the locality of incident, etc. Thus, enhancing human sufferings and create human needs that the victims cannot alleviate without assistance.

CLASSIFICATION

Disasters have been classified in various ways but the most convenient method used in classification of disasters is in two distinct categories according to their causes.

1. Natural Disaster.
2. Man-made Disaster.

Western Countries classified disasters as follows:

(1) NATURAL DISASTERS

(i) NATURAL PHENOMENON BENEATH EARTH'S SURFACE

(a) Earthquakes.
(b) Volcanic eruptions.

(ii) NATURAL PHENOMENA AT EARTH'S SURFACE

(a) Land slides.
(b) Avalanches.
(c) Metrological/Hydrological Phenomenon.
(d) Wind Storms (Cyclones, Typhoon, Hurricane).
(e) Tornadoes.
(f) Hail Storms and Snow Storms.
(g) Sea Surges, Flash Floods or Cloud Burst.
(h) Floods.
(i) Droughts.

(iii) BIOLOGICAL PHENOMENA:

(a) Locusts Worms.
(b) Epidemics of Diseases.

(2) MAN-MADE DISASTERS

(i) CAUSED BY WARFARE:

(a) Conventional Warfare.
(b) Nuclear, Biological and Chemical Warfare.

(ii) CAUSED BY ACCIDENTS:

(a) Vehicular Accidents, (Plane, Train, Ship and Motor Car, etc.).
(b) Drowning.
(c) Collapse of Building.
(d) Explosion.
(e) Fires.
(f) Biological.
(g) Chemical Including Poisoning.

Some general principals of disaster planning are:

- It should be a continuous process.
- It should reduce the unknown in a problematic situation.
- Plan must evoke appropriate action.

- Plan must foresee what is likely to happen.
- Plan must be based on valid knowledge.
- Plan must focus on general principles.
- Plan should serve as an educational activity.
- Plan for overcoming resistance.
- Plan must be tested.

These principles include following steps:

- "Prevent" the occurrence of the disaster whenever possible.
- "Minimize the Number of Casualties" if the disaster cannot be prevented.
- "Prevent Further Casualties".
- "Rescue The Victims".
- "Provide First Aid To The Injured".
- "Evacuate The Injured To Medical Installation".
- "Provide The Definite Medical Care".
- Preparedness is supported by the necessary legislation and means a readiness to cope with disaster or similar emergencies, which could not be avoided.
- Preparedness is concerned with forecasting and working, the education and training of population, staff, organisation for and management of disaster, including preparation of operational plan, training of relief group, the stock piling of supplies and the earmarking of the necessary funds.

The aims and objectives after the victims are shifted to a hospital—

- To ensure immediate medical intervention in life threatening situation.
- To expedite the care of patients through an accurate initial assessment of urgency.
- To ensure that patients are prioritized for treatment in accordance with the severity of their medical condition.
- To reduce the morbidity associated with medical conditions through early intervention.
- To assist patient requiring treatment in another hospital, department, or community health services.
- To improve public relations by communicating accurate information to friends and relatives who accompany patients.
- Sorting of dead from injured.
- Fixing of identity is a great challenge for Forensic Expert and in almost all cases autopsy is to be performed as unknown, unclaimed dead bodies.
- Post mortem examination of all the casualties is must to confirm the cause of death.

- Fixing Identity and confirmation of event by Preservation and collection of evidences for Forensic Examination (DNA Evidence, Blood Grouping, etc.).
- Almost all wounded patients need Casualty Services.
- For Post Mortem Examination, Demarcation of additional staff and space and rapid disposal of cases is the need of hour in cases of Mass Casualties.
- For creating Temporary Mortuary, use of tents, folding tables and adequate quantity of equipments may be needed.
- Mobile vans may be used for 'On the Site Post Mortem Examination'.
- Facility of 'Cold Storage Cabinets' or arrangement of Ice Cubes (blocks) for keeping the dead bodies till waiting for relatives or final disposition of dead bodies may be available.
- Provision for adequate water supply, arrangement of lights must be ensured before performing 'On the Site Post Mortem Examination'.
- Another important point needs emphasis here is to ask for adequate security arrangements to avoid 'Secondary Disaster' due to Law and Order problems.
- Removing traffic jams or road blocks so that clear passage may be available for relief vehicles, ambulance, and fire brigade vehicles, etc.
- Prevention of any untoward effects like break down of electric, water, and gas supply.
- To assist Fireman in obtaining adequate water for Fire Fighting.
- Rescue operations particularly of removing victims from under debris, etc.
- Prevention of 'Secondary Disaster': 'Disaster Over Disaster' due to law and order problems during treatment, like public outrage, conflicts between hospital staff and attendants of patient's or so called self-made local leaders, creating strike like situation.

Functions of Nursing Management

The key to efficiency and productivity is good management, that is never more true than during a crisis or disaster. All too often, the foundation functions of management are forgotten during a crisis and the system produces more chaos than was already present. The functions of nursing management should be reviewed, as they can be applied before and during a disaster.

Formal response systems tend to break down. Communication systems notoriously fail and plans are often not implemented in the expected way. Hospitals frequently plan for the wrong things, such as dealing with lots of heavy trauma. As was observed on September 11 and with previous natural disasters, the majority of victims that make it to hospitals have relatively minor injuries. The NSF study found hospital disaster planning drills are often only mandatory for nursing staff and house officers and not for all concerned. During actual disasters, however, senior medical staff and non-emergency room medical personnel who converge often do not know emergency procedures (Glass, 2001). Contingency planning for disasters or terrorism should spell out what people should do, why it will be done, where it will be done, when it will be done, how it will be done, and who will do it. The purpose of organizing during a disaster is to establish a division of labor and a chain of command (Rowland and Rowland, 1997). Organizing combines material and human resources in an orderly arrangement that provides the basic ingredients necessary for co-ordinating efforts (Rowland and Rowland, 1997). Lack of organisation at any time can spell chaos. During a disaster crisis, it is essential that a pre-identified division of duties and assignment of authority be known to all staff.

Directing the staff initiates and maintains action. Rowland and Rowland (1997) noted that successful directing depends on delegation, communication, and training. In a disaster, pre-designated staff must receive not only a list of their exact duties but the authority to fulfil their duties so action is not delayed.

Communication provides staff the information needed to perform and also feedback related to their performance. Communication problems are common during disaster (Milsten, 2000). Telephone-dependent systems may fail with loss of electrical power and congestion. Announcements not heard can lead to panic and confusion. The NSF study found that hospital disaster drills are rarely designed to include communication failure (Glass, 2001). Briggs (2001) recommends that hospitals increase reliance on multiple channels of Communication that should include cell phones and wireless communications with multiple channels.

Coordination of effort involves synchronizing activities toward desired goals (Rowland and Rowland, 1997). Needless to say, a great deal of planning must occur to ensure harmonization of actions during a disaster, or chaos will result. Coordination occurs only through strong, effective leadership and management that organizes, directs, and controls staff efforts.

Control is a manager's duty to ensure that staff performance corresponds to plan. All managers exercise control by establishing standards, measuring performance against standards, and correcting deviations from standards (Rowland, and Rowland, 1997). Cuny (1998) identified three basic conditions necessary for control during a disaster: establishment of standards and critical pathways, information showing deviations in practice, and authority to correct problems. Managers must be given flexibility in the control process, because the goal is not to ensure that everything runs strictly according to plan, but to ensure that victims are helped to the greatest extent possible (Cuny, 1999). Nothing seems to cause a breakdown in the system more than a manager who has lost control. Leadership is essential to control and to allow persons to perform in a desired manner. In a disaster staff cannot be allowed to perform contrary to set standards and procedures. Managers must evaluate and correct skills and performance during pre-disaster planning. In disasters, managers become leaders when others look to them for guidance and direction out of respect. During a crisis, when leaders must act quickly to correct problems, an autocratic, directive leadership style will be the most efficient and effective. Disasters are not the time for debate and discussion to reach consensus.

Managerial Resources

Nurse managers have accountability over five areas: human, fiscal, material, support, and system resources (Rowland and Rowland, 1997). Managing each of these resources is vital before, during, and after a disaster.

Human resources

An everyday function of nurse managers involves providing the right people for the right work, at the right place, at the right time, and in the right numbers. Health Care is in the midst of a significant personnel shortage. It is not just a shortage of nurses, but also of pharmacists, technicians, food-service workers, and housekeepers, which is affecting hospital preparedness for disaster (Bentley, 2001). An American Hospital Association (2001) study recommends that reserve staff be enlisted during a disaster. These can be physicians, nurses, or hospital workers who are retired or have changed careers. Large number of untrained volunteers, nurses, and physicians may converge upon a hospital during a disaster. This may create management problems.

The majority of hospital nurses are female and most are responsible for the care of family members in a household. The ability of staff to remain at the hospital for extended periods of time depends on the ability of their families to be cared for (Bentley, 2001). One strategy is to allow staff to bring their families to the hospital to stay. There may not be room, however, and this may not be safe during a bioterrorist attack. Another strategy is to allow staff to go home, get their family care arranged, and return to the hospital. Managers must develop a coordinated, efficient callback system that includes a wide variety of staff from multiple resources.

Fiscal and material resources

Managers must ensure fiscal and material resources are used effectively. Times of disaster are no exception. Nursing managers can make sure their own unit supplies are stocked and equipment is in constant working order. Stockpiles of antidotes and vaccines for agents identified as threats are being strategically placed and can be moved to communities in need.

Support resources

Staff will be empowered to be self-directed, control their own relationships, and work well in teams if they have a supportive, strong manager. Managers must resolve development issues, enhance learning, provide tools to problem solve, and supply access to expert resources (Rowland and Rowland, 1997). This empowerment and self-direction will provide efficiency during a disaster.

System resources

Part of the organizing function is the ability to link resources such as experts, service supports, quality measurement, data collection, outcome measurement, and competence evaluation (Rowland and Rowland, 1997). With these resources, managers can provide support that will sustain a team's efforts during a disaster. Two useful resources for staff are a bioterrorism planning and response tool published by the Association for Professionals in Infection Control and Epidemiology.

One of the best preparations a manager can make for staff is education. The American Nurses Association has been involved in the International Nursing Coalition for Mass Casualty Education (ANA, 2001). This coalition hopes to define basic nursing competencies for response to mass casualties, design continuing education programmes for practicing nurses, and identify advanced competencies for those in leadership roles.

Sheehy, Burkle, and Kinney (1993) developed a unique disaster narrative to more effectively disseminate disaster plan information. Since most disaster plan manuals sit on shelves gathering dust, the disaster narrative conceptualizes an individual's role and puts all plausible events into perspective for each employee. The narrative is similar to a theatrical script, allowing employees to fully imagine the part they would play in a disaster. One Florida agency holds a mandatory in-service designed to help staff prepare their homes and families for disaster. If their families are prepared, the staffs are more willing and able to fully participate in actual disasters and not be worried about their families.

Regular training essential for Hospital staff

In the aftermath of a disaster, severely injured persons of all ages, some screaming, and some unconscious flood the hospitals of the area; rapidly arriving on trolleys pushed by paramedics; doctors and nurses rush in. Who should be treated first—and where? The injured may be infected, carry toxic chemicals or radioactively contaminated. 'We can't admit them to the hospital just like that!' someone cries. Too late! Only a few are well versed in the effects of large scale incidents, pandemics and mass accidents. 'Training exercises or no training exercises can sometimes mean the difference between life and death. It is important to practice processes through regular training—that's the only way to ensure that in a real emergency everything runs smoothly. Well-trained staff and optimized alarm action plans can often prevent an escalation of a crisis. One of the prerequisites for this is that the hospital continuously and critically checks its concepts for their suitability for practical use. Many hospital action plans are outdated and based around threats that no longer correspond with current reality. The terrorist attacks in the US on 11 September 2001 and those in Madrid and London showed the necessity of preparation for large-scale events through more efficient rescue strategies, and this applies to Europe and Asian countries as well.' Mumbai's terrorist attack on 26th Nov. 08 is too recent to overlook.

Disaster medicine training sessions in health care institutions should be held at least once a year, although it would be desirable to hold them more frequently. It goes without saying that not every possible scenario can be provided for with training exercises right down to the last detail, but it has been repeatedly noted that participants in such simulations under real conditions develop very creative coping strategies. Efficient crisis management is characterized by three big Cs: Command, Communication and Coordination, he explained. This means that a senior management team should be appointed to take on the coordination of individual resources, and that organised reporting channels guarantee the transfer of information—if this is not done it can lead to situations where, for example, a contaminated patient contaminates all sensitive areas within a hospital because there has been insufficient preparation and structuring of his transfer through the building. In particular, the responsibilities and distribution of executive functions should be clarified before it is too late. 'The incident command team must be determined'. 'They take over the strategic management and coordination of the crisis on site. Hospitals are ethically and legally obliged to ensure the best possible medical care for patients in the case of catastrophes despite limited resources.'

The recommendations in Indian context

Justice R.C. Chopra committee observed the need for having an effective and efficient Disaster Management mechanism and that it is essential to meet situations arising out of natural disasters, accidents affecting large number, bomb blasts, riots, floods as well as conditions during war times.

1. The Disaster Management mechanism is needed to take care of the following:

A. Saving human life and providing medical help to the victims.
B. Controlling/preventing further damage to the property.
C. Restoring normal living conditions in the affected area.

2. Many times situations arising out of earthquakes, floods, fires, train accidents, bomb explosions or enemy attacks on civilian population, cannot be handled effectively by Government machinery on account of enormity of damage and as such public participation becomes essential. It has also been seen that large number of people reach the spot and try to help the victims but they are neither trained nor well equipped to render meaningful assistance and as such add to the confusion. Thus, there is a need to have

trained citizens who may give effective support to the Government machinery and supplement its efforts in the hour of need.

3. National Level Authority as well as State Level Authorities are required to draw, implement and monitor Disaster Management Plans. At District Level we need well equipped and thoroughly trained Government machinery as well as volunteers ready to come forward when the calamity strikes and take immediate steps to manage and control the situation.

Action Plan

4. The following proposals may be considered while preparing a Disaster Management Plan for Delhi:

(I) The State Level Disaster Management Authority should establish Disaster Management Units to cover all parts of the city and one way for establishing such Units is to set-up one Disaster Management Unit for one or two Police Station jurisdictions. This Unit be established in a police station itself for the reason that in case of emergency/calamity the police is the first to swing into action and this Unit being located in the police station itself can also swiftly come into action. SHO of the Police Station or the area SDM may be designated the officers Incharge of such Disaster Management Units. The District Magistrate of the area may be the overall Controlling Officer of all such Units falling within his District.

(II) Essential equipments/machines required for handling building collapse and fire fighting should be kept ready in each of these Units so that in case of a localized and smaller disaster the Disaster Management Unit of that area itself is in a position to handle the situation with the help of Fire Brigade. If the disaster be of greater magnitude additional help may be requisitioned from the Disaster Management Units of the adjoining areas. The equipment may be kept under the custody of the SHO or the officer next to him so that at the time of need these are readily available to DMU, which should start helping victims without any loss of time.

(III) All the police officers attached to a Police Station should be trained to handle rescue operations so that immediately on reaching the place of 'incident they start helping the victims'.

(IV) Each DMU should be directly linked telephonically with a Hospital in the area so that at the time of emergency the DMU as well as Doctors attached to the particular DMU may reach the spot without any loss of time and assist the victims of disaster. The DMU Incharge, Medical Officer and the Fire Officer of the area may have hotline facilities for communication round the clock so that in case of emergency they are in touch immediately.

The medical unit attached with each DMU or group of DMUs be headed by a designated Medical Officer who should have in his custody earmarked stocks of medicines/drugs and necessary equipment's required for giving immediate medical aid so that at the eleventh hour they do not start looking here and there for procuring these things.

(V) Every DMU to associate PWD Engineers of the area also so that the Engineers also reach the site of incident and guide DMU and others in the matter of rescuing victims trapped inside buildings.

(VI) For each DMU at least 150 responsible volunteers between the age group of 20 to 25 years, preferably college students, be selected for the following emergency duties:

(a) 50 volunteers be trained in fire fighting and rescue operations. At the time of crisis they should reach the spot wearing a prescribed colour jacket/cap as well as photo I-Cards and start helping the Police/Fire Brigade officials.

(b) 50 volunteers to be trained for Para-Medical help to assist the Medical Team at the spot. They should have a separate colour jacket/cap as well as photo I-Cards so that the medical team starts taking assistance from them, if required.

(c) 50 volunteers to be trained for controlling traffic as well as crowd and protect the person and property of the victims in the hour of crisis. They should wear a different color jacket/cap and should have photo I-Cards.

(d) These volunteers may be drawn preferably from the residential areas falling under the jurisdiction of a DMU with the help of RWAs so that they do not take long to reach the place of incident.

(e) After the age of 25 these volunteers be retired but should continue to be on the roll of DMU so that they can be summoned as and when required. The vacancies arising out the retirement of the volunteers should be filled up from other eligible persons so that more and more are trained and drafted into the scheme.

(VII) The Commanding Officer of the Army detailed in the area should also be a member of the State Level Disaster Management authority and he should be requested to keep in readiness a separate unit of the army officers to assist the Civil Administration in case of acute emergency. Army officers may also be requested to train the volunteers. It would be better if in due course the trainers are sent to advanced countries also for receiving training and then prepared for imparting training to the volunteers.

(VIII) The advantage of involving general public in the Disaster

Management Plan is the quick availability of the locals in the rescue operations and inculcating in them a spirit of social responsibility.

(IX) The volunteers for Disaster Management Units should be given intensive training on holidays and those who exhibit courage and grit during difficult 'situations should be honored and adequately rewarded by the State'.

(X) This Action Plan does not require heavy expenditure on the part of the Government but still makes available a large crop of trained hands for meeting an emergency. Such trained volunteers can effectively assist the Government to manage and control large-scale disasters and help in avoiding unnecessary chaos and confusions, which often take place in such situations.

USA experiences; Putting procedures in place

The Federal Emergency Management Agency's (FEMA) 'Disaster Medical Assistance Teams' (DMATs) were staged in the Gulf Region prior to Hurricane Katrina made landfall and have been on the ground treating patients ever since. The teams have treated more than 100,000 patients of Hurricanes Katrina and Rita todate, the largest population served in the teams' history. "They started out in mash-style tent operations during the immediate response and now are supporting hospitals where staff is still evacuated or were themselves victims of the hurricane. They are trained to work in disaster settings and their work has been heroic and tireless through these last four weeks." "Our team, made up of doctors, nurses and other medical support team members from Texas supported the Katrina efforts early on and we are now rotating back into Texas after a brief break," said Mona Khanna, M.D., M.P.H. Medical Officer for the Texas 4 DMAT Team, who brings expertise in internal medicine and public disaster health to FEMA medical aid efforts. Just one piece of National Disaster Medical System is FEMA's Disaster Medical Assistance Teams. These 55 teams located across the nation deploy to disaster sites to provide medical care at a fixed or temporary medical care site—a tent, a shelter, a hospital or other facility—with supplies and equipment sufficient to sustain their operations for a period of 72 hours. Additional supplies then push in behind after their immediate arrival. These teams' responsibilities include providing emergency care for serious needs from stabilizing critical care patients to administering immunizations. The teams provide high-quality medical care despite the adverse and austere environment often found at a disaster site.

In some situations, DMATs may provide primary medical care or may serve to augment overloaded local health care staffs. Under the rare circumstance that disaster victims are evacuated to a different locale to receive definitive medical care, DMATs may be activated to support patient reception and disposition of patients to hospitals.

The National Disaster Medical System assets overseen at DHS-FEMA include:

- 55 Disaster Medical Assistance Teams (DMATs), which include federal, state, local and private medical professionals. In addition, there are specialized teams to handle burns, pediatrics, crush injuries, surgery and mental health;
- 11 Disaster Mortuary Operational Response Teams (DMORTs)—which consist of private citizens with specialized training and experience to help in the recovery, identification and processing of deceased victims;
- 4 National Medical Response Teams (NMRTs), to deal with the medical consequences of incidents potentially involving chemical, biological or nuclear materials;
- 4 Veterinary Medical Assistance Teams (VMATs), which include clinician veterinarians, pathologists, animal health technicians, microbiologists and others who assist animal disaster victims and provide care to search dogs;
- 3 International Medical Surgical Teams (IMSuRTs)—one operational and two under development—highly specialized, trained and equipped to establish a fully capable free-standing field surgical facility anywhere in the world; and
- National Disaster Medical Assistance Teams have recently responded to large-scale disasters including: The World Trade Center in September 2001, Hurricane Isabel in September 2003 and treated approximately 10,000 patients during the four hurricanes that hit Florida in 2004, in addition to many other disasters.

FEMA prepares the nation for all hazards and manages federal response and recovery efforts following any national incident. FEMA also initiates mitigation activities, trains first responders, works with state and local emergency managers, and manages the National Flood Insurance Programme and the U.S. Fire Administration. FEMA became part of the U.S. Department of Homeland Security on March 1, 2003.

In October 2006 new, federally sponsored standards and guidelines for hospital incident preparedness and response were drawn up in the US. The US Department of Health and Human Services (HHS) designated the Hospital Incident Command System IV (HICS IV) as the hospital industry's route to achieving compliance with National Incident Management Systems (NIMS). "Inter-operable communications which aid cooperation between hospitals and emergency response teams in the vicinity of a disaster are now the focus." All hospitals who received federal funding to implement the plan were due to have it operational at the end of September 2008.

Los Angeles-based Port Blue is providing ICS solutions to over 200 US hospitals throughout California, Los Angeles and Texas, to meet NIMS requirements with its Command Aware hospital incident management software. Port Blue chief executive Paul Dimitruk says the heart of Command Aware is the interactive dashboard covering each role in the command structure. This includes all disaster management professionals, clinical personnel and hospital administration.

The system provides hospital managers with situation awareness, answering questions from how many ventilators an Intensive Care Unit might have available to whether the engineering department has fixed the drains. Data can be "rolled up" from the unit level, to the facility, system and regional levels and operates at all levels of incident management from preparation to mitigation, response and recovery. The system also works on a day-to-day level to track beds, supplies, equipment and personnel. Dimitruk says Command Aware has performed well in the recent surge of disasters across America, including Hurricanes Gustav, Hanna and Ike, in the recent Southern California earthquake and in the recent tragic Metro train wreck in Los Angeles. "The system has proven very effective, particularly as a communications platform when other forms of communication backed up or failed," he says. "During Ike, the mobile phone and other incident command systems were largely down, but Command Aware was up throughout." The system also offers up-to-date chemical and biological agent identification and treatment protocols. Dimitruk says because HICS IV tenets are built into the application, the education burden on staff is reduced.

"Command Aware simplifies the process of assigning different responsibilities to staff members under different hazard conditions."

"Users can apply best practices, even if they aren't disaster management experts or haven't yet received HICS IV training," he explains. "Command Aware simplifies the process of assigning different responsibilities to staff members under different hazard conditions. For example, with a few clicks, emergency management staff can establish different response teams and procedures for a tornado *versus* an earthquake." The system will get its largest test in November when it will be part of a massive six-day-long earthquake drill, "Great Southern Shakeout". The County of Los Angeles has directed all hospitals in the county to use Command Aware for the drill.

Global efforts

In the UK the NHS updated its Emergency Planning Guidance in December 2007, refreshing the section on command, control and co-ordination. The guidance focuses on co-ordination between Trusts, Special Health Authorities and Primary Care Organisations and establishes a command and response structure and guidelines.

The guidance covers health authorities within their respective regional boundaries, while also taking into account the possible need for networking between Scotland, Wales, Northern Ireland and colleagues in the wider EU on aid missions.

Nottingham University Hospitals NHS Trust is at the forefront of emergency preparedness in the UK, investing more than £1m over the last year to improve its resilience and emergency preparedness. The Trust has invested over half a million on enhancing emergency communications and site security, with new video conferencing facilities, as well as £150,000 on mass disaster equipment, £39,000 on new oxygen units and a remaining £30,000 on new flying squad equipment.

The communication facilities were provided by US-based Life Size, a high definition video communications product which allows staff to communicate and interact from distance at any bandwidth.

"Nottingham University Hospitals NHS Trust is at the forefront of emergency preparedness in the UK, investing more than £1m over the last year." "The video and audio quality of Life Size Room, and the ability to share clinical information at a much higher level than has been available in the past, is incredible," said Rob Hall from Nottingham University Hospitals NHS Trusts ICT Department at its launch. "Life Size Room has to be seen by clinicians to understand the full extent of its potential uses in health care." The hospital has also signed a multi-million pound deal with Cisco to implement a network infrastructure which will support a range of applications to help enhance health care services. One of the main benefits is access to a wireless network, providing real-time access to information at the bedside and ensuring that clinicians can be contacted anywhere on site. The project started in April 2008 and is due for completion in March 2010.

"The Cisco Medical-Grade Network connects all stakeholders in the health care system to one information and communications infrastructure as a connected health care ecosystem and provides the foundation for advanced health care solutions," said Terry Espiner, regional sales manager for Cisco, when the announcement was made.

"The Nottingham University Hospitals NHS Trust is set to become one of the UK's showcase examples of how health care providers can use networking technologies to transform the delivery of health care services."

Inter-operability is the way forward

Whether preparing for a mass antidote administration or dealing with mass casualties, in a post 9/11 environment, hospitals around the world must develop specific emergency management plans. A white paper from software giant Oracle says interoperable data sharing is the way forward for security and emergency planning, emphasizing the need to develop new ways to share data across agencies and government offices. Oracle has a series of products that can be used together to build integrated systems capable of pulling and displaying data from multiple sources. "Software giant Oracle says interoperable data sharing is the way forward for security and emergency planning." Information could then be made available to first responders and other government agencies. In some cases, the information can be provided via single sign-on systems developed specifically for incident management. Other web-based applications like mapping technology being used by the US Center for Disease Control and Prevention's Injury department will also aid preparedness. The same tool could be used by health care professionals to create regional maps illustrating illness patterns and virus movements, which in turn can help policy-makers form decisions and support public health initiatives.

As Government departments, Health Authorities and Trusts increasingly need to share information, interoperable data sharing; secure communications and reliable planning systems are becoming the vital keys to ensuring emergency preparedness. Emergencies such as the likes of Hurricane Katrina test the preparedness of hospitals and their systems to their limit. Integrated communications systems can enable interoperable data sharing and access to essential information throughout the entirety of a hospital building. Software systems such as Command Aware from Port blue can assign hospital staff to different hazards in emergency events.

One hospital's experiences; lessons to be learnt

Prudence dictates that hospitals have plans to deal with multiple casualty incidents, but few of us believe we will ever take part in an actual disaster response. Recommendations for the regular rehearsal of disaster plans often receive low priority, given the myriad of other pressing health care problems. Recently, however, when the Red Deer Regional Hospital (RDRH) was forced to deal with the aftermath of the Pine Lake tornado, the value of a well prepared disaster plan was reinforced (Hogarth and Gordon). Red Deer Regional Hospital, a 309-bed regional hospital, is located midway between Calgary and Edmonton, Alberta's 2 tertiary cardiovascular, thoracic and neurosurgical referral centres. RDRH has a substantial, but incomplete, complement of surgical specialties and accepts referrals from several smaller Central Alberta hospitals. The emergency department (ED) has 23 beds and functions at or above capacity most of the time, seeing approximately 50,000 patients annually.

On Friday, July 14, 2000, at 1900 hours, an F3 tornado touched down at Pine Lake, Alberta, just 40 kilometres from Red Deer, and destroyed a popular campground. News of the tornado reached the hospital when victims began arriving by private vehicle. Moments later, the first emergency medical services (EMS) crew reached the scene and radioed confirmation. They estimated 50 "red" and 150 "yellow" victims, but others called in estimates ranging as high as 600 casualties, with 300 walking wounded and 150 "red" victims.

At 1945 hours, the RDRH disaster plan was activated. Hospital staff was called in using the hospital's paging system and by telephone fan-outs. The ambulance bay was converted to a triage area and the ED was cleared by admitting or discharging patients. Several patients discharged themselves when they heard the scope of the disaster, and 48 ward beds were cleared by discharging stable patients and issuing passes. A command centre was established in the admitting area adjacent to the ED and a manpower pool was set-up in the auditorium. Because of the large number of severely injured patients anticipated, additional treatment areas were prepared in the OR recovery room, the day surgery and endoscopy areas, and the outpatient department. Additional supplies were brought to these areas.

Victim arrival

As is common in disasters, the first patients arrived early, by private vehicle, while the triage area was being organised and before the ED had been cleared. Close behind were the ground ambulances, carrying some of the most severely injured patients—mostly, victims of blunt trauma. An emergency physician and several ED nurses performed triage in the ambulance bay while admitting staff prepared a disaster chart for each victim. Charts stayed with patients, on the stretcher, until admission to a ward or discharge. "Red" victims (head and chest injuries), went to the ED and OR recovery room, "yellow" victims (multiple orthopedic injuries and significant wounds) went to the day surgery and endoscopy areas and "green" patients (isolated orthopedic injuries and lacerations) went to the outpatient department. These victims were moved efficiently to their defined treatment areas.

Air ambulances soon began arriving. Unfortunately, because RDRH is built on a hill and there is no suitable landing site near the ED, the helipad is at the opposite end of the hospital, necessitating long stretcher trips through the hospital—against the normal patient flow. This precluded appropriate triage and caused problems with admitting documentation. When the problem became apparent, a makeshift helipad was constructed by removing the vehicles and light standards from the ED parking; however, this work was not completed in time for the helicopters arriving from Pine Lake. In total, 85 victims, including 20 red, 35 yellow and 30 green, were seen and treated before midnight. Of these, 29 were admitted and 9 were transferred to tertiary care centres.

Hospital staff

Soon after disaster activation, ward nursing staff moved to the ED, leaving inpatient units poorly covered. An ineffective fan-out process had physicians phoning or arriving in the crowded ED, wondering what was going on and how they could help. Physicians and nurses arrived from other communities to offer their assistance—often with no means of confirming their identity or qualifications. As physicians and nurses arrived, they were assigned to specific areas. Surgeons staffed the red and yellow areas, and they triaged patients to the operating rooms. Medical consultants discharged stable patients and readied beds in the intensive care unit. Family physicians worked in the yellow and green areas. One emergency physician oversaw each treatment area and the rest were distributed as needed. In addition, an emergency physician was designated as the coordinator of physician resources and as the transfer liaison. This physician was not involved in direct patient care but this position was extremely worthwhile in maintaining patient flow. Radiologists expedited patient care by immediately interpreting all studies and writing their interpretation on the film folder.

Ancillary areas

A centre for relatives of the victims was set-up in a nearby elementary school. Unfortunately, the site had too few telephones and a poor computer link to the hospital. As a result, relatives endured long waits to use a telephone and to obtain information about their injured family members. Other areas that were outlined in the disaster plan, including a childcare centre (for children of staff) and a discharge holding area (for inpatients, ED patients and discharged disaster victims forced to rapidly vacate their beds), were never set-up. The lack of a childcare centre necessitated that the spouses of some staff members supervised the children of others who came to help.

External communication

Accurate information from the disaster scene was scarce during the early hours after the tornado strike. After the initial estimate of 50 red and 150 yellow victims there were only a few calls from the scene requesting that we accept further patients. Because there was only one telephone line into the hospital's command centre, these calls came instead to the ED.

Early on, one of the tertiary referral sites received notification from the scene that they should prepare for 150 red patients. The hospital rapidly cleared 130 inpatient beds in anticipation of these victims, then phoned to offer us physicians and nurse support. They are to be commended for their rapid mobilization.

Internal communication

Within the hospital there were several communication problems. Some ancillary areas needed computer installation and phone hookup, which led to delays. Overhead pages were not audible in all areas of the hospital. Some staff members lacked identifying hats or uniforms, therefore were not identifiable to other staff. Nursing staff who were manning the phones received incomplete information from the emergency physician coordinator, and it was difficult to get accurate information on the status of the victim treatment areas without physically visiting them. Therefore, ED staff lacked up-to-date information on hospital resource availability when requests to transfer patients from the scene arrived.

Transfers

Nine patients were transferred to tertiary care centres. In some cases, confusion arose when RDRH staff and air ambulance personnel independently made different transfer arrangements to different destinations—neither being aware of what the other was doing. For example, after arranging ground transport for some patients, hospital staff learned that helicopters were already preparing to shuttle the same patients to the local airport, where fixed-wing planes were waiting to transfer them to the tertiary care centres. On more than one occasion, relatives were told that a patient was being sent to one city when, in fact, they were routed to the other.

Crowd control and public relations

Many relatives and family members entered the hospital through the emergency and main entrances before these were secured. We were subsequently forced to remove them from the ED and sequester them in the radiology waiting room.

The RDRH command centre handled all calls from the public and the media, but shut down at 0400, only 8 hours after the disaster. Unfortunately, the telephone number that the hospital provided for the Red Cross was not their disaster number, and the line was staffed only during business hours. Consequently, the ED—already swamped—was forced to deal with large numbers of calls from relatives trying to locate victims.

Enhancing Hospital Disaster Preparedness

Better management of hospital resources and staff could greatly improve preparedness for disasters such as the tsunami that had hit South East Asia a few years ago, according to an article by J. Christopher Farmer and colleagues, published in the journal of Critical Care.

To date, disaster medical response has predominantly focused on pre-hospital issues such as triage, evacuation, and transport of casualties, and has largely assumed that hospital management would occur as planned. The intensive care unit (ICU) is an essential link in the chain of events that follow a disaster, write Farmer and colleagues. Hospitals across the world have limited bed capacity and staffs are often not prepared for critical situations.

As recent events have shown, hospitals can quickly be overwhelmed in the event of a disaster. This is also the case in countries where hospital facilities are thought to be large, modern and sufficiently equipped. For example, after the terrorist bombing in Bali in 2002, 15 patients requiring mechanical ventilation were sent to an Australian hospital, which could only care for a maximum of 12 ventilated patients. Floods in Houston Texas in 2001 quickly led to unavailability of ICU beds. Innumerable examples of attacks and environmental disasters have reinforced that hospital capacity is the major rate-limiting factor during a disaster medical response.

In the paper, Farmer and colleagues suggest improved, hospital-focused training, more detailed co-operation between hospitals, and the dual use of hospital infrastructure and resources. For example, resources currently directed for hospital patient safety could be repurposed to improve training, planning, and effectiveness of the disaster medical response. They argue that critical care professionals should be offered better, more targeted disaster medical training that includes exercises in realistic disaster situation simulations, emphasizing hospital response. In addition, web-based knowledge collections should be available to health workers for last minute, quick and easy querying at the time of an event.

Co-operation between hospitals in the vicinity of a disaster must improve, with improved communications, better training and planning, and triage algorithms that can help move hospital staff as opposed to patients. Currently, for a large-scale disaster patients are segregated to specific facilities according to condition or patient-based resource allocation. Planning and preparedness would allow for a better, more efficient exchange of material and human resources when needed.

In all, the most pressing needs are education and training, and more detailed planning that acknowledges the specific disaster medical needs of hospitals and ICU's worldwide. In the context of India and other Asian countries following questions arise.

1. In earthquake prone areas in Asia, are the hospitals structurally sound?
2. Do they have operational plans in cases of earthquake disaster, and in cases of hospital collapse?
3. Can the medical doctors in those hospitals and clinics who in normal times treat patients on an individual basis, treat the earthquake-injured people "en masse"?

Programme for Enhancement of Emergency Response (PEER) Update

The PEER programme aims to improve the search and rescue capacity and performance of emergency first responders, to conduct, effectively assess, treat and transport disaster victims, and to plan for, undertake and manage effective search and rescue operations. A two-week regional training course for Medical First Responders (MFR) was successfully conducted in April 2000 with 24 participants from the four partner countries of Indonesia, the Philippines, India and Nepal. PEER received

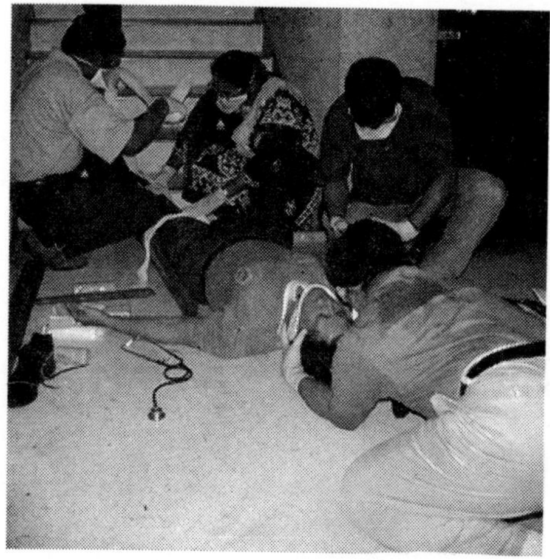

technical support from Miami Dade Fire Rescue Department which provided eight instructors to organize this interactive and performance-based course. To pass the minimum performance standard, participants had to take four skills assessment stations and written tests. Yet, it was necessary at national level to identify needs and adapt the curriculum to meet local protocol in each country. A workshop on MFR materials adaptation will be conducted by the end of 2000.

Training for Instructors (TFI) course

Disaster planning is only as good as the assumptions on which it is based. These assumptions are:

1. Dispatchers will hear of the disaster and send emergency response units to the scene.
2. Trained emergency personnel will carry out field search and rescue.
3. Trained emergency medical services personnel will carry out triage, provide first aid or stabilizing medical care, and—if necessary—decontaminate casualties before patient transport.
4. Casualties will be transported to hospitals by ambulance.
5. Casualties will be transported to hospitals appropriate for their needs and in such a manner that no hospitals receive a disproportionate number.
6. Authorities at the scene will ensure that area hospitals are promptly notified of the disaster and the numbers, types, and severities of casualties to be transported to them.
7. The most serious casualties will be the first to be transported to hospitals.

Disaster Experts from New York-Hospital Go to India; Nov. 08

While global migration to large cities has provided socio-economic opportunities to millions, it has also introduced new threats to urban populations, particularly marginalized communities. Large cities are increasingly vulnerable to manmade and natural calamities that can lead to injury, loss of life, and humanitarian crises.

Responding to this increasing vulnerability, 20 emergency medicine physicians, emergency medical services (EMS) personnel, and emergency management workers from NewYork-Presbyterian Hospital, in partnership with local and international agencies, are volunteering to conduct emergency management trainings and drills in Mumbai, India, and Colombo and Galle, Sri Lanka. The efforts, taking place Oct. 25 to Nov. 9, are aimed at improving local emergency preparedness and response by conducting trainings in pre-hospital and hospital emergency management, advanced trauma life support and public health evaluation and monitoring—and will also involve staging three large-scale disaster simulations.

"There is a tremendous need in many developing countries around the world for education and training in community-based and coordinated emergency management," says Dr. Robert Bristow, chair of the NewYork-Presbyterian Hospital's Emergency Management Committee and assistant clinical professor of medicine at Columbia University College of Physicians and Surgeons. "In 2006, Mumbai was the target of seven simultaneous bombings on its train system, killing 209 and injuring more than 700. Thousands have been killed and injured in the ongoing bombings by the separatist terrorist group in Sri Lanka. In 2004, Sri Lanka and India were hit with a deadly tsunami described as the worst disaster in its history, killing thousands. In 2005, the Maharashtra floods, the eighth heaviest ever-recorded 24-hour rainfall, crippled the city of Mumbai. We realized that much of what we have learned in emergency management post-9/11 at NewYork-Presbyterian, situated in New York City, could be beneficial in other parts of the world."

Disaster Drills

Emergency management drills have been validated in the medical literature as the single most important determinate of how well hospitals and communities respond after a disaster. As part of this two-week mission, the team is conducting large-scale emergency management drills in these two countries, simulating a mass-casualty incident. The drill will demonstrate a coordinated response between police, fire, emergency medical personnel, hospitals, clinics, government and non-governmental organisations, and other disaster responders. One hundred volunteers will act as victims and will be evaluated at the disaster site, medically triaged, and transported to hospitals where they will be evaluated and treated. At its conclusion, the drill will be evaluated for its effectiveness and used to create a road map for continued local development and coordination in emergency management.

In November of 2007, NewYork-Presbyterian's team led a similar emergency management training and drill in Ahmedabad, India, as part of a four-year grant to increase local emergency management capacity. This summer the city was struck by 17 terrorist blasts within 90 minutes. Two of the bombings involved Ahmedabad's Civil Hospital, which had participated in the drill. Government health officials reported in the Times of India that the disaster training provided by NewYork-Presbyterian's team helped improve emergency response to the attacks, expedite medical care for casualties, and armed the city with a plan that reduced panic and saved lives."This effort is unprecedented in its goals, its quality-control measures, and its scope. We are able to offer analysis using sophisticated bio-statistical tools, giving everyone a more detailed overview of the simulation's success," says Dr. Wallace A. Carter, Director of the Emergency Medicine Residency Programme at New York-Presbyterian Hospital and associate professor of clinical emergency medicine at Weill Cornell Medical College and Columbia University College of Physicians and Surgeons. "The goal is to improve disaster planning and emergency medicine around the globe and to increase public awareness about emergency management."

One such initiative in Mumbai, India, currently led by Mumbai native Dr. Satchit Balsari of NewYork-Presbyterian Hospital/Columbia University Medical Center in partnership with All India Disaster Mitigation Institute, The Harvard Humanitarian Initiative, and local partners, is the development of MumbaiVoices, a citizen-driven analysis of the disaster response to the Mumbai train blasts of 2006. Last year, Dr. Balsari and others helped to organize the first emergency medicine conference in Mumbai, and is currently helping hospitals in Mumbai start their first four-year emergency medicine residency training programme.

NewYork-Presbyterian's Emergency Medicine physicians have been involved in a number of multi-institutional, public-private and international humanitarian volunteer interventions in India, Germany, Montenegro, Darfur, Tanzania, Ghana, Dominican Republic, Guatemala and Myanmar. Among the collaborating institutions are the Harvard Humanitarian Initiative of Harvard University and AmeriCares, a disaster-response humanitarian organisation based in Stanford, Conn. The Hospital Emergency Medicine physicians have also volunteered domestically—including on the Gulf Coast, following Hurricane Katrina.

Disaster plan is a must

A. To provide policy for response to both internal and external disaster situations that may affect hospital staff, patients, visitors and the community.

B. Identify responsibilities of individuals and departments in the event of a disaster situation.

C. Identify Standard Operating Guidelines (SOG's) for emergency activities and responses.

Several types of hazards pose a threat to the hospital:

1. Internal disasters: fire, explosions, and hazardous material spills or releases.
2. Minor external disasters: incidents involving a small number of casualties.
3. Major external disasters: incidents involving a large number of casualties.
4. Disaster threats affecting the hospital or community (large or nearby fires, impending tornado, flooding, explosions,, etc.).
5. Disasters in other communities.

Important Considerations

A. Lines of Authority

The following persons, in the order listed, will be in charge:

1. Administrator.
2. Director of Nursing.
3. Nursing Supervisor on duty at time of disaster.
4. Emergency Room Supervisor.

B. Communications:

1. A Command Center will be set-up at the Security Desk to handle and coordinate all internal communications. All department heads or their designee will report to this office and call as many of their employees as needed.
2. The person in charge when the disaster happens will assign a nurse to the communications system in the E.R. This nurse will answer all radio calls from this station.
   - o The radio shall be manned immediately at the nurse's station by a unit coordinator but only for informational purposes and she should not verbally respond.
3. At least one messenger will be assigned to each radio operator to deliver messages, obtain casualty count from triage, etc.
4. Person directing personnel pool shall send a runner to all departments to advise them of the type of disaster and number of victims and extent of injuries when this information is available.
   a. Nursing will be notified by the Unit Coordinator or designated persons.
   b. Department Heads will be notified by the Supervisor or designated staff.
   c. Department Heads will notify their key personnel.
5. A "Visitor Control Center" will be set-up in the front lobby. Families of casualties will be instructed to wait there until notified of patient's condition. Normal visiting hours will be suspended during the disaster situation (orange alert).
   - o A hospital staff member will stay with the family members. (Social Services will be assigned here after reporting to the Command Center and other personnel assigned as needed)
   - o A list of the visitor's names in association with the patient they are inquiring about should be kept. Volunteers may be needed to escort visitors within the facility.
6. Telephone lines will be made available for outgoing and incoming calls. One line will be designated as the open line to the external Command Center. The person in charge will designate assigned staff to monitor the phones.

7. Assistance in providing additional radio communications to all departments within the hospital may be obtained by requesting Emergency Government RACES (Radio Amateur Civil Emergency Services) personnel from the county Emergency Government Office.

C. Supplies and Equipment

1. Extra supplies will be obtained from Purchasing personnel through runners.
2. Outside supplies will be ordered by the Purchasing Director and brought into the hospital via the loading dock.

D. Valuables and Clothing:

1. Large paper or plastic bags are available in the treatment Areas and the storeroom for patient's clothing and valuables.

E. Public Communication Center:

1. A communication center for receiving outside calls and giving information to the press, radio and relatives shall be set-up in Medical Records.
2. The press can use the restaurant as their headquarters.

F. Morgue Facilities:

1. Patients pronounced DOA will be tagged with a Disaster Tag...do not remove personal effects. The top sheet from the tag will be taken to the Command Center in Emergency Department for casualty list purposes.
2. Bodies will be stored in the hallway by Purchasing. Personnel will remain with bodies until removed by Funeral Director.
3. After bodies have been identified, the information will be filed on the Disaster Tag and Medical Records notified as to the identification of the patient.
4. The bodies will be removed via the loading dock to the Funeral Director. A complete record of all bodies must be maintained along with the name of the agency removing them, e.g., police, fire department, undertaker, etc.

   o Be sure appropriate paperwork is filled out.

Responsibilities of Individuals and Departments:

A. Administrator:

In a major disaster will do the following functions:

1. Check with local authorities to verify the disaster and obtain additional information.
2. Authorize announcement of disaster to hospital personnel.
3. Ask for help from local police and volunteer organisations as deemed necessary.
4. Stay in the area of administrative offices to be available to assist, as requested, by disaster coordinator.

B. Director of Nursing:

1. In a major disasterwill do the Administrator's functions, if he is absent.
2. Is responsible for notifying all department heads or alternates.
3. In a major disaster be responsible to see that families of victims are notified as soon as possible. These calls may be made by the physician who treats the victim, the Director of Social Services, or the Director of Nursing or her designee.
   - o The Command Center Director will coordinate these efforts and notify Medical Records personnel as to when information can be released to the press.

C. Nursing Supervisor

1. Is responsible for determining the extent of the disaster, whether it is a "major" or a "minor" disaster. If it is a major disaster, then the Administrator and Director of Nursing will be notified (if not present at time of disaster).
   - o (The Director of Nursing would then notify all department heads or alternates as noted above.)
2. Will set-up a Command Center—All department heads would report in to the supervisor before going to their departments.
3. Will attempt to find adequate numbers of nursing personnel. (This can be assigned to the Unit Coordinator or another nurse but the Supervisor must be aware of the number of nurses coming in.) Have them keep a list of those notified.
4. Leave extension "xxx" open to outside Command Center.

D. Admitting Office

1. Assign responsible person to switchboard as soon as possible.
2. Department head or designee will call in their own personnel as needed after having reported to the Command Center.

3. Notify Emergency Communications Center if internal disaster is involved.
4. After notification of disaster by authorized person, you are responsible for sounding the "Orange Alert" alarm.
5. Do not accept routine non-emergency admissions except OB's.
6. Refer all public information calls and press to desk in Reception Area.
7. Direct press to the restaurant.
8. Call local clergy as requested.
9. Assign an admissions person to aid with discharge of hospital patients from the east solarium, if requested by Med/Surg.

E. Dietary

1. Department head or designee will call in their own personnel as needed after reporting to Command Center.
2. Prepare to serve nourishments to ambulatory patients, house patients and personnel as need arises.
3. Clear hallway of all tray carts.
4. Utilize T.C. dining room and west hospital solarium for extra eating space.
5. Be responsible for setting up menus in disaster situation and maintain adequate supplies.

F. Maintenance

1. Department head or designee will call in their own personnel as needed after reporting to Command Center.
2. Maintain full operation of all facilities.
3. All doors should be locked immediately except employee entrance, Emergency Department door, and front lobby.
4. Be responsible for setting up extra beds in hospital if needed, as well as transporting storeroom supplies and bringing in extra supplies from other areas.
5. Be willing to help with movement of victims from ambulance to Triage.

G. Housekeeping and Laundry

1. Department head or designee will call in their own personnel as needed after reporting to Command Center.
2. Be available to help clean receiving area, and clean rooms between cases in treatment areas.
3. Be sure all hallways or traffic areas are clear of cleaning carts, equipment and, etc.

H. Operating Room, CSR, PAR, Anesthesia, and OP

1. Supervisor or RN will supervise Operating Room and call all needed personnel after reporting to Command Center.
2. Call additional surgeons as needed.
3. Check area for supplies and equipment.
4. Ask for additional help to carry out surgery and treatments in Operating Rooms and Recovery Room.
5. Assign and direct scrub nurses and circulate.
6. Notify Triage when Operating Rooms and Recovery Room is available for more patients.
7. Keep minimum list of supplies on hand and be prepared to process additional sterile supplies quickly.
8. Notify anesthetists who will maintain adequate anesthesia and drug supplies.

I. Hospital Unit—Supervisor will:

1. Assign nurse or unit coordinator to communications system in E.R.
2. Prepare for expansion by notifying maintenance of number of extra beds needed and where to set them up.
3. Discharge and movement of hospital patients to create more room for casualties.
4. Send for extra supplies needed from Purchasing, CSR, Laundry, and Dietary.
5. If internal, prepare for evacuation of patients to safe area.
6. Send designated personnel to Command Center with wheelchairs.
7. Periodically send messenger to Command Center to check for update.
8. The elevators will be used ONLY for the transportation of patients or equipment...all personnel will use the stairway.

J. ICU—After notification of disaster, the ICU nurse will:

1. Evaluate patients in the Intensive Care Unit for possible discharge. Use established discharge criteria as a guide. Transfer patients out if indicated.
2. Prepare to admit more critically ill patients.
3. Send runner to Command Center or phone for help.

K. Swing Bed Unit

1. Know current empty bed count and number of personnel available who could assist in other units. Send number to Command Center.

2. Remain in your unit until notified differently.
3. Will make wheelchairs available.

L. OB Unit

1. Staff from OB can be used to assist in triage if department is covered. Volunteers can be used from OB to assist in disaster.
2. Patients other than OB's will be triaged by Command Center before being transferred to OB.

M. Chemical Health Recovery Unit

1. Department Head or designee will call in their own personnel as needed after reporting to Command Center and staff holding area.
2. Department Head will send designated personnel to Triage with wheelchairs to hold in ER waiting room until needed.

N. Medical Imaging

Day Shift:

1. The department head or designee will find out the number of patients involved and any other pertinent information from the Command Center.
2. The department head or designee will be responsible for calling in any and all personnel needed to sufficiently handle the patient load.

Evening Shift:

1. The technologist on duty or on call for the Radiology Department will be alerted by the night supervisor. This technologist will be considered the designee of the x-ray department and will report to the information center for further information.
2. It will be the duty of this technologist to call in extra help as needed. All extra help called in will report directly to Radiology.

Duties of Medical Imaging Personnel:

Department Head will:

1. Call any or all personnel needed.
2. Arrange for extra supplies to be brought in if needed.
3. Coordinate flow of work and delegation of work areas.
4. Other Technologists will:

a. Perform all x-ray exams as needed and assigned.
b. Perform all clerical duties.

O. Laboratory

1. Department Head or designee will call in their own personnel as needed after reporting to Command Center.
2. Call personnel from nearby hospitals and clinics as necessary.
3. Have arrangements made to obtain additional blood, equipment and supplies from area agencies.

P. Materials Management—Purchasing

1. Department Head or designee will call in their own personnel as needed after reporting to Command Center.
2. Be prepared to supply all departments with needed supplies.
3. Director will designate assistant to supply runners or volunteers to deliver supplies.
4. Have an up-to-date list of suppliers who can quickly supply extra materials.
5. Have Kardex in Storeroom up-to-date.

Q. Pharmacy

1. Report to Command Center, then remain in department.
2. Have list of drug suppliers that can provide emergency supplies quickly (list is in Procedure Manual).
3. Keep minimum supply of emergency drugs on hand at all times.
4. Pharmacy should remain open and have a runner to deliver needed meds to areas.

R. Respiratory Therapy

1. Department Head or designee will call in their own personnel as needed after reporting to Command Center.
2. Keep adequate supply of bubblers, cannulas, masks and flowmeters available in Respiratory Therapy Department.
3. Be prepared to obtain additional respirators and equipment as needed.
4. Be prepared to assist in treatment areas.
5. Keep resuscitation equipment in good operating condition and well marked.

S. Physical Therapy

1. Department Head or designee will call in their own personnel as needed after reporting to Command Center.

2. Be prepared to accept walking wounded victims. Be prepared to provide assistance to RN's as needed.
3. Request a runner from Command Center as needed.

T. Occupational Therapy

1. Department Head or designee will call in their own personnel as needed after reporting to Command Center.

U. Stress/EKG Department

1. Reports to Respiratory Therapy Head or designee.
2. Be prepared to obtain additional equipment and supplies.
3. Be prepared to assist in treatment areas.

V. Social Services

1. Report to the Command Center and be prepared to stay with relatives of victims in hospital lobby.
2. Will provide Command Center with a list of the family members that are here.

W. Director of Community Relations

1. Department Head or designee will call in their own personnel as needed after reporting to Command Center.
2. Be prepared to call in volunteers who are familiar with physical plant of hospital to serve.
3. Have volunteers set-up downstairs classroom for babysitting personnel's children.

X. Quality Improvement/Risk Management—Utilization Review

1. Report to Command Center and assist with relatives of victims in hospital lobby. Also assist Education Coordinator with press information.

Y. Security

1. Report to Command Center.
2. Assist RN's as needed.

Z. Infection Control

1. Report to Command Center.
2. Be prepared to assist in Pharmacy as needed.

AA. Nursing Personnel Assigned to Disaster Victims

1. Obtain information and fill out available information and time on disaster tags. Even if no information is available as to identity, give information as to condition, types of injuries, etc.
   - o If top sheet on tag has already been picked up, use O.P. record (may use ER Nurses notes) to record changes in patient's condition, additional information, etc.
   - o Be sure to use hospital disaster tag number for identification (the tag is in triplicate).
2. BE SURE top sheet of disaster tag is made available to Medical Records with pertinent information.
3. DO NOT leave your patient unattended. Patient may be signed off to person in charge when admitted to a unit.
4. Give aggressive first aid treatment.
5. Make out the appropriate lab slips and x-ray requisitions with disaster number. It is essential that they have these slips made out.
6. Patients who have been admitted to the hospital should have the information slips placed with the Command Center in the Emergency Department.
7. If a patient is transferred, be sure to indicate on the tag to which hospital he has been sent.
8. If a patient is admitted to our hospital, be sure and send all oxygen equipment to his room with him.
9. Sign disaster tags.

AB. Medical Records

1. Department Head or designee will call in their own personnel as needed after reporting to the Command Center.
2. Assign person to be responsible for maintaining casualty lists and assist with paperwork as needed at Command Center.
3. Supply extra forms as needed.
4. Be responsible for releasing information to the press after the families of the victims have been notified.

World Health Organisation's (WHO) call

Calling on Member-States to support the 2008-09 World Disaster Reduction Campaign, the World Health Organisation's Regional Office for the Western Pacific said structural safety of hospitals need to be ensured to allow continuous services in times of disaster. The campaign, with the theme "Hospitals Safe from Disasters: Reduce Risk, Protect Health Facilities, Save Lives", aims to raise awareness about why and how to redouble efforts to protect health facilities and staff and how hospitals can ensure their function during and in the aftermath of disasters. WHO noted that the world has recently witnessed accounts of destroyed health facilities:

1. In 2008, Typhoon Fengshen destroyed or damaged 89 hospitals and health facilities in central and southern Philippines, further aggravating the suffering of disaster victims and their families due to lack of medical services. Similarly terrorists attacked several hospitals in Mumbai on 26th Nov. 08.
2. In 2005, the South Asian earthquake destroyed almost 50% of health facilities in the worst affected region of Pakistan.
3. In December 2004, the earthquake and tsunami damaged or totally destroyed more than 360 hospitals and health facilities were in Indonesia, Sri Lanka, Maldives, and India.
4. In 2001, the Gujarat earthquake in India destroyed 3812 health facilities, requiring US$60 million for reconstruction.

The damages that disasters can incur to health facilities reach millions of dollars and may range from 15% to 60% of annual government health spending. Studies have shown that retrofitting—bracing, reinforcement or other engineering interventions—of health facilities are cost-effective and can protect up to 90% of the value of the hospital. For some hospitals, however, retrofitting may have cost implications which would require the commitment from policy-makers. "Preparedness and response can be reinforced so that human suffering is prevented or minimized," said Dr Arthur Pesigan, head of the WHO Emergency and Humanitarian Action. "This can only be achieved by structures that will not collapse in disasters, with an organised contingency plan, and with a trained health workforce to continue and provide its services during critical situations."

News and Views about some Disaster Events in Recent Times

Mumbai serial blasts

A routine working day for the surgery registrar on call; attending to the emergency admissions. Suddenly, one patient, with his arm blown away, lands in the Emergency Ward. Even before he is examined, five others arrive with somewhat similar presentations and then the flow continues. Each one has come from a different location Matunga ...Mahim ....Khar—all western suburbs of the city. Within a span of 45 minutes, around 50 patients entered the Casualty Department. Twenty-one dead bodies were brought in. Of the 76 patients who came in with injuries related to the bomb blast, 54 were admitted to the hospital with severe injuries.

Within 5-10 minutes of the arrival of the victims, two lecturers from the department of surgery undertook triage of victims and the institutional Disaster Management Programme (DMP) was activated. As per the international accepted norms on disaster management, the waiting area outside casualty was quickly converted into a makeshift patient examination area from where stable patients were directly transferred to two general wards. These were managed by three resident doctors posted in each of these wards. Other patients including the ones who were critically ill were managed in the ESW. Resident doctors and faculty members of various other specialties like orthopedics, anesthesiology, oto-rhinolaryngology, plastic surgery and pediatric surgery joined their colleagues from the General Surgery department in management of these patients. They were supported by interns and medical students, nurses, lab technicians and support staff. The Dean, Dr Nilima Kshirsagar visited the ESW several times during the night giving every bit of support. The other senior administrative staff ensured that adequate material and manpower were available in the wards. This helped in providing simultaneous multi-specialty evaluation and treatment, which most patients needed. The Radiology department carried out 327 investigations over 8 hours, which included plain radiographs, CT scans and ultrasound examinations. Eighteen major surgical interventions were carried out; sixteen of these were completed within 18 hours of the event. One hundred and seventy-five units of blood and blood products were transfused; over 90% of these were carried out during the same night. Head injury, chest trauma (pneumothorax and hemothorax), fractures, tympanic membrane perforations, tinnitus, giddiness and varying degrees of hearing loss were the common injuries encountered. Patients requiring exclusive specialty care (orthopedic, cardiovascular or respiratory medicine) were transferred to the respective wards. This helped ease the burden on ESW. There was no mortality within 24 hours subsequently two out of the 54 patients admitted to the hospital expired.

Social support

A number of dignitaries including the honorable President Shri APJ Abdul Kalam and the honorable Prime Minister Dr. Manmohan Singh visited the institution and spoke to the grieving victims and relatives. Officials of the Municipal Corporation and Railways also offered valuable assistance. The spirit of Mumbai was evident in the 1000-odd volunteers who turned up to help the patients, care-providers and hospital. The blood bank received 1165 blood donors over 8-10 hours and finally had to stop accepting blood donations. Restaurants in the nearby areas worked through the night ensuring a steady flow of food and beverages for all the workers and pharmaceutical companies supplied drugs free of cost.

Winter weather can bring winter disaster

If a bad storm hits your area, you need to be prepared to be snowed in and go without electricity for at least a week. How to Survive a Winter Storm and Survive for a Week:

- Stay away from down power lines. If you're in your car and a falling wire hits your car, stay in your car. Call emergency, but don't get out of the car.

- Get a generator. If you live up north and your area tends to get a lot of winter storms, then a generator is a must.
- Don't use your generator inside! The fumes are dangerous. Keep it in the garage or on the front porch.
- Do not use unsafe heating appliances in your house. Catalytic propane, kerosene, or wood burning heaters are safe when used properly. They must be ventilated and kept away from small children. Carbon monoxide is a quick and silent killer.
- Don't use extension cords brought from another location to power your house, it's not safe and the chances are that if your power went out, so will theirs.
- Before or soon after the storm hits, call someone outside your area and let them know where you are or where (what shelter or other location) you might go to if the storm worsens.
- Be prepared with supplies that can last a week. Don't wait to stock up on supplies the day of the storm, the stores will be picked over and chaotic, and the storm could hit before you get back home. Helpful supplies include water, a weather radio with batteries, small-sized sterno stoves that can be used to heat up canned goods, non-perishable foods such as crackers and peanut butter, emergency blankets, lighters or waterproof matches, a first aid kit, a roll of plastic and duct tape to seal a broken window or help seal drafts are also helpful.
- Stay calm and pay extra attention to those who are particularly vulnerable to cold weather conditions. Young children and the elderly (and your pets) get colder faster and cannot always communicate their needs. Be sure everyone is dressed in layers, and it's smart to pack a deck of cards and other simple games to keep everyone entertained.

Staying Safe and Warm in a Blizzard

1. Get a generator. If you're not near a city, then this is a must. It's great to enjoy a few hours by candlelight, but as night falls, temperatures drop. A generator isn't for running your chandelier, it's for survival.
2. Stock up on flashlights, candles, batteries and a battery operated radio.
3. Keep your cell phones charged. Towers may go down, but it may be possible to get a signal and let someone know where you are.
4. Before the storm hits, dress in layers and have your supplies nearby. Get out those extra blankets and be prepared.
5. Have water and non-perishable foods on hand.
6. Know where needed prescriptions or other medical devices such as oxygen are so you won't have to hunt in the dark.

7. Make sure your pipes are insulated. A busted pipe is a mess when it's freezing and can cause major water damage.
8. If there's ice, be aware of falling limbs and trees—and power lines.
9. If your electricity goes out, bring your family together, including the pets. Conserve your supplies since you don't know how long you'll be in this state. Call someone on your cell and tell them where you are and that you're okay. If your power is out for more than a few hours, turn-off your cell and conserve your battery.
10. Don't open the doors—keep the house as warm as possible and cover any drafts. Don't open your frig unless you have to. If you need to move meats and other frozen goods outside, do it all at once.
11. Be very careful what heating appliances you use in the house. Carbon monoxide poisoning is a very real danger.
12. Know the signs of frostbite and hypothermia. Watch for teeth chattering, slurred speech, shaking followed by lethargic behavior.

Even if you have a generator, plenty of water and food, winter storm conditions can be dangerous.

Being prepared is the best way to take care of those you love.

Motorists scrambled from their cars to avoid being crushed as car after car plowed into each other. No deaths were attributed to the pileup, but several were trapped in their cars and more than a dozen were injured with broken bones, and abrasions, stated Chief Jack Webb of the Derry Fire Battalion. The incident occurred between exits 3 and 4 on I-93 at around 9 a.m. on Sunday morning where 46 cars, three buses, two tractor trailers and eight trucks piled into each other in a continuous collision causing cars to be wedged under buses and caused cars to be pinned under jack-knifed trailers in the debris. Emergency crews spent hours trying to untangle victims from being pinned in their cars.

The accident began when a charter bus of Boy Scouts from Boston, Massachusetts tried to avoid a car that was skidding on the ice and overturned. A busload carrying the women's hockey team from the University of Massachusetts was also in the pileup. I-93 was reopened later Sunday evening, but officials warned motorists to take extreme caution and be aware that a winter storm advisory is still in place.

Fighting in Gaza

As the fighting in Gaza continues, human suffering increases. The International Committee of the Red Cross states that 4,000 people have been injured and close to 600 people have been killed in the Palestinian territory. Civilian casualties continue to rise as supplies dwindle. The fighting in Gaza is considered a humanitarian crisis because of the countless innocent lives who live and work in the region have no place to go and are in the midst of rocket and land fighting. Many of these families have no way to leave the region. This disaster has left many without food, electricity, water, or medical supplies as the raids continue.

The ICRC (International Committee of the Red Cross) states that there is a shortage of everything from medical personnel, medical supplies, and as well as the need for generators and generator parts to keep the hospital running since basic necessities such as electricity and running water are not always available. In response to the crisis, the American Red Cross has contributed $250,000 to the ICRC to help support the work humanitarian work being carried out in the Gaza Strip.

The ICRC said that Israeli authorities have given them permission to bring in medical supplies, blood, and plasma in the Gaza region, as well as tetanus vaccinations that will be given to the wounded and could save countless lives. They are also allowing Red Cross war surgeons access to Gaza to help the doctor's at Shifa hospital to treat those in need of medical care.

Flood Zones and How to Prevent Disaster

Have you ever wondered what it costs to insure a home that's located on the beach? Have you considered a river or lake front home and wanted to know how much of a risk you were taking–if a flood were to occur?

There are different types of flood zones, and each zone presents varying risks which determine the insurance premium rate required. FEMA's rating system is divided into a V flood zone and an A flood zone. The V flood zone is considered to be a secial hazard flood area and include low lying areas such as beach front properties and are indicated as VE, V-1, and V-30 zones. This area is also exposed to "wave velocity," or tsunami type conditions which make flood insurance mandatory for this zone.

The V zone structures require that the lowest portion of the home or business be at or above BFE, Base Flood Elevation, meaning that it cannot be below sea level. The lowest level cannot be used for living space (that's why you will see homes built on "stilts" with ony parking underneath) and the building must be placed on piles, piers, posts, or column foundations. Also, the electrical heating, plumping and other home equipment must be elevated. Make sure that the home or business you buy or build meets FEMA's V zone requirements in order to qualify for the insurance and more importantly, keep you and your loved ones safe.

The A flood zone area is still in the flood zone, but is considered less of a risk and includes residences and businesses that can be effected by rising waters. This includes homes and communities near a river, lake, or other types of water. Flood insurance is still mandatory in all A zones because potential rising flood waters and are indicated as A zones AE, AH, AO, AR, and A99 to reflect various flooding conditions. Those who live in the A zone are also required that their lowest floor be at or above BFE, Base Flood Elevation, that their lowest floor cannot be used for living space, and that their electrical, heating, and various equipment be elevated as well. There is also a flood zone x, but it is not required to carry flood insurance and is less defined.

The best way to prevent a flood disaster is by knowledge and taking the proper steps to prepare. Don't risk your safety. Make sure your family is safe and your belongings are properly insured. Water damage can be dealt with, but lives should not be lost.

Winter Wildfires

Boulder County, a community about 25 miles outside of Denver, Colorado continues to battle the Neva fires that have burned close to 4,000 acres and has caused the evacuation of more than 11,000 residents. Several residential homes and businesses have been lost to the blaze as well as two injured firefighters. No deaths are reported at this time.

Crews have now a 30 percent containment field around the fires and are using back burning tactics to control the burn. Close to two hundred firefighters are working to douse the flames. The fires are believed to have started when high winds toppled a power pole that sparked the first blaze and was quickly followed by a second pole that fell and added to the flames. These two fires joined in a crescent shape and were named the Neva fire after Neva Road, the location of the first blaze. The Boulder County area is home to many animals livestock, and the city has responded by opening the Boulder County Fairgrounds as an emergency shelter for horses, sheep, goats and other animals to be housed until the wildfires are contained.

Hurricanes

In light of the recent series of hurricanes, organisations should be proactive in protecting their information technology assets in case they are faced with a natural or man-made disaster. This means that it is critical for organisations to have a solid disaster recovery plan in place, prior to an incident occurring. To illustrate the threat, back-to-back hurricanes and tropical storms, such as Gustav, Hanna and Ike, have had devastating effects on entire regions of the country. And the threat is not over as hurricane season begins June first and ends on November 30th, with most hurricanes occurring mid August through mid October.

"It is critical that organisations ensure they have measures in place to swiftly respond to adverse affects of natural disasters, such as hurricanes and man-made disasters," said Al Tirevold, director of security architecture at SecureWorks. "Safeguarding critical customer or member data is not just an IT issue; it's a business continuity issue, and the opposite can cause you financial loss and an inability to serve your customers."

"We checked on our clients in Texas after Hurricane Ike hit because our clients' well-being is always our first concern," said Tirevold. "We were pleased to find out they were doing well and in good spirits despite the circumstances, and they were in full disaster recovery mode. One client reported 13 of their 29 centers in Houston had power, and they were open for business. They had disaster recovery trailers equipped with computers and generator power in place. They had ample fuel capacity for their data center, and they were able to shift personnel to other locations because of a damaged call center and damages to their corporate headquarters. This is an organisation that minimized business disruption because of a well-thought out and well-executed disaster recovery plan," explained Tirevold.

Although hurricanes originate in the Atlantic and Eastern Pacific oceans before making landfall along coastal states, organisations in other geographical areas should be concerned with preventing business disruptions as well. According to news reports, the affects of Hurricane Ike, for example, reached areas like Illinois, Ohio, Kentucky and New York, causing floods, wind damage and power outages. Kentucky alone saw winds of up to 75 mph and had four deaths attributed to the storm.

Many organisations and regulating bodies have guidelines on how companies should handle data loss prevention, response and recovery. The Federal Financial Institutions Examination Council (FFIEC), which prescribes uniform principles and standards for financial institutions, outlines key areas of a business continuity plan (BCP) in its Business Continuity Planning IT Examination Handbook. Additionally, the National Institute of Standards and Technology (NIST), a non-regulatory federal agency within the U.S. Department of Commerce, offers guidance on preparing for disasters as well.

For companies who have not yet formalized their BCP plans, here are some guidelines which are aligned with some of today's common regulations:

- Make sure your business continuity plan has a section for disaster recovery, and make sure your BCP is enterprise-wide, considering every critical aspect of your business including personnel and physical workspace. The BCP should include a sequence of tasks and responsibilities that are clearly spelled out.
- Do a thorough business impact analysis (including a security business impact analysis) and risk assessment.
- Test your BCP for its effectiveness, and make adjustments/ updates to reflect changes in your organisation. Testing is recommended at least on an annual basis, and you should include third parties like data processors, managed security service providers and core processors.
- Identify alternate locations to operate from in the event you are no longer able to conduct business from your office. This should include a capacity for data centers, computer operations and telecommunications.
- Back up data, operating system configurations, applications and utility programmes, and identify alternate telecommunications.

- Identify off-site storage for back up media, supplies and documents such as your BCP, inventory list, operating and other procedures, etc.
- Make sure you have alternate power supplies in case you are without electricity (uninterruptible power supplies [UPS] and back-up generators).
- Assemble a team in advance and designate people who are responsible for various tasks in the event of a disaster. All personnel should be trained in their contingency-related duties and new personnel should be trained as they join your organisation.

Preparedness makes a huge difference when the unexpected strikes, from a tornado to a flood, a gunman to terrorists, says Harry Nolan, PhD, chief loss-control engineer for Bowman Specialty Services. Clients receive a customized emergency preparedness manual, a safety video and technical support. "Safety for Life" can supplement the efforts of in-house safety staff or be used by organisations that do not have their own safety professionals. "The emergency preparedness manual is designed as a working plan that's regularly updated and always ready to be implemented at a moment's notice," Nolan says. It also outlines setting up a crisis management team (CMT), creating an emergency evacuation plan, showing how to test the plan, addressing employee training and motivation and more. Evacuation planning is often overlooked, but planning can make a difference between life and death in an extreme emergency like a high-rise fire or an attack by terrorists or a murderous gunman.

The approved safety video, in DVD or computer format, shows employees how to respond in emergencies, while covering the key safety concerns in any organisation, whether it's a manufacturer, a service business, hospital, government agency or utility.

It has been said that disasters can turn hospitals into casualties. As the world around us appears beset by threats from hurricanes to terrorism, for hospitals—where the business model is built on dealing with emergencies—managing the fallout from a mass event requires secure and reliable communication.

"Recent events have shown that hospitals can quickly be overwhelmed in a disaster."

Increasingly the technology required is coming from the internet and software applications designed to help hospitals prepare for, manage and recover from disasters.

In the past, emergency preparedness focused on the readiness of medical response, covering issues like triage, evacuation and transport of casualties. However, there was the unproven presumption that hospital management would just continue to flow automatically. Recent events, however, have shown that hospitals can quickly be over-whelmed in a disaster. Incidents like those of Hurricanes Katrina and more recently

Hanna, Gustav and Ike have illustrated that even in countries where facilities are thought to be large, modern and sufficiently equipped, emergency preparedness is tested to its limit.

Following the terrorist attacks of 11 September 2001, the US established the National Incident Management Plan which dictates a national template for government and private sector organisations to: "work together effectively and efficiently to prepare for, prevent, respond to and recover from domestic incidents, regardless of cause, size or complexity, including acts of catastrophic terrorism."

As a result, interoperable communications which aid cooperation between hospitals and emergency response teams in the vicinity of a disaster are now the focus. These are set to work alongside better training and planning which can help move hospital staff as opposed to patients.

Bomb blasts

The Australian health care system was exposed to mass casualties on 12 October 2002 as a result of bomb blasts at two popular tourist bars in Bali in which 202 people were killed and 196 injured. Another bomb attack in Bali on 1st October, 2005 killed 23 and injured 108. Interagency communication and cooperation, civilian and military responses, evacuation systems and the in-hospital care of these patients were tested, and all have improved as a result.

However, the response to the Bali bombings is not equivalent to the response that would be required for a major terrorist event occurring on our own soil. Thus, state and federal agencies continue to gather the most up-to-date expert advice to further improve the level of preparedness for casualties resulting from terrorist attacks. Although bomb blasts are a currently preferred method of terrorist attack, our field and hospital systems should also have the capacity to decontaminate large number of people exposed to unconventional types of chemical, biological and radiation injury.

Bomb explosions cause combinations of burns, baro-trauma, and penetrating, blunt crush injuries. These injuries, collectively and for the individual, are much more severe than those usually seen in Australian hospitals. Blast victims (especially those with major burns) consume more resources, in volume and time, than civilian trauma victims. Treating children and pregnant women with bomb-blast trauma presents particular challenges.

Here we discuss some issues related to hospital preparedness for mass casualties after terrorist attacks.

Arriving at hospital

Disasters in urban areas are characterized by many of the injured making their own way to hospital. A US Centers for Disease Control and Prevention overview of explosions and blast injuries warns that, in the event of an urban disaster, half of all casualties will arrive at hospital seeking medical care over a 1-hour period.

Recent terrorist incidents have been characterized by multiple explosions targeting civilians in urban areas. Many of the victims, although sustaining significant soft-tissue trauma, burns and pulmonary injury, have left the scene quickly, making their own way to hospitals. This was the case both in Bali in 2002 (eyewitness accounts reported to MF) and in New York in 2001. In the case of large, urban blasts (involving over 60 casualties), victims remaining at the scene for transport have, in some respects, self-triaged themselves as more severely injured. Their arrival at hospital via ambulance follows those patients who have already been able to make their own way there. However, it should be noted that most of the Madrid and London casualties were evacuated by ambulance.

Assessing the injured

There are several clinical indicators for determining which blast victims are likely to need critical care. These include tachypnoea, tachycardia, confusion, multiple penetration wounds and multiple areas of soft-tissue damage. Patients with penetrating injury to the head or torso, burns to more than 10% of the body and skull fractures are more likely to have blast lung injuries. Tympanic membrane rupture does not always correlate with significant barotrauma, although its absence does not exclude significant trauma. Clinical manifestations of pulmonary barotrauma evolve over time. Injured patients may require a minimum of 6 hours' observation before being considered safe for discharge. This makes it imperative that we build a surge capacity into our major trauma centers.

It is critical that experienced and trained senior medical officers perform the triage of casualties in emergency departments. The flow of received casualties should be unidirectional. Frequent reassessment of the casualties by a senior surgeon enhances the detection of missed injuries and diagnosis of pulmonary blast injury. Digital photographs of the victims' faces should be taken soon after arrival to help in identification, as the face rapidly becomes un-recognizable in many cases. The liberal use of ultrasound can assist in initial surgical triage. Computed tomography scans are frequently required, but are a potential cause of bottleneck in moving patients out of the emergency department. Intensive care units, operating theatres and wards need to be cleared sufficiently to make way for the mass casualties. Explosion victims often need interventional angiography treatment. The distribution of mass casualties across multiple hospitals improves access, but we recommend provision of resources for additional surge capacity in the major trauma centres, including a boost in intensive-care-unit bed capacity.

Disaster planning

Any large terrorist event would require a response from both federal and state governments. To ensure that there are adequate resources to cope with terrorism, each state and territory health department has reviewed its disaster plan for the initial management of casualties. Emergency services have concentrated on pre-hospital response, scene triage and casualty distribution.

As already noted, in the event of a disaster, many people travel to hospital unassisted. Initially there is chaos as mass casualties arrive, but the more prepared hospitals and trauma systems are the more quickly order can be restored and the more lives can be saved. Terrorist bombings that result in mass civilian casualties will seriously challenge even the most experienced and prepared medical centers. Major hospitals in large urban centers in Australia should plan for large numbers of undifferentiated and potentially contaminated casualties arriving with minimal warning. While no hospital can be fully prepared or resourced for mass casualty events, currently most Australian hospitals would be unlikely to be able to cope with any more than small numbers (10–24) of seriously injured patients.

Some countries enforce regular exercises focusing on mass casualty management. The only way to test the system—apart from a real event—is by "table-top" exercises (in which simulated disaster scenarios are played out in a room by senior personnel from various departments) and real-time drills for staff, with modulated casualties and sometimes "smart" simulated victims. The importance of hospital training drills was highlighted during the response to the 7 July 2005 bomb blasts in London, where rehearsal and drills were ingrained. It is further emphasized by the Hadassah University Hospital in Jerusalem (which arguably sees the largest number of terrorist events and victims of any hospital in the world). This hospital takes part in mandatory regular exercises with the Israeli emergency services, and even senior medical students are required to attend a 2-week course on managing casualties after a terrorist attack. The Australian health care system should review the model of training conducted in Israel and consider including a mandatory component of disaster management training for all health care workers, medical students and student nurses.

It is vital that there be well developed and accessible standard operating procedures for mass casualty events and disaster response at each hospital, and that regional and national trauma systems be put in place. Australian doctors and nurses who would be receiving and treating victims of terrorist attacks must be up to date with their knowledge of the types of injuries and the treatments required after bomb blasts. Consideration should also be given to training hospital staff to treat injuries resulting from weapons of mass destruction (such as nuclear, chemical or biological weapons). Australian military medical and nursing personnel who are currently serving with the 332nd Expeditionary Medical Group of the US Air Force in Iraq are obtaining a great deal of experience in managing bomb blast victims and mass casualties. Their knowledge and experience would be invaluable to pass on to Australian health professionals who may be required to treat such victims in Australia.

Hospital administrators should be an integral part of the in-hospital response to a major incident and should also be involved in training exercises, with a clear chain of command and communication established as a priority. An operational room set-up for coordinating the in-hospital response and liaison with other hospitals and emergency services is a key component of current external disaster plans. Trained personnel should be assigned to telephones to assist with victim identification and family liaison. Assigning experienced nurses and social workers to coordinate a family/relative centre has been an extremely effective initiative within the Israeli health system.

It is essential that security be enhanced immediately after a mass casualty incident, especially as hospitals themselves may become targets for terrorism. Media management and public information centres need to be set-up. Stress management services should be made available for staff, and regular management debriefings should be held after normality is partially restored (usually within 12–18 hours).

A longer-term perspective

Beyond the initial crisis, there is a need for long-term planning, as each injured person may take 6 weeks or more to recover and be transferred for rehabilitation. Multiple surgical procedures (especially orthopaedic surgery) are usually required for bomb blast victims. These may proceed over several weeks and have a major impact on the routine activities of a hospital.

Management of the impact of terrorist events on the long-term psychological well-being of the community—and, in particular, emergency-services and health care workers—needs to be rigorously reviewed within the Australian health system. There are lessons to be learnt from countries, such as Israel, that have dealt with this on an ongoing basis. The long-term squeal of terrorist attacks on victims will place extra burdens on our rehabilitation system. Bomb blast victims who have suffered neuro-trauma pose particular challenges as a result of their cognitive, behavioral and physical injuries.

Mental health care of disaster victims

Mental health is defined as the successful performance of mental function, resulting in productive activities, fulfilling relationships, the ability to adapt to change, and successful coping with adversity. Among the findings reported in the US surgeon general's mental health report are that mental disorders are common but treatable and that stigmatization, poor material circumstances, and lack of access are major barriers to successful treatment of mental disorders.

An estimated 450 million people worldwide have mental or behavioral disorders, accounting for 12% of the global disease burden. Worldwide, 40% of countries have no mental health policy, and for the majority of countries, mental health budgets constitute less than 5% of total health expenditures. As is the case for many health conditions, there are disparities in mental health between groups defined socially, economically, geographically.

Some disaster victims do need additional attention from a professional therapist, but most will not. Much of the initial mental health disaster response involves two primary goals:

(1) "Normalizing feelings: reassuring victims that the strange and upsetting feelings they experience after a disaster (as following other traumatic events) are normal—given what happened, and
(2) Helping victims find effective ways of coping with their stress.

Disaster Mental Health Handouts as prepared by US health department

Adult Victims

Victim Emotional Health

Emotional health issues for victims, from the American Red Cross.

Warning Signs

Warning signs of trauma-related stress, from the American Psychological Association.

Critical Incident

Critical incident stress information sheet, from Los Angeles County Department of Mental Health.

Normalizing Emotions

You are not alone! description of normal emotions following a disaster, from the American Red Cross.

Building Safety

Reducing fear about building safety, by Dan Friedman, American Society of Home Inspectors.

Coping Suggestions

Coping suggestions, from Los Angeles County Department of Mental Health.

Steps to Take

After a disaster: Steps you can take, from Los Angeles County Department of Mental Health.

Families and Child Victims

Family Coping

Coping suggestions for families, from the Los Angeles County Department of Mental Health.

Helping Children after a Disaster

Child behaviors to watch and suggestions to help, by the American Academy of Child and Adolescent Psychiatry.

Helping Children Cope

Helping children cope with disaster, from FEMA and the American Red Cross.

Children's Reactions

Children's reactions to disaster; author unknown.

Talking with Children about the Bombing

Suggestions for parents or other adults about what to tell children about terrorist bombings, by Eitan Schwartz MD.

Disasters dreams

In addition to real disasters the dream of disaster may also haunt many people who have seen or heard about one or more disasters. The psychiatrist may help these people. The following Questions may arise:

Earthquake or disaster variation:

- What situations in your waking life feel at risk?
- What did you do in the dream to escape destruction?
- How can you get the help you need in the waking world to stabilize the situation and yourself?
- Is there any possible benefit from the drastic change that's underway?

Flood variation:

- What situation in waking life is making you feel overwhelmed?
- Do you feel profoundly sad about current life circumstances?
- What did you do in the dream to save yourself?
- What can you do in the waking situation to improve it or get support? Tornado or great wind variation:
- What is it in waking life that is making you feel storm-tossed?
- What did you do in your dream to protect yourself from the storm?
- How can you improve your waking life situation?
- How can you resolve your inner turmoil and return to a stable state?

Fire or volcano variation:

- What is waking life is making you feel hotly aroused right now? Anger? Passion? Fever? Inflammation?

- What did you do to cope with the destructive fire in the dream?
- What do you need to do about the waking circumstances?
- How can you calm your internal fire?

Snowstorm or ice storm variation:

- What situation in your waking life might be making you feel frozen out or loveless at this time?
- Is there any circumstance at present that makes you feel frozen with grief?
- Is there something in your environment making you feel cold with fear?
- How did I cope with the ice and cold in my dream? Did I take action?
- What can I learn about my waking life situation to thaw out any icy feelings or invite warm, loving ones?

War and explosion variations:

- What is making me feel under angry attack at the moment?
- What did you do in the dream to protect yourself and others?
- What could you have done in the dream to protect yourself and others better?
- How can you best resolve or cope in the waking state with the anger present in you or others?
- What might you learn from this period of inner and/or outer conflict?

References

Aasted A, Darre E, Wolf HC. Mustard Gas: Clinical, Toxicological and Mutagenic Aspects Based on Modern Experience. *Ann Plastic Surg,* 1987; 19:330-333.

Acad Emerg Med. 2002; 9(3): 255-6 B.R. Sharma. Development of pre-hospital trauma-care system-an overview. *International Journal of the Care of the Injured.* 2005; 36:570-587.

Ali J *et al.* Trauma patient outcome after the prehospital trauma life support programme. *Journal of Trauma,* 1997, 42:1018–22.

Almogy G, Belzberg H, Mintz Y, *et al.* Suicide bombing attacks: update and modifications to the protocol. *Ann Surg* 2004; 239: 295-303.

Almogy G, Luria T, Richter E. *et al.* Can external signs of trauma guide management? Lessons learned from suicide bombing attacks in Israel. *Arch Surg* 2005; 140: 390-393.

American College of Surgeons, Committee on Trauma. *Resources for optimal care of the injured patient.* Chicago, IL, American College of Surgeons, 1999.

American Nurses Association. (2001). Are we ready to respond? Assessing nursing's bioterrorism preparedness. The American Nurse. Retrieved May 2, 2002 http://www.nursingworld.org/tan/01novd ec/respond.htm

Anandan S. Manic Monday Revives '9's Memories. *Hindustan Times,* 26th August 2003: 9.

Anderson PB. A comparative analysis of the emergency medical services and rescue responses to eight airliner crashes in the United States, 1987-1991. *Prehospital Disaster Med.* 1995;10:142-53.

Anderson PB. A comparative analysis of the emergency medical services and rescue responses to eight airliner crashes in the United States, 1987-1991. *Prehospital Disaster Med.* 1995;10:142-53.

Angus DC *et al.* Recommendations for life-supporting first-aid training of the lay public for disaster preparedness. *Prehospital Disaster Medicine,* 1993, 8:157–60.

Arreola-Risa C *et al.*Trauma care systems in urban Latin America: the priorities should be prehospital and emergency room management. *Journal of Trauma,* 1995, 39:457–62.

Asaeda G., MD. The Day That the START Triage System Came to a STOP: Observations from the World Trade Center Disaster.

Asaeda G., MD. The Day That the START Triage System Came to a STOP: Observations from the World Trade Center Disaster. *Acad Emerg Med.* 2002; 9(3): 255-6.

Australian Government Attorney-General's Department. Emergency Management Australia. EMA disasters database. Available at: http://www.ag.gov.au/ema/emadisasters.nsf (accessed Nov 2005).

Avitzour M, Libergal M, Assaf J, *et al.* A multicasualty event: out-of-hospital and in-hospital organisational aspects. *Acad Emerg Med* 2004; 11: 1102-1104.

B.R. Sharma. Development of pre-hospital trauma-care system-an overview. *International Journal of the Care of the Injured.* 2005; 36:570-587.

Bagian JP,Allen RC.Aeromedical transport. In:Auerbach PS, ed.*Wilderness medicine: management of wilderness and environmental emergencies,* 4th ed. St. Louis, MO, Mosby, 2001:660–72.

Balani-mood M. Sulfur Mustard poisoning in the Iran-Iraq War. *Clin Pharmaco Ther,* 1990; 47: 183-184.

BBC News. London attacks: 21 July attacks. Available at: http://news.bbc.co.uk/1/hi/in_depth/uk/2005/london_explosions/default.stm

Benson DO, Keonig KL, Schultz CH. Disaster triage: START then SAVE—a new method of dynamic triage for victims of a catastrophic earthquake. *Prehosp Disaster Med.* 1996;11:117-124.

Benson DO, Keonig KL, Schultz CH. Disaster triage: START then SAVE—a new method of dynamic triage for victims of a catastrophic earthquake. *Prehosp Disaster Med.* 1996;11:117-124.

Bentley JD (2001). Hospital preparedness for bioterrorism. *Public Health Reports,* 116 (Suppl. 2), 36-39.

Bettina SM (2001). Responding to the threat of bioterrorism: Practical resources and references, and the importance of preparation. *Journal of Emergency Nursing,* 27(5), 471-475.

Beyersddorf SR, Nania JN, Luna GK. Community medical response to the Fairchild mass causualty event. *Am. J. Surg.* 1996;171:467-470.

Beyersddorf SR, Nania JN, Luna GK. Community medical response to the Fairchild mass causualty event. *Am. J. Surg.* 1996;171:467-470.

Bioterror readiness plans available as a template. (2001). *Health Care Risk Management,* 23(11), 125-127.

Briggs B. (2001). Hospitals recheck: Are they ready for anything? *Health Data Management,* 9(12), 42-44.

Brown LH, Prasad M, Whitley TW. Adverse lighting condition effects on the assessment of capillary refill. *Am. J. Emerg. Med.* 1994;12:47-47

Brown LH, Prasad M, Whitley TW. Adverse lighting condition effects on the assessment of capillary refill. Am. J. Emerg. Med. 1994;12:47-47.

Bur A *et al.* Effects of bystander first aid, defibrillation and advanced life support on neurologic outcome and hospital costs in patients after ventricular fibrillation cardiac arrest. *Intensive Care Medicine,* 2001, 27:1474–80.

Bwale P, Husum H, Gilbert M. Prehospital trauma care: a training model in less resourced countries: examples from Angola, Cambodia, and Mozambique. In: 6th.

"9 Climbers Killed In Avalanche"; *Hindustan Times;* 23rd September 2003: "41 Feared Killed In Himanchal Cloud Burst"; *Hindustan Times;* 9th, August 2003: 1.

Caldicott DG, Edwards NA. Medical preparation for terrorism in Australia. Is luck running out for "the lucky country"? *Prehospital Disaster Med* 2003; 18: 57-65. <PubMed>

Callaham M. Quantifying the scanty science of prehospital emergency care. *Annals of Emergency Medicine,* 1997, 30:785–90.

Chaloner E, Blast injury in enclosed spaces. *BMJ* 2005; 331: 119-120.

Chapman AJ, White C. Death Resulting From Lacrimating Agents. *J Forensic Sci,* 1978; 23: 527-530.

Comunicato relativo al decreto del Ministro dell'interno per il coordinamento della protezione civile concernente: Adozione dei "Criteri di massima per l'organizzazione dei soccorsi sanitari nelle catratrofi". (Supplemento Ordinario G.U., Serie generale 12 maggio 2001 n°109).

Cone DC *et al.* Field triage systems: methodologies from the literature. *Prehospital Emergency Care,* 2004, 8:130–7.

Consultants, AH (2001). How to best create a plan for terrorism: 'Think of crowds of desperate people' and don't assume anything. *Health Care Risk Management,* 23(11), 121-124.

Cooke MW. How much to do at the accident scene? *British Medical Journal,* 1999, 319:1150.

Cuny FC (1998). Principles of disaster management lesson 1: Introduction. *Prehospital and Disaster Medicine,* 13(1), 80-85.

Cuny FC (1999). Principles of disaster management lesson 5: Programme supervision, monitoring, and control. *Prehospital and Disaster Medicine,* 14(3), 198-210.

Cuny FC (2000). Principles of disaster management lesson 7: Management leadership styles and methods. *Prehospital and Disaster Medicine,* 15(1), 78-86.

Deep Joshi. Center to Offer Lessons on Disaster Management. *Hindustan Times;* 2nd August 2003: 7.

Della Corte F., Olliveri F., Enrichens F. (2002). Manuale di Medicina d'Emergenza. (pp. 1024-1026) Milano: Mc Graw-Hill.

DePalma RG, Burris DG, Champion HR, Hodgson MJ. Blast injuries. *N Engl J Med* 2005; 352: 1335-1342.

Donna J. Middaugh, MSN, RN, is Clinical Assistant Professor, University of Arkansas for Medical Sciences, College of Nursing, Little Rock, AR.

Eckert WG. Mass Deaths by Gas or Chemical Poisoning: A Historical Perspective. *Am J Forensic Med Pathol* 1991; 12: 119-125.

Eckert WG. Mass Deaths by Gas or Chemical Poisoning: A Historical Perspective"; Am *J Forensic Med Pathol,* 1991; 12: 119.

Eckstein M. *et al.* Effect of prehospital advanced life support on outcomes of major trauma patients. *Journal of Trauma,* 2000, 48:643–8.

Eiseman B. Combat casualty management for tommorow's battlefield: Urban terrorism. J. Trauma, Injury, Infection, and Critical care. 2001;51(5):821-823.

Eiseman B. Combat casualty management for tommorow's battlefield:Urban terrorism. *J. Trauma, Injury, Infection, and Critical Care.* 2001;51(5):821-823.

Ellenhorn MJ, Schonwald S, Ordog G, Wasserberger J. Chemical Disasters.In: Ellenhorn's Medical Toxicology, 2nd Edition-1997; Williams and Wilkins, USA: 1236-1266.

Emergency and Disaster Management, Inc. The London bombing attack on 7 July 2005. Available at: http://www.emergency-management.net/london_bomb.htm

Employment News; 10th-16th January, 2004: 8.

Express Disaster. *Hindustan Times,* 16th May 2003: 1.

Fawcus S *et al.*A Community-based investigation of avoidable factors for maternal mortality in Zimbabwe. *Studies in Family Planning,* 1996, 27:319–27.

Fries GR, McCalla G, Levitt MA, *et al.* A prospectic comparison of paramedic judgement and the trauma triage rule in the prehospital setting. *AnnEmerg Med.* 1994; 25:885-889.

Fries GR, McCalla G, Levitt MA, *et al.* A prospectic comparison of paramedic judgement and the trauma triage rule in the prehospital setting. *AnnEmerg Med.* 1994; 25:885-889.

Frykberg ER. Terrorist bombings in Madrid. *Critical Care,* 2005, 9:20–2.

Gans L, Kennedy T. Management of unique clinical entities in disaster medicine. *Emerg. Med. Clin North Am.* 1996; 14:301-326.

Gans L, Kennedy T. Management of unique clinical entities in disaster medicine. *Emerg. Med. Clin North Am. 1996;* 14:301-326.

Garner A, Lee A, Harrison K, *et al.* Comparative analysis of multiple-casualty incident triage algorithms. *Ann Emerg Med.* 2001; 38: 541-548.

Garner A, Lee A, Harrison K, et all: Comparative analysis of multiple-casualty incident triage algorithms. *Ann Emerg Med* 2001; 38: 541-548.

Gearhart PA, Wuerz R, Localio AR. Cost-effectiveness analysis of helicopter EMS for trauma patients. *Annals of Emergency Medicine,* 1997, 30:500–6.

Glass TA (2001). Understanding public response to disasters. *Public Health Reports,* 116 (Suppl. 2), 69-73.

Gofrit ON, Leibovici D, Shemer J, *et al.* The efficacy of integrating "smart simulated casualties" in hospital disaster drills. *Prehospital Disaster Med* 1997; 12: 26-30.

Goldfrank LR, Flomenbaum NE, Lewin NA, Weisman RS, Howland MA, Hoffman RS. Toxicologic Plagues and Disasters in History. In: Goldfrank's Toxicologic Emergencies, 6th Edition-1998, Appleton and Lange, USA: 19-28.

Gove S *et al.*Development and technical basis of simplified guidelines for emergency triage assessment and treatment in developing countries. WHO Integrated Management of Childhood Illness (IMCI) Referral Care Project. *Archives of Disease in Childhood,* 1999, 81:473–7.

Gutierrez de Ceballos JP, Turegano Fuentes F, Perez-Diaz D, *et al.* Casualties treated at the closest hospital in the Madrid, March 11, terrorist bombings. Crit Care Med 2005; 33 (1 Suppl): S107-S112.

Haines JA. Technological Disasters: Global Trends. Regional Symposium on Chemical Disasters, Addis Ababa; From ICPS/WHO Geneva, Switzerland, May 30, 1991.

Hauswald M,Yeoh E. Designing a prehospital system for a developing country: estimated cost and benefits. *American Journal of Emergency Medicine,* 1997, 15:600–3.

Hischberg A, Holcomb JB, Mattox KL: Hospital trauma care in multiple-casualty incident: a critical view. *Ann Emerg Med* 37: 647-652, 2001 G.F.T. Gruppo Formazione Triage (2000). Triage Infermieristico. Milano:Mc Graw-Hill.

Hodgetts TJ. Mackaway-Jones K, eds. Major Incident Medical Management and Support, the Practical Approach. Plymouth, MA: BMJ Publishing Group; 1995

Hodgetts TJ. Mackaway-Jones K, eds. Major Incident Medical Management and Support, the Practical Approach. Plymouth, MA: BMJ Publishing Group; 1995.

Hodgetts TJ. Triage. Prehosp Immediate Care. 1997;1:104-111 Janet T. Ihlenfeld, RN, PhD. A primer on triage and Mass casualty Events. *Dimensions of Critcal Care Nursing,* 2003; 22(5): 204-209.

Hodgetts TJ. Triage. Prehosp Immediate Care. 1997;1:104-111 Janet T. Ihlenfeld, RN, Ph.D. A primer on triage and Mass casualty Events. *Dimensions of Critcal Care Nursing,* 2003; 22(5): 204-209

Husum H, Gilbert M,Wisborg T. *Save lives, save limbs*.Penang, Malaysia,Third World Network, 2000.

Joshipura M *et al.* Essential trauma care: strengthening trauma systems round the world. *Injury*, 2004, 35:841–5.

Kennedy K, Aghababian RV, Gans L, *et al.* Triage: techniques and applications in decision-making. *Ann Emerg Med*. 28:136-144, 1996.

Kennedy K, Aghababian RV, Gans L, *et al.* Triage: techniques and applications in decision-making. *Ann Emerg Med* 28:136-144, 1996.

Kirschenbaum L, Keene A., O'Neill P, *et al.* The experience at St Vincent's Hospital, Manhattan, on September 11, 2001: preparedness, response, and lessons learned. *Crit Care Med* 2005; 33 (1 Suppl): S48-S52.

Kobusingye O, ed. Emergency care saves lives. *Injury Control News: Newsletter of the Injury Control Centre-Uganda*, 2002, 3:3.

Lanoix R. Wiener DE, Zayas VD. Concepts of disaster triage in the wake of the World Trade Center 'terrorist attack. *Top Emerg. Med*. 2002;24(2):60-71.

Lanoix R. Wiener DE, Zayas VD. Concepts of disaster triage in the wake of the World Trade Center terrorist attack. *Top Emerg. Med*. 2002;24(2):60-71.

Leibovici D, Gofrit ON, Shapira SC. Eardrum perforation in explosion survivors: is it a marker of pulmonary blast injury? *Ann Emerg Med* 1999; 34: 168-172.

Levitin H, Siegelson H. Hazardous materials. Disaster medical planning and response. *Emerg Med Clin North Am* 1996; 14: 327-348. <PubMed>

Liberman M, Mulder D, Sampalis J. Advanced or basic life support for trauma:meta-analysis and critical review of the literature. *Journal of Trauma*, 2000, 49:584–99.

Lundy PM, Hansen AS, Hand BT, Boulet CA. Comparison of Several Oximes against Poisoning. *Toxicol*, 1992; 72: 99-105.

Mehta PS, Mehta AS, Mehta SJ, Milkijani AB. Bhopal Tragedy's Health Effects: A Review of Methyl iso-cyanate Toxicity. *JAMA* 1990; 264: 2781-2787.

Meredith W, Rutledge R, Hansen AR *et al.* Field triage of trauma patients based upon the ability to follow commands: A study in 29,573 injured patients. J. Trauma 1995;38:129-35

Meredith W, Rutledge R, Hansen AR *et al.* Field triage of trauma patients based upon the ability to follow commands: A study in 29,573 injured patients. *J. Trauma* 1995;38:129-35.

Mhasawade SC, Unnikrishanan C. Mahyem in Mumbai"; *Hindustan Times;* 26th August 2003: 01.

Milsten A. (2000). Hospital responses to acute-onset disasters: A review. *Prehospital and Disaster Medicine*, 15(1), 40-53.

Mock C *et al.Guidelines for essential trauma care*. Geneva, World Health Organisation, 2004.

"NHRC Calls For Restructuring Emergency Medicare Facilities" Daily Excelsior, 6th September 2003: 8.

Mock C, Joshipura M, Goosen J. Global strengthening of the care of the injured. *Bulletin of the World Health Organisation*, 2004, 82:241.

Mock CN *et al.*Improvements in prehospital trauma care in an African country with no formal emergency medical services. *Journal of Trauma*, 2002, 53:90.

Mock CN *et al.*Trauma mortality patterns in three nations at different economic levels: implications for global trauma system development. *Journal of Trauma*, 1998, 44:804–12.

Mortia H, Yanagisawa N, Nakajima T, *et al.* Sarin Poisoning In Matsumoto, Japan. *Lancet* 1995; 346:290-293.

Munro I. Silence at dusk: surfers pay a heartfelt tribute. The Age (Melbourne) 2005; 9 Oct. Available at: http://www.theage.com.au/news/war-on-terror/silence-at-dusk-surfers-pay-a-heartfelt-tribute/2005/10/08/1128563036528.html?oneclick=true (accessed Nov 2005).

Murray JA *et al.* Prehospital intubation in patients with severe head injury. *Journal of Trauma,* 2000, 49:1065–70.

Nicholl J *et al. A review of the costs and benefits of helicopter emergency ambulance services in England and Wales: final report to the Department of Health,* 2003.

Okie S. Traumatic brain injury in the war zone. *N Engl J Med* 2005; 352: 2043-2047.

Okumura T, Takasu N, Ishimatsu S, *et al.* Report on 640 victims of the Tokyo subway sarin attack. *Ann Emerg Med* 1996; 28: 129-135. <PubMed>

Osterwalder JJ.Insufficient quality of research on prehospital medical emergency care– where are the major problems and solutions? *Swiss Medical Weekly,* 2004, 134:389–94.

Pelinka LE *et al.* Bystander trauma care—effect of the level of training. *Resuscitation,* 2004, 60:289–96.

Peterson TD *et al.* Bystander trauma care training in Iowa. *Prehospital Emergency Care,* 1999, 3:225–30.

Phillips S, Rond PC, Kelly SM, *et al.* The need for pediatric-specific triage criteria results from the Florida trauma triage study. Pediatric Emerg Care. 1996;12:394-399

Phillips S, Rond PC, Kelly SM, *et al.* The need for pediatric-specific triage criteria results from the Florida trauma triage study. *Pediatric Emerg Care* 1996;12:394-399.

Plan now for the disaster that is soon to come: Disasters bring unanticipated problems. (2001, May). *Health Care Risk Management,* 23 (Suppl.), 1-2.

Pozner CN *et al.* International EMS systems. The United States: past, present, and future. *Resuscitation,* 2004, 60:239–44.

Prasad NH, Brown LH, Ausband SC *et al..* Prehospital blood pressures: inaccuracies caused by ambulance noise? Am. J. Emerg. Med. 1994;12:617-20.

Prasad NH, Brown LH, Ausband SC *et al..* Prehospital blood pressures: inaccuracies caused by ambulance noise? *Am. J. Emerg. Med.* 1994;12:617-20.

Razzak JA, Kellermann AL. Emergency medical care in developing countries: is it worthwhile? *Bulletin of the World Health Organisation,* 2002, 80:900–5.

Rediff.com. El Deeb S. 88 die in Egyptian resort blast. 24 July 2005. Available at: http://us.rediff.com/news/2005/jul/23egypt.htm (accessed Nov 2005).

Rodoplu U., Arnold JL, Tokyay R, *et al.* Mass-casualty terrorist bombings in Istanbul, Turkey, November 2003: report of the events and the prehospital emergency response. *Pre-hospital Disaster Med* 2004; 19: 133-145.

Ross SE, Leipold C, Terregino C, *et al.* Efficacy of the Glasgow Coma Score in trauma triage. *J Trauma* 1998;45:42-44.

Ross SE, Leipold C, Terregino C, *et al.* Efficacy of the Glasgow Coma Score in trauma triage. *J Trauma* 1998;45:42-44.

Rowland HS, and Rowland BL (Eds.). (1997). Nursing administration handbook (4th ed.). *Gaithersburg,* MD: Aspen Publishers, Inc.

Rubin J (2001). Institutional networks: Regional response to disasters. *Public Health Reports,* 116 (Suppl. 2), 45-48.

Sandhu K. Mobilization Disaster Stares Nation in Face. *Hindustan Times;* 2nd August 2003:11.

Sarkisian AE, Khondkarian RA, Amirbekian NM, *et al.* Sonographic screening of mass casualties for abdominal and renal injuries following the 1988 Armenian earthquake. *J Trauma* 1991; 31: 247-250. <PubMed>

Satendra Gupta A. Managing Disaster Must For Sustainable Development. *Employment News,* Vol. XXVIII No. 30, 25th-31st Oct. 2003: 1,

Schmid T *et al.* Transportation for maternal emergencies in Tanzania: empowering communities through participatory problem solving. *American Journal of Public Health,* 2001, 91:1589–90.

Shapira SC, Mor-Yosef S. Applying lessons from medical management of conventional terror to responding to weapons of mass destruction terror: the experience of a tertiary university hospital. Stud Conflict Terrorism 2003; 26: 379-385.

Shapira SC, Mor-Yosef S. Terror politics and medicine: the role of leadership. *Stud Conflict Terrorism* 2004; 27: 65-71.

Shapira SC, Shemer J. Medical management of terrorist attacks. *Ist Med Assoc J* 2002; 4: 489-492. <PubMed>

Sheehy SB, Burkle Jr. RM. and Kinney ML (1993). The personalized disaster plan narrative: An effective teaching tool for hospitals. *Journal of Emergency Nursing*, 19(3), 254-257.

Sidell FR. Chemical Agent Terrorism. *Ann Emerg Med*, 1996; 28: 223-224.

Smith GCS, Pell JP. Parachute use to prevent death and major trauma related to gravitational challenge:systematic review of randomised controlled trials. *BMJ*, 2003, 327:1459–61.

Sodemann M *et al.*High mortality despite good care-seeking behaviour:a community study of childhood deaths in Guinea-Bissau. *Bulletin of the World Health Organisation*, 1997, 75:205–12.

Souvenir "DISMAN-2003", released on "Workshop on Development of Contingency Plan for Management of Mass Casualties during Disaster of Jammu Province, 14th-16th March 2003.

Spengler C. The Oklahoma City bombing: A personal account. *J. Child Neurol.* 1995;10:392-398

Spengler C. The Oklahoma City bombing: A personal account. *J. Child Neurol.* 1995;10:392-398

Stockinger ZT, McSwain NE. Prehospital endotracheal intubation for trauma does not improve survival over bag–valve–mask ventilation. *Journal of Trauma*, 2004, 56:531–6.

Tan, G., Fitzgerald M. Chemical–biological–radiological (CBR) response: a template for hospital emergency departments. Med J Aust 2002; 177: 196-199. <eMJA full text> <PubMed>

The Lowa Persian Gulf Study Group. Self-Reported Illness and Health Status among Gulfwar Veterans. *JAMA*, 1997; 227: 238-245.

Tikoo A. CBSE Chairman Asks Jammu Schools To Make Effective Changes In Education System. 6th May 2003: 4.

Tur-Kaspa I., Lev E.I., Hendler, I., *et al.* Preparing hospitals for toxicological mass casualties events. *Crit Care Med* 1999; 27: 873-874. <PubMed>

United States National Highway Traffic Safety Administration. *First there, first care.* Washington, DC, US Department of Transportation, 2000.

"Vajpayee to Convene C.M.'s Meeting on Disaster Management"; *Hindustan Times;* 5th June 2003: 7.

Van Rooyen *et al.* International emergency medical services: assessment of developing prehospital systems abroad. *Journal of Emergency Medicine*, 1999, 17:691–6.

Varghese M, Mohan P. *When someone is hurt: a first aid guide for lay persons and community workers.* New Delhi, The Other Media Communications, 1998.

Wesson DE, Scorpio R: Field triage:Help or Hindrance? *Can. J. Surg* 1992;35:19-21

Wikipedia. 11 March 2004 Madrid train bombings. Available at: http://en.wikipedia.org/wiki/11_March_2004_Madrid_attacks

Wikipedia. List of wars and disasters by death toll. Available at: http://www.answers.com/topic/list-of-wars-and-disasters-by-death-toll (accessed Nov 2005).

Wiseman Barrett D, MD, Ellenbogen, MD, and Shaffrey I. MD: Triage for the neurosurgeon. *Neurosurgeon Focus* 2002; 12(3): article 5.

Wiseman Barrett D, MD, Ellenbogen, MD, and Shaffrey I. MD: Triage for the neurosurgeon. *Neurosurgeon Focus* 2002; 12(3): article 5.

World Health Organisation.*Surgical care at the district hospital.* Geneva, WHO, 2003 (http://www.who.int/surgery/publications/en/SCDH.pdf, accessed 18 May 2005).

Zuthsi M. The agony doesn't end with Death. *Hindustan Times*, 17th May 2003:11.

Appendix I

DEFINITIONS

1. STANDBY ORANGE ALERT: Prepare for the possibility of an ORANGE ALERT. Usually precedes the alert. Dispense in-house employees to the Personnel Pool for sign in, call in on-call staff, and lock all doors except the Front Entrance and the Emergency Room doors.

2. ORANGE ALERT: Impending disaster with a count of victims being rescued and transferred to the hospital. Organize treatment and triage areas, continue with Disaster Plan assignments, initiate calling of employees, prepare to triage and treat victims. Establish Control Center.

3. ALL CLEAR: Discontinue Disaster Plan. Disaster is finished. All victims have been treated. Disaster treatment areas can be dismantled.

4. MESSENGER: Writes down messages and transports them to the intended receiver.

5. TRANSPORTER: Transports victims by carts, wheelchairs or accompanies them ambulatory and remains with the victims until released by the person in charge of the area.

6. GUARD: Stationed at doors and checks identification of persons attempting to gain entrance to the facility. Sends people without proper identification to Control Center for identification.

7. INTERNAL DISASTER: A need for extra hospital personnel to care for patients and possible evacuation of them due to an accident within the facility such as fire, tornado or explosion. (See specific Standard Operating Guidelines)

8. EXTERNAL DISASTER: A disaster which occurs outside the hospital, somewhere in the community, when there is a disproportionate amount of hospital staff to care for the incoming Emergency Room patients or victims.

9. ON-CALL STAFF: The members of the various hospital departments who are on call for hospital business on a 24 or 48 hour basis.

10. CRITICAL: Vital signs are unstable and not within normal limits. Patient is acutely ill or unconscious. Indicators are questionable or unfavorable.

11. NONCRITICAL: Vital signs are stable and within normal limits. Patientis conscious and can be either comfortable or uncomfortable. Indicators are favorable or excellent.

Appendix 2

SOME OF THE MAJOR DISASTER EVENTS

Year	*Place of Disasters World Wide*	*Casualties Reported*
1348	Epidemic (Bubonic Plague) World Wide	25,000,000
1556	Earthquake China	8,30,000
1919	Epidemic (Influenza) World Wide	20,000,000
1949	Mini disaster Germany	3,000
1956	Hurricane China	2,000
1962	Avalanches Ranrahivca Peru	3,500
1963	Air Crashes Canada	118
1963	Dam Collapse Valout, Italy	3,000
1985	Volcanic Eruption Colombia, USA	23,000
1985	Air Crashes (Air India) Montreal, Canada	348
1987	Nuclear Plant Disaster Chernobyl, USA	29
1988	Earthquakes Armenia, USSR	55,000
1988	Train Accident South-West, London (Injured)	36(115)
1988	Earthquakes Unan, China	900
1988	Earthquakes Tazakistan, USSR	1,415
2001	Terrorist's Attack on WTC, USA	3,000
2003	Earthquake Bam, Iran	20,000
2004	MEENA, NEAR MACCA SAUDI ARABIA	244
2004	MADRID BLAST, SPAIN	198 (1400 Injured.)

Year	*Place of Disasters in India*	*Casualties Reported*
1737	Earthquake Calcutta, India	3,00,000.
1961	Floods India	1,000
1977	Cyclone Andhra Pradesh, India	10,000
1979	Flash Flood Gujarat, India	2,500
1984	Chemical Disaster Bhopal, India	2,500
1988	Train Accident Quilon, India (Injured)	300(500)
1988	Air Crash Ahmedabad, India	135
1993	13 Bomb Blasts in Mumbai, India	250
1998	Train Accident Khanna, Pusa, India	211
2001	Earthquake Bhuj, Gujarat, India	10,000
2003	Frontier Mail Fire Ludhiana, Punjab, India	36 (14)
2003	2 Bomb Blasts in Mumbai, India	45
2003	Cloud Burst Himanchal Pradesh, India	41
2003	Stampede At Kumbh, Nasik, India	35 (75)

Year	*Place of Disasters in J & K*	*Casualties Reported*
2002	Terrorist's Attack Kaluchak, Jammu	23

2003	Terrorist's Attack on Railway Station, Jammu	20
2004	Terrorist's Attack on Railway Station, Jammu	08
2008	Bombay terror attacks	183

Some International terrorist attacks involving bombings in recent years

Date	*Place*	*Type of Incident*	*Number injured*	*Number killed*
11 Sep. 2001	New York, USA1	A series of suicide bomb attacks involving four hijacked commercial aircraft, three of which were crashed into intentionally targeted major buildings	> 2100	> 2986
12 Oct. 2002	Bali, Indonesia	A small explosion in a bar followed by a large car-bomb explosion outsidea club	196	202
15 and 20 Nov. 2003	Istanbul, Turkey	Improvised explosive devices in trucks exploded outside two synagogues (15 Nov.) and a bank and the British Consulate (20 Nov.)	> 750	63
6 Feb. 2004	Moscow, Russia	A bomb explosion in the underground railway system	> 129	> 39
11 Mar. 2004	Madrid, Spain	A series of coordinated bombings on commuter trains	1460	191
7 and 21 July 2005	London, UK	Three large bomb blasts in the underground railway system and one in a bus (7 July); four small attempted train and bus bomb attacks (21 July)	> 700	52
23 July 2005	Sharm el-Sheik, Egypt	A series of car bombs and another blast in a hotel and coffee shop in a tourist resort	> 116	> 88
1 Oct. 2005	Bali, Indonesia	A series of bomb blasts in restaurants in Bali	108	23

2

First Receivers of Disaster Casualties in Hospitals

Health care workers risk occupational exposure to chemical, biological, or radiological materials when hospitals receive patients contaminated with these substances during mass casualty incidents (Horton *et al.*, 2003). Such incidents could be associated with manmade or natural disasters and can involve a wide range of hazardous substances-from chemical weapons agents to toxic industrial chemicals. Health care workers at a hospital receiving contaminated victims for treatment may be termed first receivers (Koenig, 2003). This group is a subset of first responders. However, most first responders typically act at the site of disaster. In contrast, inherent to the definition of first receivers, is an assumption that the hospital is not itself the primary incident site, but rather is remote from the location where the hazardous substance release occurred. Thus, the possible exposure of first receivers is limited to the quantity of substance arriving at the hospital as a contaminant on victims and their clothing or personal effects. First receivers typically include personnel in the following roles: clinicians and other hospital staff who have a role in receiving and treating contaminated victims (e.g., triage, decontamination, medical treatment, and security) and those whose roles support these functions.

The United States Occupational Safety and Health Administration (OSHA) is an agency of the United States Department of Labor. It was created by Congress under the Occupational Safety and Health Act, signed by President Richard M. Nixon, on December 29, 1970. Its mission is to prevent work-related injuries, illnesses, and deaths by issuing and enforcing rules (called standards) for workplace safety and health. As of March 2006, the agency is headed by Assistant Secretary of Labor Edwin Foulke. Most of the observations given below are based on recommendations of OSHA. See various appendices attached to this chapter for more detailed guidelines.

OSHA's best practices

By implementing those prerequisites, hospitals can reduce the exposures of their own first receivers. The best practices indicate the minimum PPE that OSHA anticipates generally will be needed to protect first receivers faced with a wide range of unknown hazards. However, as with any generalized protection, OSHA's PPE for first receivers offers more protection against some hazards than others. When a hospital determines that first receivers could reasonably anticipate encountering a specific known hazard, the hospital also must determine whether this generalized protection must be supplemented to more fully address that specific hazard. JCAHO requires that hospitals also consider their anticipated roles and coordinate activities with other emergency response agencies and hospitals within the community. When these sources point to a specific substance or situation from which the hospital should protect its first receivers, the hospital must confirm that PPE selection provides effective protection against that hazard.

Personal protective equipment (PPE) and other essential equipment

PPE selection for first receivers has been a topic of significant discussion. At the root of this discussion is the need for hospitals to provide adequate protection for the reasonably anticipated worst-case employee exposure scenario, despite having limited information regarding the nature of the substance with which victims may be contaminated (OSHA, 2002b). This lack of information challenges hospitals' abilities to conduct the hazard assessments on which PPE selection must be based.

Despite many hospitals' strong interest in powered air-purifying respirators (PAPR) as a practical form of respiratory protection for first receivers in the Decontamination Zone, many knowledgeable sources avoid making specific PPE recommendations. OSHA requires Level B protection or self-contained breathing apparatus (SCBA) for unknown hazards, but points out there are substantial difficulties for health care workers who attempt to care for patients while wearing this type of equipment and also addresses the hazards of wearing SCBAs (e.g., slips, trips, falls, and overexertion, particularly for infrequent users).

A key factor supporting OSHA's PPE best practices is the limited amount of toxic substance to which first receivers might be exposed. Many recent sources note that the quantity of contaminant on victims is restricted. Horton *et al.* (2003) stated that, during victim decontamination procedures, the hazard to health care workers is strictly from secondary exposure and "depends largely on the toxicity of the substance on the victims' hair, skin, and clothing; the concentration of the substance; and the duration of contact with the victim." The quantity of contaminant that health care workers might encounter can be dramatically less than the amount to which the victim was exposed or that was originally deposited on the victim. Gas or vapor releases can expose victims to toxic concentrations, but tend to evaporate and dissipate quickly. Horton *et al.* agree, stating that substances released as gas or vapor "are not likely to pose a secondary contamination risk" to first receivers.

Removal of victim's clothing or, better yet, decontamination of victims before they arrive at the hospital has a marked effect on the quantity of contaminant that first receivers encounter. Pre-hospital decontamination can eliminate the risk of secondary contamination. Removing contaminated clothing can reduce the quantity of contaminant associated with victims by an estimated 75 to 90 percent (Macintyre *et al.*, 2000; Vogt, 2002; USACHPPM, 2003a). The clothing is cut away using blunt-nose shears to eliminate stretching, flapping, wringing, or excessive handling of fabric that might contribute to worker exposure. Showering with tepid water and a liquid soap with good surfactant properties is widely considered an effective method for removing the remaining hazardous substance from victims' skin and hair (Goozner et al, 2002; Macintyre *et al.*, 2000). As a final step in minimizing first receiver exposure to hazardous substances, the accepted industrial hygiene practice is for the health care workers also to shower following contact with contaminated victims and cleanse equipment as part of decontamination procedures. Hospitals use a strict protocol for personnel to decontaminate themselves while removing gloves, protective suits, boots, and hooded powered air-purifying respirators (PAPRs). Those workers who experienced symptoms were unprotected and tended to have close, extended contact with the contaminated victims. Respiratory tract and eye irritation were the primary symptoms and no employees required hospitalization.

More than 70 percent of the hazardous materials incidents involved flammable materials (e.g., methane gas, diesel fuel, gasoline, and hydraulic oils). Approximately 7 percent of the incidents involved highly toxic materials, all of which fell into the categories of mercury, pesticides, and cyanides. An additional 5 percent of the events were associated with toxic gases (primarily carbon monoxide, with a few cases of anhydrous ammonia or chlorine exposure). Corrosive materials accounted for another 10 percent of the incidents and primarily involved mineral acids and basic materials such as lime and sodium hydroxide. Walter found that those patients transported to the hospital were usually treated for inhalation exposure to airborne toxicants, for which few required hospitalization.

If correctly selected, fitted, used, and maintained, respiratory protective equipment reduces significantly the effective exposure level that an employee experiences. An employee wearing a respirator that offers a protection factor of 1,000 will breathe air that contains no more than 1/1,000 (or 0.1 percent) of the contaminant level outside the respirator. The combination of high efficiency (HE) particulate filters plus organic vapor (OV) cartridges currently available for PAPRs will protect against many of the airborne hazards that first receivers might encounter (e.g., toxic dusts, biological agents, radioactive particulates, organophosphates and other pesticides, and solvents). Acid gas cartridges add an additional level of protection from gases such as chlorine, which generally will dissipate before victims arrive at the hospital.

Gloves and Boots

No single glove or boot material will protect against every substance. Most glove manufacturers offer detailed guides to glove materials and their chemical resistance. Butyl rubber gloves generally provide better protection than nitrile gloves for chemical warfare agents and most toxic industrial chemicals that are more likely to be involved in a terrorist incident, although the converse applies to some industrial chemicals. Foil-based gloves are highly resistant to a wide variety of hazardous substances and could also be considered when determining an appropriate protective ensemble. Hospitals must select materials that cover the specific substances that the hospital has determined first receivers reasonably might encounter. However, given the broad scope of potential contaminants, OSHA considers it of vital importance for hospitals also to select materials that protect against a wide range of substances. A double layer of gloves, made of two different materials, or foil-based gloves resist the broadest range of chemicals.

In general, the same material selected for gloves will also be appropriate for boots. Because boot walls tend to be thicker than gloves, boots of any material are likely to be more protective than gloves of the same material. Butyl gloves worn over inner nitrile gloves are often the best option for use by hospital workers during emergencies and mass casualties involving hazardous substances. However, hospitals are advised to select the combination that best meet their specific needs. Depending on the dexterity needed by the hospital worker, the glove selection can be modified to allow for the use of a glove combination that is thinner than that usually recommended for the best protection. With increased thickness comes greater loss of manual dexterity. When advanced medical procedures must be performed before decontamination, thicker gloves might be too awkward, and, therefore, it might be necessary to use a butyl rubber glove of 7 mil over the nitrile glove, or a 14 mil butyl rubber glove alone. If sterility is required and decontamination is not possible before procedures, a double layer of disposable 4 to 5 mil nitrile gloves might be the best option (USACHPPM, 2003a).

Protective Garments

The optimal garment material for first receivers will protect against a wide range of chemicals in liquid, solid, or vapor form. Because first receivers might become contaminated with liquid or solid contaminants through physical contact with a contaminated victim, the ideal fabric will repel chemicals during incidental contact. Additionally, the optimal garment will restrict the passage of vapors, both through the suit fabric and through openings in the suit. Finally, optimal clothing is also sufficiently flexible, durable, and lightweight for long-term wear (up to several hours) during physically active work. The ability of protective garment fabric to withstand physical abrasion and tearing is also important. When assisting non-ambulatory victims, first receivers might subject the protective garments to physical stresses that should be considered in garment selection. Hospitals should select PPE (e.g., respirators, suits, gloves, face and eye protection) based on a hazard assessment that identifies the hazards to which employees might be exposed.

OSHA's Personal Protective Equipment Standard also requires that employees be provided with equipment that fits appropriately. Some hospitals assign a set of protective equipment (except the PAPR respirator) to a specific individual. The equipment is stored in a container marked with the individual's name. Suits do not need to fit as closely and excess fabric can be taped or rolled to fit. To prevent protective suits from tearing at the crotch, hospitals should order over-sized suits (SBCCOM, 2003). Loose-fitting PAPR respirator hoods offer a universal fit, thus are not included in individual or size-based PPE sets; however, tight fitting face pieces do require fit testing.

The respirators can be integrated into the hospitals existing respiratory protection programme, which should include the following elements:

- Procedures for selecting respirators for use in the workplace.
- Medical evaluations of employees required to use respirators.
- Fit testing procedures for tight-fitting respirators.
- Procedures for proper use of respirators in routine and reasonably foreseeable emergency situations.
- Procedures and schedules for cleaning, disinfecting, storing, inspecting, repairing, discarding, and otherwise maintaining respirators.
- Procedures to ensure adequate air quality, quantity, and flow of breathing air for atmosphere-supplying respirators.
- Training of employees in the respiratory hazards to which they are potentially exposed during routine and emergency situations.
- Training of employees in the proper use of respirators, including putting on and removing them, any limitations on their use, and their maintenance.
- Establishing and implementing respirator chemical cartridge change schedules.
- Procedures for regularly evaluating the effectiveness of the programme.

The Hospital Decontamination Zone

It includes any areas where the type and quantity of hazardous substance is unknown and where contaminated victims, contaminated equipment, or contaminated waste may be present. It is reasonably anticipated that employees in this zone might have exposure to contaminated victims, their belongings, equipment, or waste. This zone includes, but is not limited to, places where initial triage and/or medical stabilization of possibly contaminated victims occur, pre-decontamination waiting (staging) areas for victims, the actual decontamination area. This area will typically end at the ED door.

Conditions Necessary for Hospitals to Rely on the PPE

1. Thorough and complete hazard vulnerability analysis (HVA) and emergency management plan (EMP), which consider community input, have been conducted/developed, and have been updated within the past year.
2. The EMP includes plans to assist the numbers of victims that the community anticipates might seek treatment at this hospital, keeping in mind that the vast majority of victims may self-refer to the nearest hospital.
3. .Preparations specified in the EMP have been implemented (e.g., employee training, equipment selection, maintenance, and a respiratory protection programme).
4. The EMP includes methods for handling the numbers of ambulatory and non-ambulatory victims anticipated by the community.
5. The hazardous substance was not released in close proximity to the hospital, and the lapse time between the victims' exposure and victims' arrival at the hospital exceeds approximately 10 minutes, thereby permitting substantial levels of gases and vapors from volatile substances time to dissipate.
6. Victims' contaminated clothing and possessions are promptly removed and contained (e.g., in an approved hazardous waste container that is isolated outdoors), and decontamination is initiated promptly upon arrival at the hospital. Hospital EMP includes shelter, tepid water, soap, privacy, and coverings to promote victim compliance with decontamination procedures.
7. EMP procedures are in place to ensure that contaminated medical waste and wastewater do not become a secondary source of employee exposure.
8. The decontamination system and pre-decontamination victim waiting areas are designed and used in a manner that promotes constant fresh air circulation through the system to limit hazardous substance accumulation. Air exchange from a clean source has been considered in the design of fully enclosed systems (i.e., through consultation with professional engineer or certified industrial hygienist) and air is not re-circulated.

Minimum Personal Protective Equipment (PPE)

SCOPE AND LIMITATIONS

This applies when:

- The hospital is not the release site.
- Prerequisite conditions of hospital eligibility are already met
- The identity of the hazardous substance is unknown.

ZONE	MINIMUM PPE
Hospital Decontamination Zone • All employees in this zone (Includes, but not limited to, any of the following employees: decontamination team members, clinicians, set-up crew, cleanup crew, security staff, and patient tracking clerks).	• Powered air-purifying respirator (PAPR) that provides a protection factor of 1,000. The respirator must be NIOSH-approved. • Combination 99.97% high-efficiency particulate air (HEPA)/organic vapor/acid gas respirator cartridges (also NIOSH-approved). • Double layer protective gloves. • Chemical resistant suit. • Head covering and eye/face protection (if not part of the respirator). • Chemical-protective boots. • Suit openings sealed with tape.
Hospital Post-decontamination Zone. • All employees in this zone.	• Normal work clothes and PPE, as necessary, for infection control purposes (e.g., gloves, gown, and appropriate respirator).

Training first receivers

OSHA recognizes that hospital staffs who decontaminate victims at the hospital are removed from the site of the emergency (OSHA, 2002a, 2002b, 19992b). In each case, the training must be effective, that is, be provided in a manner the employee is capable of understanding.

Training requirements for First Responder Operations Level indicates a minimum training duration of 8 hours and outlines topics to be covered (competencies the employee must acquire). OSHA, however, allows these topics (but not the minimum training time) to be tailored to better meet the needs of first responders. For example, the training might omit topics that are not directly relevant to the employee's role (e.g., recognition of Department of Transportation placards), but instead should include alternative training on hazard recognition (e.g., signs and symptoms of contamination or exposure), on decontamination procedures provided by the hospital, and on the selection and use of PPE (OSHA, 1992c).

"...employees with sufficient experience may objectively demonstrate the required competencies instead of completing eight hours of training" (OSHA, 2003). However, it is important to note that in most hospital settings it might be difficult to ensure that employees have sufficient experience to waive the training requirement. Most hospital employees do not have extensive experience with hazardous materials or PAPRs, and decontamination activities are performed infrequently.

Training core elements must include:

- Understanding the hospital emergency operations plan and their roles in the response.
- Site safety, including risks to receiving personnel.
- Appropriate selection and use of PPE.
- Decontamination procedures.

At a minimum, that training must cover the following:

- When PPE is necessary
- What PPE is necessary
- How to properly put on, remove, adjust, and wear PPE
- Limitations of PPE
- Proper care, maintenance, useful life, and disposal of PPE.

Employees must demonstrate their understanding of the training by showing they can use the PPE properly, prior to using the protective equipment in the workplace. Refresher training is warranted when the employee cannot demonstrate proficiency in the proper care and use of the PPE, when changes in the workplace render the previous training obsolete, or when changes in the type of PPE to be used render the previous training obsolete. OSHA specifies that the hospital must maintain a written record of employee PPE training.

Specifically, any employee who must wear a respirator must be trained in the proper use and limitations of that device prior to its use in the workplace. The training must be comprehensive enough that the employee is able to demonstrate knowledge of the seven training topics specified in the standard and outlined below. The employee also must be able to demonstrate competence in wearing the complete PPE ensemble, including respirator, protective garment, gloves, boots, and other safety equipment required for the employee's role. Refresher training is required at least annually or sooner if changes in the workplace or type of respirator render previous training inadequate. Refresher training is also required if the employee does not demonstrate proficiency in the proper care and use of the respirator, or any other time when retraining appears necessary to ensure safe respirator use.

At a minimum, training under OSHA's Respiratory Protection Standard must cover the following topic areas:

- The nature of the respiratory hazard, and why a respirator is needed.
- Respirator capabilities, limitations, and consequences, if the respirator is not used correctly.
- How to handle respirator malfunctions and other emergencies.
- How to inspect, put on, remove, use, and check seals on the respirator.
- Maintenance and storage procedures.
- When to change cartridges on APRs.
- How to recognize medical signs and symptoms that may limit or prevent effective use of a respirator.
- General requirements of the respiratory protection programme.

Awareness level training

First Responder Awareness Level training is required even for those employees who work in the contaminant-free Hospital Post-decontamination Zone, but might be in a position to identify a contaminated victim who arrived unannounced. This group includes ED clinicians, ED clerks, and ED triage staff who would be responsible for notifying hospital authorities of the arrival, but would not reasonably be anticipated to have contact with the contaminated victims, their belongings, equipment, or waste.

First Responder Awareness Level training also is required for hospital security guards who work away from the Hospital Decontamination Zone, but who may be involved tangentially in a mass casualty event. Training can be waived if the employee has had sufficient experience to objectively demonstrate competency in specific areas. Annual refresher training is required for employees trained at the Awareness Level. A member of the staff who is unexpectedly called on to attend to a contaminated victim, or perform other work in the Hospital also requires awareness training. Examples include a medical specialist or a trade person, such as an electrician. These individuals must receive expedient orientation to site operations, immediately prior to providing such services (OSHA, 1997). The orientation must include:

- Nature of the hazard (if known).
- Expected duties.
- Appropriate use of PPE.
- Other appropriate safety and health precautions (e.g., decontamination procedures).

As part of the briefing, these personnel also must be medically cleared for respirator use and properly fit tested (if wearing a tight-fitting respirator), as required for Respiratory Protection. Thus, hospitals should diligently consider the broad range of skills/capabilities that may be required within the Decontamination Zone during a mass casualty event and attempt to identify, and train, all persons who may be called to work in the Decontamination Zone prior to a mass casualty event.

Training for First Receivers

MANDATORY TRAINING	FIRST RECEIVERS COVERED	REFERENCE
First Responder OPERATIONS LEVEL	All employees with designated roles in the Hospital Decontamination Zone. This group includes, but is not limited to:	OSHA, 2003, 1992c, 1999
Initial training Annual refresher Both initial and refresher training may be satisfied by demonstration of competence	• Decontamination staff, including decontamination victim inspectors; clinicians who will triage and/or stabilize victims prior to decontamination; security staff [e.g., crowd control and controlling access to the emergency department (ED)]; set-up crew; and patient tracking clerks.	OSHA, 1997
Briefing at the time of the incident	Other employees whose role in the Hospital Decontamination Zone was not previously anticipated (i.e., who are called in incidentally). (e.g., a medical specialist or trade person, such as an electrician)	
First Responder AWARENESS LEVEL Initial training Annual refresher Both initial and	a. Security personnel, set-up crew, and patient tracking clerks assigned only to patient receiving areas proximate to the Decontamination Zone where they might encounter, but are not expected to have contact with, contaminated victims, their belongings, equipment, or waste.	OSHA, 1991a, 1991b

RECOMMENDED TRAINING	PERSONNEL COVERED	REFERENCE
refresher training may be satisfied by demonstration of competence.	b. ED clinicians, clerks, triage staff, and other employees associated with emergency departments, who might encounter self-referred contaminated victims (and their belongings, equipment, or waste) without receiving prior notification that such victims have been contaminated.	
Training similar to that outlined in the Hazard Communication Standards	Other personnel in the Hospital Post-decontamination Zone who reasonably would not be expected to encounter or come in contact with unannounced contaminated victims, their belongings, equipment, or waste. T,U (e.g., other ED staff, such as housekeepers)	

Donning Procedures

Use a room with privacy and plenty of sitting space to facilitate donning of PPE—

1. It is preferable that a scrub suit be worn in lieu of regular street clothes. Clothing should be suitable for preserving comfortable body temperature.
2. Remove all jewelry and leather material and place in plastic bag with your name on it-place in secure location for Security to maintain. Persons needing to wear glasses or with beards or mustaches are NOT to use a face mask device.
3. Persons with long hair should apply a hairnet or place up in a braid.
4. Hydrate with 8-16 ounces of fluid.
5. If time allows have blood pressure (BP), pulse, respiration rate, and temperature taken and recorded on Medical Surveillance form.
6. Obtain appropriate sized PPE ensemble pack or individual pieces, APR/PAPR, battery, and appropriate cartridges (2-3 depending on APR/PAPR being used).
7. Layout PPE pieces and confirm they are right size and in working order.

8. Apply appropriate type of cartridges (most incidents will require HEPA/organic vapor cartridge set) and remove all pull-tabs. DO NOT OVERTIGHTEN the cartridges on the mask.
9. Put on latex or plastic inner glove-consider placing light circular band around top of glove to lessen chance of premature removal during doffing.
10. While sitting, remove shoes and place on foot covers (foot protection should not present tear risk to the suit nor be heelless).
11. Pull on chemical/biological protective suit to waist.
12. Place outer booties/boots on over the foot portion of the suit.
13. Using duct tape, seal top of booties to protective coverall (use a flap of tape at the end and place facing front to ease removal).
14. For chemical incident, place one set of nitrile gloves and one set of butyl rubber gloves on hands. For biological incident, use double plastic/latex gloves or plastic/latex and nitrile gloves.
15. Seal seam of protective suit and gloves with duct tape (use a flap of tape at the end and on the front of the wrist area to ease removal of tape).
16. Zip up protective suit to neck and close zipper securing and covering zipper seal.
17. If using PAPR, put on vest. Cinch up vest to snug fitting around with motor unit riding above the buttocks. Secure battery to the belt (side of the dominant hand is suggested) and plug in the PAPR. The air hose should come over the shoulder not under the arm.
18. Position APR/PAPR face piece to ensure full visibility and comfortable fit. Tighten all bands in pairs by pulling them backwards and not up. Confirm tight seal by covering cartridge opening with hand and taking deep breaths-face shield should pull tight against face. If faulty seal is found, then retighten all bands and repeat seal test. If tight seal cannot be obtained, then seek second provider assistance or use hooded devise.
19. Pull suit hood up and over the head maximizing the coverage of the head, neck, and ears and covering the APR/PAPR seal edge around the face—ensure the suit is pulled up and fully under the chin and zipper is closed and covered. There should be NO exposed skin.
20. Turn PAPR on, also making sure that all cartridge tabs are removed to allow airflow.
21. Have someone place a 3 in. piece of Velcro or tape across shoulders with staff member's last name and function (e.g., Jones RN) written with magic marker.
22. Have second person perform safety check before proceeding to assigned work area.
23. Note time personnel left the dress out area.

24. Have patient remove all valuables and place in the small plastic bag.
25. Clothing is removed and placed in the larger plastic bag. Place both bags into the red biohazard plastic bag. Place identifying tag with unique patient number on bag and seal off top. Place outside on ramp area for future disposition by Safety and Security.
26. Patient will do head-to-toe gross decontamination wash using mild soap and water. Have patient place ID band around wrist. This ID band will have the same identifying number that has been placed on the red biohazard plastic bag holding the patient's personal effects.
27. Special attention should be paid in the washing process to hair and all body crevices. Wash time cycle should be 5 (five) minutes per person under a single stream of water.
28. Water temperature should be tepid.
29. Washing should be gentle to avoid abrading skin.
30. Open wounds should be washed first with sterile water and covered with occlusive dressing prior to remainder of body decontamination.
31. Upon completion of wash cycle, patient should step away from the immediate wash area, towel dry, and put on a supplied Tyvek® gown from the Patient Redress Kit.
32. All ED towels and wash cloths used by patients in the showering process should be placed in a marked contaminated container for later clean up and decontamination.
33. Patient may then enter the ED, where the receiving RN can obtain vital signs, complete secondary triage, complete decon paperwork, and transport to an assigned bed in ED.
34. Decon team personnel should be decontaminated prior to entering the ED as described in Personnel (Technical) Decon section.
35. Soap should be changed out every five patients or whenever needed.
36. The Decon team for non-ambulatory patients must include a minimum of four (4) providers, two of whom will be responsible for turning the patient on the backboard and one who will be responsible for maintaining cervical spine precautions.
37. If the patient has not had a primary gross decon in the field (defined as the removal of clothing and first wash), visible particulate matter should be removed by gently brushing or dusting, and clothing should be cut and rolled away from the center of body, in order to contain the contaminants on the clothing.
38. Follow procedure for removal and bagging of personal valuables.

39. Follow procedure for head-to-toe decontamination wash cycle.
40. Irrigate open wounds with irrigation syringe and copious amounts of saline and cover with occlusive dressings. Any existing dressing must be removed and placed in bio-hazard trash container.
41. Eye irrigation may be done with Morgans lens and NS and/or IV tubing alone, if gross contaminants on the face are suspected. Otherwise, perform manual irrigation with copious fluids.
42. Gentle ear and nasal irrigation with frequent suctioning from portable suction may be done if such contamination is suspected.
43. C-collars as well as backboards must be washed or changed if they are still required for patient immobilization.
44. Patient should be transferred to a clean stretcher for entry into the ED.

References

ACGIH. 2001. Heat Stress and Strain. Documentation of Threshold Limit Values and Biological Exposure Indices. American Conference of Governmental Industrial Hygienists (ACGIH), Cincinnati, OH.

Ali J *et al.*Trauma patient outcome after the prehospital trauma life support programme. *Journal of Trauma,* 1997, 42:1018-22.

American College of Surgeons, Committee on Trauma. Resources for optimal care of the injured patient. Chicago, IL,American College of Surgeons, 1999.

Arreola-Risa C *et al.* Low cost improvements in prehospital trauma care in a Latin American city. *Journal of Trauma,* 2000, 48:119-24.

Arreola-Risa C *et al.*Trauma care systems in urban Latin America: the priorities should be prehospital and emergency room management. *Journal of Trauma,* 1995, 39:457-62.

ATSDR. 2000. Managing Hazardous Materials Incidents: Hospital Emergency Departments - A planning guide for the management of contaminated patients, Volume II (revised). Agency for Toxic Substances and Disease Registry, U.S. Department of Health and Human Services. Last accessed April 21, 2003: http://www.atsdr.cdc.gov/mhmi.html

ATSDR. 2003. Managing Hazardous Materials Incidents: Medical Management Guidelines (MMGs) for Unidentified Chemical, Volume III. Agency for Toxic Substances and Disease Registry, U.S. Department of Health and Human Services. Last accessed April 21, 2003: http://www.atsdr.cdc.gov/mmg.html

Auf der Heide, E. 2002. Principles of hospital disaster planning (Part II (8)). In Disaster Medicine. Hogan, D. and J.L. Burstein, editors. Lippincott Williams and Wilkins. pp. 57-89.

Barbera J.A., Anthony G. Macintyre. 2003. Mass Casualty Handbook: Hospital, Emergency Preparedness and Response, First ed: Jane's Information Group, Ltd.

Beatty J. 2003. Decontamination procedures (personal e-mail correspondence). Central Arkansas Veterans Health Care System, Little Rock, AR. October 23.

Blackwell T.Principles of emergency medical services systems.In:Marx JM,ed.Rosen's emergency medicine concepts and clinical practice, 5th ed. St. Louis, MO, Mosby, 2002:2616-25.

BNA. 2003. Hospitals low on protective suits in event of bioterrorist attack, report says. Daily Labor Report Banner, Bureau of National Affairs. August 13.

Burgess J.L. 1999. Hospital Evacuations Due to Hazardous Materials Incidents. *Am J Emerg Med* 17:50-52. January.

CA EMSA. 2003a. Personal communication between Cheryl Starling of the California Emergency Medical Services Authority and Eastern Research Group, Inc. July 21.

CA EMSA. 2003b. Recommendations for Hospitals: Chemical Decontamination, Staff Protection, Chemical Decontamination Equipment and Medication List, Evidence Collection. Hospital and Health Care System Disaster Interest Group (DIG). California Emergency Medical Services Authority. June.

Callaham M. Quantifying the scanty science of prehospital emergency care. *Annals of Emergency Medicine,* 1997, 30:785-90.

CDC. 2003. Interim Guidelines for Hospital Response to Mass Casualties from a Radiological Incident. Center for Disease Control and Prevention (CDC), U.S. Department of Health and Human Services. December.

Cone DC *et al.* Field triage systems: methodologies from the literature. *Prehospital Emergency Care,* 2004, 8:130-7.

Cooke MW. How much to do at the accident scene? British Medical Journal, 1999, 319:1150.

Department of Homeland Security. 2003. Working document from Department of Homeland Security Working Group on Radiological Dispersal Devices (RDD) Preparedness Response Subgroup. Version: May 1.

DuPont. 2002. Technical Data Sheet. DuPont Tychem F: Helps protect against chemical warfare agents. E.I. DuPont de Nemours and Company.

DuPont. 2003. Permeation Guide for DuPont Tychem Protective Fabrics. E.I. du Pont de Nemours and Company.

Eckstein M *et al.* Effect of prehospital advanced life support on outcomes of major trauma patients. *Journal of Trauma,* 2000, 48:643-8.

Eckstein M. *et al.* Effect of pre-hospital advanced life support on outcomes of major trauma patients. Journal of Trauma, 2000, 48:643-8.

ECRI. 2002. ECRI Advisor—Selecting personal protective equipment for chemical and bioterrorism preparedness: risks and costs. Center for Health Care Environmental Management, Emergency Care Research Institute (ECRI), Plymouth Meeting, PA. March.

Environmental Technologies. (undated). Product literature for APD 2000. Environmental Technologies Group, Inc. Baltimore, MD.

Federal Register. 2003. Assigned Protection Factors; proposed rule. Occupational Safety and Health Administration (OSHA). 68 FR 34035. June 6.

Georgopoulos, P.G., P. Fedele, P. Shade, P.J. Lioy, M. Hodgson, A. Longmire, M. Sands, and M.A. Brown. 2004. Hospital response to chemical terrorism: personal protective equipment, training, and operations. *American Journal of Industrial Medicine* 46(5):432-445. November.

Goozner B., L. Lutwick, E. Bourke. 2002. Chemical Terrorism: a Primer for 2002. *Journal of the Association for Academic Minority Physicians.* 13(1):14-18. January.

HAZMAT for Health Care. 2003. Haz Mat for Health Care—An Operations Course. EnMagine, Diamond Springs, CA. Available at www.hazmatforhealth care.org. Last accessed September 16.

HCA. (undated). Disaster Readiness: Guidelines for Emergency Management Planners. Hospital Corporation of America (HCA). Nashville, TN.

Hendler *et al.* 2000. The Effect of Full Protective Gear on Intubation Performance by Hospital Medical Personnel. *Military Medicine,* Volume 149. [As cited in USACHPPM 2003a]

Hick J.L., D. Hanfling, J.L. Burstein, J. Markham, A.G. Macintyre, J.A. Barbera. 2003a. Protective equipment for health care facility decontamination personnel: regulations, risks, and recommendations. *Annals of Emergency Medicine* 42(3):370-380. September.

Hick J.L., P. Penn, D. Hanfling, M.A. Lapp, D. O'Laughlin, J.L. Burstein. 2003b. Establishing and training health care facility decontamination teams. *Annals of Emergency Medicine* 42(3):381-390. September.

Hodgson, M.J., A. Bierenbaum, S. Mather, M.A. Brown, J. Beatty, M. Scott, and P. Brewster. 2004. Emergency management programme operational responses to weapons of mass destruction: Veterans Health Administration, Volumes I and II (NIJ Guide 100-00). National Institute of Justice, U.S. Department of Justice. June. http://ncjrs.org/pdffiles1/nij/184449.pdf

Husum H, Gilbert M,Wisborg T. Save lives, save limbs.Penang, Malaysia, Third World Network, 2000.

Joshipura M *et al.* Essential trauma care: strengthening trauma systems round the world. *Injury,* 2004, 35:841-5.

Kobusingye O, ed. Emergency care saves lives. *Injury Control News: Newsletter of the Injury Control Centre-Uganda,* 2002, 3:3.

Mock C *et al.*Guidelines for essential trauma care. Geneva, World Health Organisation, 2004.

Mock C, Joshipura M, Goosen J. Global strengthening of the care of the injured.
Bulletin of the World Health Organisation, 2004, 82:241.

Mock CN *et al.*Improvements in prehospital trauma care in an African country with no formal emergency medical services. *Journal of Trauma,* 2002, 53:90-7.

Mock CN *et al.*Trauma mortality patterns in three nations at different economic levels: implications for global trauma system development. *Journal of Trauma,* 1998, 44:804-12.

Murray JA *et al.* Prehospital intubation in patients with severe head injury. *Journal of Trauma,* 2000, 49:1065-70.

NIOSH. 2003. NIOSH Pocket Guide to Chemical Hazards and Other Databases (online edition). National Institute for Occupational Safety and Health (NIOSH), Department of Health and Human Services (DHHS), Cincinnati, OH. Last accessed April 20, 2004 at: http://www.cdc.gov/niosh/npg/npg.html

Nozaki H., S.O. Hori, Y. Shinozawa *et al.* 1995. Secondary exposure of medical staff to sarin vapor in the emergency room. *Intensive Care Med* 21:1032-1035.

Okumura, Takasu, Ishimatsu *et al.* 1996. Report on 640 victims of the Tokyo subway sarin attack. *Annals of Emergency Medicine* 28(2):129-135. August.

OSHA. 1991a. Letter of Interpretation Addressed to Mr. Edward McNamara, Executive Director, Central Massachusetts Emergency Medical Systems Corporation, Re: Training Requirements for emergency medical service personnel. June 14. Accessed April 6, 2004 at http://www.osha.gov/pls/oshaweb/owadisp.show_document?p_table=INTERPRETATIONS&p_id=20302

OSHA. 1991b. Letter of Interpretation Addressed to Mr. Eugene D. McCoy, Police Department, City of Ft. Lauderdale, FL. Re: Minimum number of hours required for awareness level for police officers. June 17. Accessed April 6, 2004 at http://www.osha.gov/pls/oshaweb/owadisp.show_document?p_table=INTERPRETATIONS&p_id=20307

OSHA. 1991c. Letter of Interpretation Addressed to Mr. William Borwegen, Service Employees International Union, AFL-CIO, Re: HAZWOPER EPA and OSHA jurisdictional issues. December 18. Accessed April 6, 2004 at http://www.osha.gov/pls/oshaweb/owadisp.show_document?p_table=INTERPRETATIONS&p_id=20500

OSHA. 1992a. Letter of Interpretation Addressed to Randy Ross, Re: Medical personnel exposed to patients contaminated with hazardous waste. March 31. Accessed April 6, 2004 at http://www.osha.gov/pls/oshaweb/owadisp.show_document?p_table=INTERPRETATIONS&p_id=20609

OSHA. 1992b. OSHA Letter of interpretation from C.K. O'Toole to L. Bloomfield. Occupational Safety and Health Administration (OSHA), U.S. Department of Labor. Various questions on HAZWOPER. October 21. Accessed April 6, 2004 at http://www.osha.gov/pls/oshaweb/owadisp.show_document?p_table=NTERPRETATIONS&p_id=20890

OSHA. 1992c. Letter of Interpretation Addressed to Howard W. Levitin, Re: Training requirements for hospital personnel involved in an emergency response of a hazardous substance. October 27. Accessed April 6, 2004 at http://www.osha.gov/pls/oshaweb/owadisp.show_document?p_table=INTERPRETATIONS&p_id=20911

OSHA. 1993. Letter of Interpretation Addressed to Mr. Edward E. Hartin, Vice-President of Operations, HAZMAT Training Information Services, Inc., Re: Post-emergency response and medical surveillance requirements of HAZWOPER. August 5. Accessed April 6, 2004 at http://www.osha.gov/pls/oshaweb/owadisp.show_document?p_table=INTERPRETATIONS&p_id=21222

OSHA. 1997. Letter of Interpretation Addressed to Mr. Thomas Whittaker, New England Hospital Engineer's Society, Re: Emergency response training requirements for hospital staff. April 25. Accessed April 6, 2004 at http://www.osha.gov/pls/oshaweb/owadisp.show_document?p_table=INTERPRETATIONS&p_id=22393

OSHA. 1999. Letter of Interpretation Addressed to Daniel Burke, Safety Coordinator, St. John's Medical Center, Re: Emergency response training necessary for hospital physicians/nurses that may treat contaminated patients. March 10. Accessed April 6, 2004 at http://www.osha.gov/pls/oshaweb/owadisp.show_document?p_table=INTERPRETATIONS&p_id=22710

OSHA. 2002a. Letter of Interpretation Addressed to Mr. Francis J. Roth, Supervisor, Loss Protection, Princeton Insurance, Re: Level of respiratory protection required for hospital staff members. September 5. Accessed April 6, 2004 at http://www.osha.gov/pls/oshaweb/owadisp.show_document?p_table=INTERPRETATIONS&p_id=24516

OSHA. 2002b. Letter of Interpretation Addressed to Captain Kevin J. Hayden, Acting Commanding Officer, State of New Jersey Emergency Management Section, Re: Personal protective requirements for hospital employees. December 2. Accessed April 6, 2004 at http://www.osha.gov/pls/oshaweb/owadisp.show_document?p_table=INTERPRETATIONS&p_id=24523

OSHA. 2002c. Memorandum for Regional Administrators (RAs) regarding enforcement policy change for respiratory protection for select respirators for use in the pharmaceutical industry. May 30. Accessed April 6, 2004 at http://www.osha.gov/pls/oshaweb/owadisp.show_document?p_table=INTERPRETATIONS&p_id=24248

OSHA. 2003. Letter of Interpretation Addressed to Mike Bolt, Re: HAZWOPER training requirements for hospital staff whole decontaminate chemically contaminated patients. April 22. Accessed April 6, 2004 at http://www.osha.gov/pls/oshaweb/owadisp.show_document?p_table=INTERPRETATIONS&p_id=24605

Osterwalder JJ. Insufficient quality of research on prehospital medical emergency care-where are the major problems and solutions? *Swiss Medical Weekly*, 2004,134:389-94.

Penn P. 2002. Hospital Hazardous Material Emergency Response: The Devil is in the Details. National Disaster Medical Systems Conference. Atlanta, GA. April 14.

Peterson TD *et al.* Bystander trauma care training in Iowa. Prehospital Emergency Care, 1999, 3:225-30.

Pozner CN *et al.* International EMS systems.The United States: past, present, and future. *Resuscitation*, 2004, 60:239-44.

Razzak JA, Kellermann AL. Emergency medical care in developing countries: is it worthwhile? Bulletin of the World Health Organisation, 2002, 80:900-5.

San Mateo County HAS. 1998. HEICS—The hospital emergency incident command system (Volumes I and II). San Mateo County Health Services Agency. June. Accessed August, 2003 at www.emsa.cahwnet.gov.

Saruwatari. 2003. Personal communication between M. Saruwatari of Kaiser Permanente, and Eastern Research Group, Inc. August 18.

SBCCOM. 2000a. Guidelines for Responding to a Chemical Weapons Incident. Domestic Preparedness Chemical Team, U.S. Army Soldier and Biological Chemical Command. http://www2.sbccom.army.mil/hld/downloads/cwirp/cwirp_guidelines_responding_cw_incident.pdf

SBCCOM. 2000b. Guidelines for Mass Casualty Decontamination During a Terrorist Chemical Agent Incident. U.S. Army Soldier and Biological Chemical Command. January. http://hld.sbccom.army.mil/downloads/cwirp/cwirp_guidelines_mass_casualty_decon.pdf

SBCCOM. 2001a. Swatch Test Results of Commercial Chemical Protective Gloves to Challenge by Chemical Warfare Agents: Executive Summary. Domestic Preparedness Chemical Team, U.S. Army Soldier and Biological Chemical Command. February. http://www2.sbccom.army.mil/hld/downloads/reports/protective_gloves_summary_report.pdf

SBCCOM. 2001b. Swatch Test Results of Phase 2 Commercial Chemical Protective Gloves to Challenge by Chemical Warfare Agents: Executive Summary. Domestic Preparedness Chemical Team, U.S. Army Soldier and Biological Chemical Command. June. http://www2.sbccom.army.mil/hld/downloads/reports/protective_gloves_phase2_ca_exec_sum.pdf

SBCCOM. 2003. Guidelines for Use of Personal Protective Equipment by Law Enforcement Personnel During a Terrorist Chemical Agent Incident. U.S. Army Soldier and Biological Chemical Command. Original June 2001. Revised July 2003. http://www2.sbccom.army.mil/hld/downloads/cwirp/ppe_law_enforcement_ca_incident.pdf

Schmid T *et al.*Transportation for maternal emergencies in Tanzania: empowering communities through participatory problem solving. *American Journal of Public Health,* 2001, 91:1589-90.

Schultz, M., J. Cisek, and R. Wabeke. 1995. Simulated exposure of hospital emergency personnel to solvent vapors and respirable dust during decontamination of chemically exposed patients. Annals of Emergency Medicine. 26(3):324-329. September.

Smith GCS, Pell JP. Parachute use to prevent death and major trauma related to gravitational challenge:systematic review of randomised controlled trials. *BMJ,* 2003, 327:1459-61.

Stockinger ZT, McSwain NE. Prehospital endotracheal intubation for trauma does not improve survival over bag-valve-mask ventilation. *Journal of Trauma,* 2004, 56:531-6.

Sutter Health. 2002. Training materials: First Responder Operations. Sutter Health, Sacramento, CA. October 1.

Thorne C.D., Curbow B., Oliver M. *et al.* 2003. Terrorism preparedness training for nonclinical hospital workers: empowering them to take action. *J Occup Environ Med.* 45:333-337. March.

Tiska M *et al.*Appropriate prehospital trauma care training:a model devised in Ghana. In: 6th world conference on injury prevention and control: abstract. *Montreal, Les Presses de l'Université de Montréal,* 2002: 1003-4.

U.S. Army, U.S. Marine Corps, U.S. Navy, and U.S. Air Force. 2001. Multiservice Tactics, Techniques, and Procedures for Nuclear, Biological, and Chemical Aspects of Consequence Management. AFTTP (I) 3-2.37. December.

U.S. EPA. 2000. First responders' environmental liability due to mass decontamination runoff (EPA 550-F-00.009). U.S. Environmental Protection Agency, Office of Solid Waste and Emergency Response. July. http://yosemite.epa.gov/oswer/Ceppoweb.nsf/vwResourcesByFilename/onepage.pdf/$File/onepage.pdf

USACHPPM. 2003a. Personal Protective Equipment Guide for Military Medical Treatment Facility Personnel Handling Casualties from Weapons of Mass

Destruction and Terrorism Events (Technical Guide 275). U.S. Army Center for Health Promotion and Preventive Medicine. August. http://chppm-www.apgea.army.mil/documents/TG/TECHGUID/TG275new.pdf

USACHPPM. 2003b. Chemical Risk Assessment and Exposure Guidelines (and how AEGLs fit in). U.S. Army Center for Health Promotion and Preventive Medicine, Directorate of Health Risk Management. March. http://www.osha.gov/SLTC/emergencypreparedness/chemical/ppt/csepp-aegl_march_2003.ppt.

VA. 2003. VHA Decontamination Training Programme—Train the Trainer Participant Manual. Little Rock Employee Education Resource Center, Employee Education System, Department of Veterans Affairs (VA), Little Rock, AR. April.

Varghese M, Mohan P. When someone is hurt: a first aid guide for lay persons and community workers. New Delhi, The Other Media Communications, 1998.

Vogt, B.M. and J.H. Sorrensen. 2002. How clean is safe? Improving the effectiveness of decontamination of structures and people following chemical and biological incidents - Final Report (ORNL/TM-2002/178). Prepared by Oakridge National Laboratory for the U.S. Department of Energy. October. Accessed September 2004 at http://emc.ornl.gov/EMCWeb/EMC/PDF/How_Clean_is_Safe.pdf

Walter F.G., Bates G., Criss E. A. *et al.* 2003. Hazardous materials responses in a mid-sized metropolitan area. Prehosp Emerg Care 7:214-218. Apr-Jun.

World Health Organisation.Surgical care at the district hospital.Geneva, WHO, 2003. (http://www.who.int/surgery/publications/en/SCDH.pdf, accessed 18 May 2005).

Young Bruce H., Ford Julian D., Rusek Josef I. *et al.* Disaster Mental Health Services: A Guidebook for Clinicians and Administrators. National Center for PTSD. Last Accessed: 2002. Available from: http://www.ncptsd.org/treatment/disaster/index.html.

APPENDIX A

BACKGROUND, LITERATURE REVIEW, AND SITE VISIT EXAMPLES

This Appendix supplements the Best Practices from OSHA by providing useful background information on how various aspects of a hospital's preparation, response, and recovery impact employee protection during hazardous substance emergencies. Look in Appendix A for:

Preparation

- Examples of roles that hospitals fill in their communities and the benefits hospitals can derive from playing an active role in community emergency preparedness.
- Suggestions for coordinating Emergency Response Plans (EMPs) with other organisations.
- Tips for designating staff for decontamination teams.
- Discussion of the different levels of training for first receivers filling various roles, plus information on training requirements for the team members.
- Medical monitoring considerations for first receivers before, during, and after a response.

Response

- Discussion of the benefits associated with different types of decontamination facilities and examples of factors hospitals consider when selecting a system.
- Outline of the basic steps typically involved in victim decontamination procedures.
- Examples of several organisations' shower flush times and practices used for victim decontamination.
- Review of OSHA requirements for employers whose employees wear respirators and other personal protective equipment (PPE).

Recovery

- Discussion of management practices for contaminated solid waste.
- Examples of arrangements hospitals have made to manage wastewater during and after a response.
- Strategies for decontaminating surfaces and equipment.

The following discussion provides examples of ways hospitals have attempted to enhance employee protection as part of general preparedness for mass casualty emergencies involving contaminated victims. This discussion is designed to further worker health and safety by referencing practices and procedures considered and/or adopted in the health care community. However, statements in this appendix cannot create nor diminish obligations under the occupational safety and health (OSH) Act.

In making preparations, hospitals must consider key assumptions regarding communication, resources, and victims. When developing plans, hospitals should anticipate:

- Victims will arrive with little or no warning to the hospital.
- Information regarding the hazardous agent(s) will not be available immediately.
- A large number of victims will be self-referred victims (as much as 80 percent of the total number of victims).
- Victims will not necessarily have been decontaminated prior to arriving at the hospital.
- A high percentage of people arriving at the hospital will have experienced little or no exposure and this eventuality should be considered in decontamination plans.
- Most victims will go to the hospital closest to the site where the emergency occurred.
- Victims will use other entrances in addition to the emergency department (ED).

The hospital emergency management plan (EMP) outlines how the facility will respond to an emergency. The plan should address the hazards the hospital will encounter, identify the hospital's role in the response, and serve as a road map for incident preparation, response, and recovery.

No organisation can prepare fully for every conceivable emergency. To use resources effectively, a hospital requires information that will help emergency planners make informed decisions about the type, probability, severity, and impact of specific hazards to which the hospital might be subject. A hazard vulnerability analysis (HVA) assists a hospital in organizing this information, which is used to customize the hazard assessment for personal protective equipment (PPE) selection (a critical aspect of the EMP). The Joint Committee for Accreditation of Health Care Organisations (JCAHO) requires an HVA as the first step in emergency planning (JCAHO, 2004). Specific information on conducting HVAs may be obtained directly from JCAHO.

The HVA and resulting preparations are only as specific to the individual hospital as the information on which preparation decisions are based. Important modifying factors include the hospital's role in the community, how up-to-date the hospital EMP is, and formal planning agreements between the hospital and other organisations that have roles in emergency response activities. With knowledge of these details, hospitals can customize EMPs and effectively tailor preparedness (including employee protection) to address the circumstances relevant to that hospital.

Using Information from a Hazard Vulnerability Analysis

As noted previously, an HVA helps hospitals organize information and guide decision-making. A thorough HVA can serve as the basis for informed decisions regarding the training and equipment employees will require to protect themselves under foreseeable emergency scenarios.

A popular HVA, an electronic spreadsheet, prompts the user to enter a numerical rating (e.g., 1 to 3) for various factors associated with each of numerous listed threats (both from a standard list and additional hazards added by the user). JCAHO (2002) offers a matrix of threats that hospitals might consider. The user generates (or the spreadsheet calculates) a hazard vulnerability score based on the inputs. The inputs may be weighted to reflect the importance of certain information to the final score. Hospitals use both the final score and the individual numerical rating inputs to identify and rank priority areas that should receive administrative attention or resources.

Other hospitals use a tabular format HVA and more descriptive text input to guide the user through the analysis. The tables can provide more information, but are also more cumbersome for evaluating a large selection of threats. Because these formats are more likely to have been developed in-house, they tend to be more diverse.

None of the HVA formats have been validated to determine whether the inputs and final assessment accurately reflect hazard vulnerability. Nevertheless, an informal qualitative review conducted by the developer of one HVA spreadsheet tool suggested that independent users, when operating in similar hospital and community environments, do generally arrive at similar conclusions regarding vulnerability and priorities for improvement (Saruwatari, 2003).

The hospitals interviewed for this project agree that the HVA should be updated frequently and reviewed at least annually, as required by JCAHO (2004). By collaborating with Local Emergency Planning Committees (LEPCs), hospitals can keep current with information on changes in threats in their localities. Hospital D noted that, if appropriate, resources could be reallocated sooner if emergency managers are able to update the HVA as new information arrives (e.g., emerging threats), rather than waiting for an annual review cycle. These changes can also modify the local hospital's vulnerability to those hazards. As an example, Hospital D had rated "preparation for chlorine-related emergencies" as a top priority. When the local potable water facility changed processes, the threat of a large-scale chlorine emergency was eliminated from the community. Upon revising the HVA, Hospital D was able to redirect resources to address the next most urgent threat without waiting until the next annual review cycle.

Characteristics of the community (e.g., businesses, chemical inventory, population, transportation lines, clandestine drug labs, and possible targets of terrorism) influence the type of hazardous substance-related emergencies that a hospital might reasonably anticipate. This information should be considered in the HVA. These factors range from the number and condition of victims that the hospital might reasonably anticipate, to the rate at which hazard information could become available during an emergency.

Identifying the Hospital's Role in the Community

The community in which a hospital is located and the hospital's role in that community impact emergency preparations on several levels. Hospital D's emergency manager suggested that the real objective of emergency planning is "community preparedness, and a hospital's preparedness represents only one component." For the purposes of this discussion, "community" is defined as the local population center that the hospital serves on a day-to-day basis, as well as any additional population centers from which the hospital would reasonably expect to receive victims in the event of a mass casualty emergency involving hazardous substances.

Fully coordinated planning helps hospitals identify their roles in their communities. Roles vary considerably with individual circumstances, but ultimately have a strong impact on the conditions and hazards for which a hospital must plan employee protection. Examples of roles some hospitals fill (or expect to fill) in their communities include:

- Providing decontamination and treatment for any and all victims.
- Promoting wider level of preparedness in the community by providing low-cost hazard communication or hazardous waste operations and emergency response (HAZWOPER) training for local government and business emergency response personnel.
- Providing information and services related to emergency preparedness (e.g., respirator medical clearance).
- Participating actively in multi-disciplined community-based planning and preparedness activities, such as LEPCs (e.g., Hospital D reports devoting a minimum of 12 man-hours per week to its active role in community preparedness. This time is in addition to the hours spent managing the hospital's internal preparations).

The hospitals interviewed for this project also note that, in addition to a better coordinated community emergency response plan, they receive additional financial, informational, and business benefits from active participation in community-focused emergency preparedness and planning. The following list indicates benefits that hospitals can derive from an active role in community emergency preparedness:

- Increased access to community records, which help managers improve the accuracy of the HVA and help the hospital customize its EMP.
- Increased access to grants and other financial resources.
- Group buying power that allows for volume discounts or

government rates (including reduced sales tax) for equipment and supplies.

- More opportunities to contain costs by sharing or trading expertise, training resources, equipment, and services.
- Greater opportunity to tailor community drills so they test the hospital's emergency plans.
- Increased opportunities to network and develop useful alliances with emergency first responders and other emergency planners (particularly useful for resolving complex issues that emerge as groups coordinate their activities under difficult circumstances).

Coordinating Emergency Plans with Other Organisations

Well-coordinated EMPs ensure that hospitals are aware of the capabilities of first responders and other hospitals, as well as what the local professional and response community expects from them. Coordinated plans encourage open lines of communication and improve the safety of both victims and health care workers. The following example demonstrates the value of coordinated EMPs. After problems were identified during a drill, Hospital D determined that health care workers needed faster access to information from hazardous materials incident sites. Initially, the fire department felt Hospital D's request for more timely information would be too burdensome during life-threatening emergencies. When the two organisations met, however, they each learned the reasons behind the other's needs. As a result, the first responders recognized that, by coordinating efforts, they could enhance the first receivers' ability to provide rapid and appropriate care to victims. The fire department was able to modify its own EMP to incorporate direct communication between the hospital and a representative of the incident commander at the scene.

The hospitals interviewed for this project mentioned several methods by which they improve EMP coordination and communication:

- Use an incident command system compatible with the National Incident Management System (NIMS) structure.
- Get to know members of the other organisations and the details of their plans. Seek opportunities to improve communication.
- Seek input from other organisations (such as local emergency planning groups) when developing or updating plans.
- Use compatible forms of communication, such as radios capable of operating on the same frequency. Keep compatibility in mind when purchasing equipment.
- Participate in multi-organisational drills. Execute multi-organisational drills that test the way organisations interact under adverse conditions.
- Analyze drills to identify areas that need improvement and meet directly with the other organisations to develop action plans that provide mutually agreeable, practical solutions to problems.

Bear in mind that a solution suggested by one party might not be feasible for another organisation to implement.

- Test inter-organisational communication systems at every opportunity (e.g., fire department, law enforcement, emergency medical services, environmental management, and other hospitals).

Barbera and Macintyre (2003) suggest the following organisations with which hospitals should coordinate:

- Public health groups (including special laboratories).
- Local emergency management organisations (e.g., LEPCs).
- Emergency medical services.

Law enforcement, at all levels.

PREPARING STAFF AND MANAGEMENT

Organisations, such as OSHA, those states operating OSHA-approved State Plans, JCAHO, the National Fire Protection Association (NFPA), and other state or local government agencies, set standards that govern employee preparation, particularly regarding employee training and medical evaluations. OSHA standards, or the parallel State Plan standards, relevant to the training of first receivers include the HAZWOPER, Personal Protective Equipment, Respiratory Protection, and Hazard Communication Standards. Hospitals with decontamination facilities should also comply with the requirement for medical evaluations contained in the HAZWOPER and Respiratory Protection Standards.

JCAHO (2004) requires "an orientation and education programme for all personnel, including licensed independent practitioners, who participate in implementing the emergency management plan." When plans involve management of chemical hazards, OSHA's HAZWOPER and hazard communication (HAZCOM) Standards complement the JCAHO requirements by providing specific topics that should be addressed during the training. Other requirements of these standards might also apply (e.g., training duration, demonstration of skills, and retraining), depending on whether the HAZWOPER (Hospital Decontamination Zone) or HAZCOM (Hospital Post-decontamination Zone) standard is in effect. NFPA (2002) suggests competencies for incident commanders and others responding to hazardous materials incidents.

Maintaining Decontamination Teams

A challenge for any hospital is the need to maintain a decontamination team, without compromising the ability of hospital departments to provide medical treatment for patients.

Hospitals interviewed for this project use employees from a range of specialties to maintain minimal staffing levels in patient care areas. In addition to drawing limited staff from the ED, Hospital A suggests including individuals from departments such as mental health, facilities and engineering, and security on decontamination teams.

The hospitals also indicate that it is often possible to identify individuals in unrelated departments who are uniquely qualified to serve on the team due to previous military experience, work history, or volunteer service. Hospital A staffs a particularly large decontamination team (over 100 members) by drawing from employees with relevant skills from past experience in fire departments, emergency medical services, rescue units, HAZMAT or hazardous waste handling, National Guard, and military reserve units. In these cases, the previous experience might be a more important selection criterion than the individual's day-to-day role in the hospital. Hospital A avoids assigning unwilling staff to their team, citing the advantages of volunteer team members' enthusiasm and willingness to participate in training and drills.

Decontamination teams might include individuals who perform the following functions:

- *Decontamination team leader—responsible for management of the decontamination operation.
- *Decontamination safety officer—responsible for monitoring the decontamination area for developing hazards and for ensuring team safety.
- *Pre-decontamination triage—responsible for assessing medical status and prioritizing victims for decontamination.
- Decontamination system set-up.
- Security.
- Decontamination hospital attendants.
- Post-decontamination inspection.
- Cleanup and decontamination crew (surfaces, equipment, human and hazardous wastes).
- Other roles that might be performed in the Hospital Decontamination Zone under some circumstances (e.g., patient tracking, assistants helping team members with PPE).

The size of the decontamination team depends on the minimum number of people required to operate the decontamination system and implement the hospital's decontamination procedures. Activities involving a few victims and small decontamination systems usually require only a few staff members, each of whom might fill several functional roles. Hick *et al.* (2003b) suggest that a small hospital might have a 2-person team available at all times, while a metropolitan hospital might need a 5-person team available to work in the Hospital Decontamination Zone, with additional personnel on-call to allow for staff rotation. According to Hick, the 5-person team would include one person handling triage and coordinating pre-decontamination treatment, two people working with non-ambulatory victims, and two team members working with ambulatory victims. During a major emergency in a metropolitan area, hospitals might be required to continue operations "at maximum capacity for at least 2 to 4 hours, with appropriate staff rotations" (Hick *et al.*, 2003b).

Another hospital organisation advocates a 12-member (minimum) decontamination team, all wearing PPE. Although it is recognized that smaller hospitals would not be able to staff such a robust team, the rationale may illustrate useful points. Under this model, the Northern Virginia Hospital Alliance calls for a single "team leader," three team members responsible for conducting ambulatory decontamination (one to assist in the undressing, one to supervise showering, and one to assist in the re-dressing), four team members to participate in the care of non-ambulatory patients, and four security personnel to preserve the perimeter of the Hospital Decontamination Zone.

Orienting and Training Personnel

First Responder Operations Level training is required for employees (including security staff) who have a role in the Hospital Decontamination Zone, as well as the hospital's contamination cleanup crew.

First Responder Awareness Level training is required for ED clerks and ED triage staff who might identify unannounced contaminated victims (then notify the proper authority) and security staff working outside the Hospital Decontamination Zone.

A briefing at the time of the incident is required for employees whose roles in the Hospital Decontamination Zone could not be anticipated before the incident ("skilled support personnel", e.g., a medical specialist or a trade person, such as an electrician).

Information similar to hazard communication training is recommended for ED staff and other employees who work in the ED (Hospital Post-decontamination Zone), provided contaminated victims would not have access to them.

Competencies for First Responder Operations Level Training

The HAZWOPER Standard, requires that employees trained at the First Responder Operations Level shall have received at least eight hours of training or have had sufficient experience to objectively demonstrate competency (e.g., in exercises and drills) in the following areas:

- An understanding of what hazardous substances are, and the risks associated with them in an incident.
- An understanding of the potential outcomes associated with an emergency when hazardous substances are present.
- The ability to recognize the presence of hazardous substances in an emergency through signs and symptoms of exposure.
- The ability to identify the hazardous substances, if possible.
- An understanding of their role in the hospital's emergency

response plan, including site security and control, and decontamination procedures (OSHA, 1992c).
- The ability to realize the need for additional resources and to make appropriate notifications to the communication center.
- Knowledge of the basic hazard and risk assessment techniques.
- Know how to select and use proper PPE.
- An understanding of basic hazardous materials terms.
- Know how to perform basic control, containment, and/or confinement operations within the capabilities of the resources and PPE available.
- Know how to implement basic decontamination procedures.
- An understanding of the relevant standard operating procedures and termination procedures.

Several examples of HAZWOPER First Responder Operations Level training curricula are available for hospitals preparing employees to conduct decontamination activities (HAZMAT for Health Care, 2003; CA EMSA, 2003a; VA, 2003; Sutter Health, 2002). However, these curricula are not necessarily designed as 8-hour presentations (some are longer, others are shorter and intended for use when employees are able to demonstrate specific areas of competency).

Hospital A and Hospital G opt to provide more than 8 hours of training to decontamination team employees. Hospital A requires staff that will have a direct role in decontamination activities to undergo 24 hours of initial training and an additional 16 hours of refresher training annually. Employees can satisfy some of the training requirement by attending monthly educational team meetings. Other training is provided using a standard course curriculum developed by the Department of Veterans Affairs.

Hospital G is in the process of changing from a single yearly 8-hour course curriculum to a programme that provides twelve 1-hour sessions. The emergency planner believes that an annual training day is not the best condition for learning and skills retention. Under the new system, Hospital G divides the required training topics into 12 modules, one for each month, including several opportunities to don PPE over the course of a year. The monthly module will be presented several times on each shift. Although the net hours of training per student will be greater annually, the departments might find it less burdensome to release students for the shorter classes. Thus, instructors will teach fewer classes, resulting in a net savings in man-hours.

As mentioned earlier, 8 hours of First Responder Operations Level training might not be necessary for employees who have sufficient experience. These employees are allowed to demonstrate competency as an alternative to 8 hours of training. In most hospital settings, however, it might be difficult to ensure that employees have sufficient experience to waive the training requirement. Most hospital employees do not have extensive experience with hazardous materials and decontamination activities are performed infrequently, thus more than 8 hours of training may be helpful to ensure competence. Employees particularly benefit from the practical experience they gain during training provided as part of exercises and drills. These events also offer employees an opportunity to demonstrate competence in critical areas

Competencies for First Responder Awareness Level Training

First responders at the awareness level shall have sufficient training or have had sufficient experience:

- An understanding of what hazardous substances are, and the risks associated with them in an incident.
- An understanding of the potential outcomes associated with an emergency created when hazardous substances are present.
- The ability to recognize the presence of hazardous substances in an emergency.
- The ability to identify the hazardous substances, if possible.
- An understanding of their role in the hospital's emergency response plan, including site security and control, and decontamination procedures (OSHA, 1992c).
- The ability to realize the need for additional resources and to make appropriate notifications to the communication center.

In addition to the HAZWOPER training topics, staff who might identify contaminated victims that arrive unannounced require specific instructions for handling the situation. Once ED clerks or staff suspect a patient is contaminated, they should be well trained in the following procedure:

1. Avoid physical contact with the patient.
2. Immediately notify supervisor and safety officer of possible hospital contamination.
3. Allow other properly trained and equipped staff to isolate and decontaminate the victim according to EMP.

All the hospitals interviewed for this project provide Awareness Level training for staff who have a role during decontamination activities, but are not directly involved in patient decontamination. As with First Responder Operations Level training, there is considerable variability in the extent of training provided at the Awareness Level. The hospitals use curricula that range from 2 to 4 hours and most require an annual refresher course of 1 to 4 hours

OSHA recommends some form of basic training for employees who work in the Hospital Post-decontamination Zone and who would not be expected to come in contact with unannounced contaminated victims, their belongings, equipment, or waste. This training could take a format similar to hazard communication which might include at least the following:

- Methods and observations that may be used to detect the presence of a hazardous substance in the work area (e.g., an odor or announcement by staff trained to identify possible contamination).
- General information on victims as a possible source of hazardous substances.
- The measures employees can take to protect themselves during an incident, including specific procedures the hospital has implemented to protect employees from exposure to hazardous substances (e.g., emergency procedures for leaving the area).

In developing a training programme of this type, hospitals should consider which specific topics would best help this group of employees respond appropriately during an incident.

Monitoring Performance During Drills

All hospitals interviewed for this project conduct several types of drills. The hospitals note that the greatest value occurs when their EMPs are tested rigorously as part of the drill, when realistic scenarios are involved (including interaction with outside organisations), and when the hospital follows the drill with a detailed evaluation and post-drill action plan for improvement.

It is essential to the success of the EMP that drills are conducted and that they reflect the actual conditions, resources, and personnel that would be available during a real incident.

In addition to self-assessments, some hospitals find it helpful to receive a performance evaluation from an outside organisation. Hospital C participated in a community-wide drill that was observed by a contractor hired specifically for that purpose. The hospital used the contractor's observations and comments to help prioritize the emergency management team's activities. Alternatively, organisations that share post-drill analysis can critique each other. Any of these methods of assessment can lead to corrective actions and improved response, particularly if the process is formalized with hospital administrators.

Prior to an Incident

Hospitals A through G all indicate that they typically conduct a thorough baseline evaluation of an employee's health at the time the person is hired. Based on hospital policy, the employee's job category, or the hazards associated with tasks the employee performs, additional periodic health monitoring might also be provided. Most of the hospitals interviewed for this project indicate that they have no special additional requirements for members of the decontamination team, unless the individual might wear a respirator. In that case, the employee receives a baseline evaluation and any follow-up evaluations needed to obtain the necessary medical clearance, as discussed below.

One of the hospitals interviewed follows a somewhat more rigorous medical monitoring programme. Under this programme, each member assigned to the decontamination team receives a periodic physical exam (often every 1 or 2 years), which includes a basic health screening. Evaluations for medical clearance to wear a respirator are incorporated into these exams.

The HAZWOPER Standard requires that employees be provided periodic medical evaluations (annual or bi-annual) if they exhibit signs or symptoms of exposure, or if it is anticipated that the employee would be exposed to hazardous substances, in excess of the established permissible exposure limit (PEL), for 30 days per year or more. Drills and practice sessions that do not involve hazardous substances would not count toward the 30 days.

The hospitals interviewed for this project also mentioned that prophylactic vaccinations and antidotes should be stockpiled for employees in case the need arises.

During a Response

The combination of first receivers' activities and PPE often create a greater physical workload for employees than they experience during their normal daily jobs. Thermal stress (heat and cold stress) also impacts the period for which first receivers can perform their duties. Some hospitals monitor employee vital signs as one method of tracking employee response to these stressors. For example, Hospital A evaluates each employee's vital signs before that individual dons PPE. Prior to a team member donning a protective suit and hooded PAPR respirator, a technician records the individual's weight, vital signs, and recent medical history. This information is obtained as other team members assist the individual into the protective gear. If vital signs exceed predetermined limits set by the hospital organisation, the individual is prohibited from wearing PPE that day and the team member's activities are restricted accordingly. Decontamination safety officers at Hospital A report that during every drill conducted, they have rejected at least one participant (out of a dozen or more) due to elevated vital signs. When PPE is removed, vital signs and weight are recorded again. The employee's time in PPE is also recorded and tracked. Decontamination team members at Hospital A are generally permitted to wear a protective suit and hooded PAPR for 30 minutes at any one time, although this period can be adjusted up or down depending on workload, weather, and the condition of the first receiver.

Hospital A uses two-way headset radios to communicate with and monitor the health status of individuals who are wearing hooded PAPRs and protective suits in hot weather. This hospital found that a behind-the-head "temple transducer" style headset is more practical under PAPR hoods than "over-the-head" models, which tend to dislodge and are difficult to reposition without removing the hood.

Thermal Stress

Both heat and cold stress can decrease first responders' ability to work safely for extended periods. Hospital A believes that in its hot, humid southern climate, heat stress presents the greatest threat to employee health. To combat this hazard, the hospital uses a combination of administrative controls and cooling devices. As noted above, team members whose vital signs are outside prescribed starting parameters are not allowed to don respiratory protection. To further reduce the risk of heat stress, the team makes extensive use of icepack vests. Freezers for icepacks are located in the Safety Office, fire department, and elsewhere for easy access. Although Hospital A recognizes that use of icepacks to combat heat stress is somewhat controversial, this hospital reports no problems among the many team members who have drilled over the years. Additionally, team members report that they find the icepack vests to be a comfortable asset in hot weather.

The American Conference of Governmental Industrial Hygienists (ACGIH) offers guidance for managing heat stress in employees wearing heavy protective clothing (ACGIH, 2001). This conservative approach uses a combination of common-sense administrative controls (e.g., good hydration) and physiological measures of heat strain (remove worker if body core temperature exceeds 100.4 degrees Fahrenheit or heart rate exceeds 180 beats per minute (bpm) minus the employee's age, or is greater than 110 bpm one minute after peak exertion).

Evaluating Existing Resources

Hospitals are challenged to identify spaces that will support decontamination activities (including equipment storage) and ensure operations can continue in the event one area of the hospital becomes contaminated. Hospitals planning additions or remodeling projects have a unique opportunity to design spaces appropriately. Other hospitals should use creative planning to identify existing architectural features that they can use to their advantage. Several examples follow:

- Hospital F has two existing physical characteristics that have proven advantageous: (1) in the event that one side of the ED became contaminated by an unannounced victim, doors between two sections of the ED can be closed and normal ED activities can continue on the uncontaminated side; and (2) a pair of unused, canopy-covered ramps leading to one entrance of the ER (left from a period of construction when the ER was used as the main entrance to the hospital) is being converted into a permanent decontamination shower for ambulatory patients. When considering use of divided spaces, hospitals should determine whether the ventilation systems are also separate and whether they recirculate air. If a space becomes contaminated, it might be necessary to shut down the area's ventilation system to prevent circulation of contaminated air to other spaces.

- While looking for an appropriate location for its large portable decontamination system, Hospital A (in a hot humid climate) considered the advantages of a particularly large shade tree for preventing heat stress. The tree shades the entire shower system and all support features (extensive mechanical systems, triage and victim inspection stations, and victim waiting areas).

Equipment

Hospital A, which trains other hospitals to offer decontamination services, notes that it is critical to match the decontamination equipment purchased to the needs of the hospital and the community it serves. Hospital advisors recommend that any hospital with an emergency room should be prepared to decontaminate victims. However, facilities such as long-term care facilities and specialty clinics do not necessarily need decontamination capability. A hospital with a minimal risk of receiving multiple contaminated victims should consider acquiring a small system that can be handled by a few employees. According to Hospital A, "every hospital should have a well-coordinated plan for arranging [timely] decontamination of any patients who may show up at the door, without putting staff at undue risk." The plan should include medical triage and treatment capability with proper precautions.

Hospitals may select from an array of decontamination shower options. Portability is an advantage if the system might be required at different locations. A wide variety of portable, temporary decontamination systems are commercially available. Durable portable systems are designed to be cleaned and reused (if the type of contaminant is not highly toxic or persistent), while other systems are intended to be disposable and, thereby, simplify the post-incident recovery phase. The systems need to be stored in an easily accessible location. There is considerable variety in the sizes of portable decontamination systems available and the number of people required setting up the system. All require some set-up time.

Permanent decontamination facilities are generally recommended over temporary equipment because these facilities can be activated quickly (some permanent models may be activated by simply unlocking the doors and turning on the water) and offer reliable long-term service. They also function well in harsh climates. Although permanent facilities require a dedicated space and more maintenance than disposable systems, Hospital A finds that permanent decontamination showers can generally be installed for the same (or lower) cost than a portable system with comparable features.

Enclosed decontamination facilities should provide for fresh air circulation. When constructing a fully enclosed system, hospitals should consult a ventilation engineer or Certified Industrial Hygienist early in the system design phase.

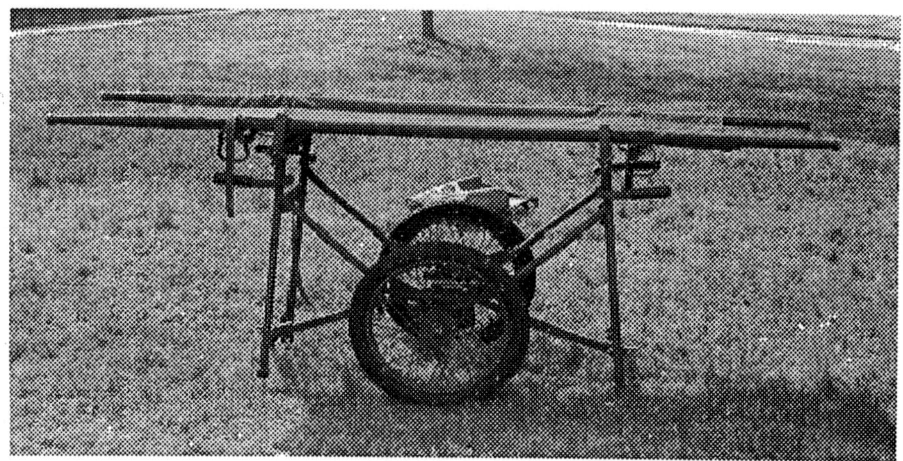

Because of the time it takes first receivers to put on PPE and to set-up decontamination facilities, hospitals may want to consider arranging for alternate rapid forms of decontamination until more sophisticated decontamination facilities are up and running. For example, some hospitals use high capacity, low-pressure hoses or showerheads, connected to high capacity, temperature-controlled water sources. These hoses and showers allow rapid preliminary drenching of multiple victims. Where multiple shower heads can be activated, ensure that the available water flow into, and through, the system is adequate to provide rapid decontamination at each shower head.

A field stretcher for transferring non-ambulatory victims from arriving vehicles to the decontamination facility

Decontamination procedures can have a large impact on first receiver exposure to hazardous substances. All the hospitals interviewed agree that the basic steps include:

1. Activate the EMP.
2. Learn as much as possible (as soon as possible) about the number of victims, the contaminant, and associated symptoms. Previous arrangements with first responder organisations can improve the timeliness and quantity of information received.
3. Activate the decontamination system and assemble the decontamination team and site security staff.
4. Perform any medical monitoring (e.g., vital signs), if specified by the EMP.
5. Put on PPE.
6. Triage victims to determine which individuals require decontamination and provide critical medical treatment to stabilize them before decontamination (e.g., atropine).

7. Assist victims (ambulatory and non-ambulatory) in removing contaminated clothing and securing personal property as soon as possible (within minutes of arrival).
8. Place clothing and other contaminated items in an approved hazardous waste container that is isolated outdoors so the items are not a continuing source of exposure.
9. Wash victims using soap, with good surfactant properties, and water (preferably tepid water to improve victim compliance). This step should include copious rinsing. [See discussion below.]
10. Inspect victims to evaluate the effectiveness of decontamination and guide decontaminated victims to the medical treatment area (Hospital Post-decontamination Zone). Return inadequately decontaminated victims to the shower area and repeat cleansing.
11. Decontaminate equipment and the decontamination system (if not disposable).
12. Staff remove PPE and decontaminate themselves.

All of the steps above can influence the extent of health care workers' exposure to the contaminant. However, certain steps should be highlighted for their direct impact on the concentrations of contaminant first receivers will encounter. For example, disrobing might remove as much as 75 to 90 percent of the contaminant arriving on a victim (Macintyre *et al.*, 2000; Vogt, 2002; USACHPPM, 2003a). By isolating (in an approved hazardous waste container) the contaminated clothing, staffs prevent these materials from off-gassing into the work area. To minimize first receiver exposure levels, these steps should be implemented immediately as victims arrive.

Non-ambulatory victims can require a substantial proportion of first receivers time and efforts. First receivers are likely to experience the greatest exposures while assisting these victims. Staff should take steps to identify possible sources of contamination and limit their exposure to those sources. For example, Hospital A uses specific procedures for removing victims clothing to minimize first receiver and victim exposures. Assistants use blunt-nose scissors to cut away clothing, rather than pulling it off. Tugging on clothing can produce a wringing action that might distribute contaminant on the victim, health care workers, and the surrounding area. Once removed, the clothing is immediately placed into a sealed container.

Unless a hospital uses detection equipment with demonstrated accuracy and reliability, victim washing procedures and visual inspection offer the only practical way health care workers can conclude that victims are definitively decontaminated. Staff in the ED might become exposed if contaminated victims are permitted to enter the Hospital Post-decontamination Zone. All the hospitals interviewed for this project indicated that they currently require victims to soap and shampoo completely and spend 5 to 6 minutes under a flow of running water. Some hospitals time the individual victims' total wash periods, while others observe the victims to ensure they wash thoroughly. It may be advantageous to start the victim cleansing process with a full minute under a drenching shower to rinse away as much contaminant as possible, followed by subsequent soaping and rinsing steps, repeated as necessary (USACHPPM, 2003a). Hospital G has a progressive shower, in which each victim spends one minute at each of several wash stations.

Most of the hospitals interviewed also provide victims with written or pictorial instructions. In addition, tepid water, security of personal effects, single-gender facilities, shelter, and replacement clothing influence how quickly and completely victims comply with requirements to undress, shower appropriately, and wait for medical treatment until they are completely decontaminated. In cold climates, heated spaces and blankets might be necessary. Victim inspection provides a final check to ensure contaminant is not carried into the ED.

Victims from some incidents may arrive at the hospital after having been decontaminated at the incident site (Release Zone) or elsewhere. Before admitting a victim to the ED, first receivers should evaluate each individual to ensure the patient was adequately cleansed.

While there is little definitive published information available regarding optimal shower procedures (for victims or staff), the following sections summarize information provided by organisations with some expertise in this area. These procedures apply to a wide variety of contaminants and are appropriate for unknown contaminants that could arise from a release of toxic chemicals, biological agents, or radiological particulates. Decontamination procedures, like PPE use, c n be modified once the contaminant is identified; hospitals that are cleansing victims to remove known contaminants can tailor procedures as appropriate. For example, a longer rinse might be beneficial for corrosive substances or contamination in the eyes. Organisations such as the Center for Disease Control and Prevention (CDC) and the Department of Homeland Security offer specific recommendations for decontaminating victims exposed to individual hazards, such as ionizing radiation (CDC, 2003; Department of Homeland Security, 2003). After cleansing with soap and water, certain residual chemical warfare agents (sarin, mustard gas, and others) can be neutralized on the skin using a substance such as the reactive skin decontamination lotion (RSDL), used by the US Army and other military organisations.

Shower Flush Time and Practices

Numerous agencies and organisations recommend a shower time of approximately five minutes for contaminated victims brought to a hospital. Despite the fact that there is no empirical data, operational procedures deem this time as adequate.

- The U.S. Army Center for Health Promotion and Preventive

Medicine (USACHPPM) recommends one-minute rinsing from head to toe with tepid water (slightly warm, not hot) after removal of contaminated clothing, followed by a more thorough decontamination of washing with a soap with good surfactant properties (e.g., hand dishwashing detergent), tepid water, and soft sponges. Avoid stiff brushes and vigorous scrubbing, which can damage the skin and increase the chance the contaminant would be absorbed by the victim. USACHPPM recommends these procedures for most classes of contaminants, except certain reactive metal dusts (USACHPPM, 2003a).

- The U.S. Army Soldier and Biological Chemical Command's (SBCCOM) Mass Casualty Decontamination Research Team (MCDRT) states that actual showering time will be an incident-specific decision but might be as long as 2 to 3 minutes per individual under ideal circumstances (SBCCOM, 2000b).
- The Agency for Toxic Substances and Disease Registry (ATSDR) recommends that patients contaminated with an unidentified chemical should flush exposed or irritated skin and hair with plain water for 3 to 5 minutes. For oily or otherwise adherent chemicals, mild soap on the skin and hair followed by a thorough rinse with water is also recommended (ATSDR, 2003).

A technical expert for Hospital A's Emergency Mass-Casualty Decontamination Programme stated that research regarding how long it takes to decontaminate an individual is scarce. This organisation recommends a 5-minute shower time, based on operational experience.

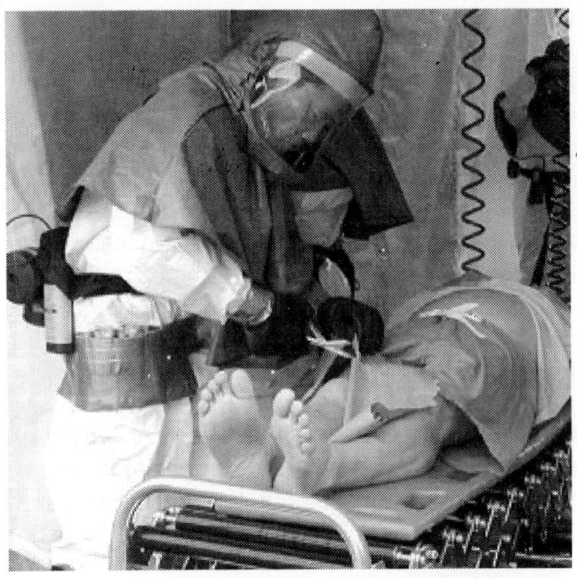

Use blunt scissors to cut away clothing. Avoid stretching or wringing cloth.

However, in some cases the total decontamination period could last longer than five minutes, depending on the agent, its viscosity, the quantity on the victim, and the amount of clothing removed.

Ionizing Radiation Meters

Experts suggest that alpha or beta emitting particles may be the more likely contaminants in mass casualty events involving the release of radiological particles (CDC, 2003). Relatively reliable and easy to use instruments are available for measuring ionizing radiation. Hospitals that offer patients nuclear medicine services generally have access to specific types of radiation meters used in that department. For example, the Radiation Safety Office for Hospital F indicated that such meters would be available for post-decontamination evaluation of victims, staff, and hospitals, as deemed appropriate. It is important that meters used by first receivers be selected based on the types of radiological particles with which victims could be contaminated. To ensure more immediate access to appropriate equipment, Hospital B has obtained micro-roentgen per hour (μR/h) survey meters for the dedicated use of the decontamination team. In the event of a radiological emergency, the team will use the meters as they evaluate the effectiveness of victim decontamination.

To evaluate the effectiveness of decontamination procedures and also to help identify possible embedded fragments of radioactive materials, Hospital G obtained a pair of radiological monitoring devices (Ludlum Model 3 Survey Meters, with Model 44-7 End Window G-M Detectors and headphones). This choice was based on reports of good experiences with the instrument, price, and versatility (the equipment can be used for estimating exposure rate as well as detecting contamination). The hospital also acquired Radiagem-4 Personal Portable Radiometers, which are small hand-held gamma source meters that will potentially serve the dual purpose of screening victims for contamination and simultaneously recording the accumulated exposure of the employee using the equipment. These user-friendly detectors integrate the reading and will alarm after reaching a preset threshold.

Ionizing radiation detection equipment could also be useful for identifying contaminated individuals that might enter the ED unannounced. Hospital G is in the process of obtaining and testing radiation detection meters (Syrena Gamma Source Finder) that will be located at patient entrances to the hospital. These portable devices-about the size of an attaché case-will be tested at an entrance to determine whether they are useful for detecting radioactivity. The hospital hopes to use this type of equipment to avoid the spread of contamination by identifying contaminated individuals as they enter the hospital. The hospital also plans to evaluate equipment that could be used to screen victims by moving them past an instrument (e.g., at the entrance and exit of a shower system) eliminating the need for an employee in this position.

Chemical and Biological Agent Detection Equipment

User-friendly equipment of adequate sensitivity is also becoming available for specific agents typically used as chemical weapons (Environmental Technologies, undated). For example, two of the interviewed hospitals (Hospitals B and C) obtained the same make and model ("APD 2000" from Environmental Technologies) of hand-held detection meters designed to detect parts per billion levels of specific chemical "nerve and blister agents" used as chemical weapons (e.g., organophosphates, and mustard agent). However, a third hospital (Hospital A) felt that this type of equipment might be more useful for evaluating an incident site than for declaring victims to be thoroughly clean after decontamination efforts.

Equivalent equipment for detecting industrial chemicals and biological agents remains problematic. Although the interviewed hospitals indicated that they are interested in obtaining comparable detection equipment that would identify and measure low levels of industrial chemicals or biological agents, none of the hospitals feel the instruments currently available are practical for this purpose. Experts do agree, however, that some of the current broad-spectrum detection devices are capable of detecting classes of agents (although not the individual agent) with reasonable sensitivity and accuracy. Hospitals should determine the availability and utility of these instruments for the specific categories of substances identified in the hospital's HVA.

Hospital A indicated that optimal detection instruments would be: (1) sensitive at low concentrations to a wide range of substances, (2) have a rapid response time (preferably a few seconds), (3) be easy to operate, (4) be rugged and portable enough to function outdoors under emergency conditions, (5) require only occasional routine maintenance, and (6) be reasonably priced. Macintyre *et al.* (2000) point out that the currently available detectors and monitors "would only complicate and lengthen the decontamination process," without providing substantial value.

Pre-decontamination triage serves three purposes

- Distinguish contaminated individuals from other patients arriving at the hospital (e.g., by identifying symptoms and victim's proximity to a known chemical release).
- Identify victims who require immediate stabilization before they enter the decontamination system (e.g., shock and respiratory arrest).
- Identify injuries or critical pre-hospital treatment materials that will require special handling inside the decontamination system (e.g., a tourniquet that must be replaced with an uncontaminated compression device).

A plan for pre-decontamination triage should be included in the EMP. Post-decontamination triage for medical treatment should occur in the

Hospital Post-decontamination Zone, after victims are inspected and found to be free of contamination. Some hospitals combine decontamination and initial medical treatment (such as antidotes), which means either the health care worker attempts medical triage while wearing PPE (preferred) or the worker is at risk of exposure from victims that have not been adequately decontaminated

Wastewater Management

During an emergency, first receivers should take all necessary steps to save lives, protect the public, and protect themselves. Once imminent threats to human health and life are addressed, first receivers should make all reasonable efforts to contain contamination and avoid or mitigate environmental consequences (U.S. EPA, 2000).

Wastewater from decontamination showers can contain low-level concentrations of the substance(s) with which victims are contaminated. Given the opportunity to plan for decontamination activities (by designing and installing or purchasing decontamination facilities, developing procedures, and preparing staff), hospitals should consider the management of decontamination shower water as part of the plan. To determine appropriate wastewater management practices, hospitals should consult with LEPCs, whose members "can work together creatively using available resources to minimize the environmental impact of [hazardous materials] incidents" (U.S. EPA, 2000).

The hospitals interviewed follow several strategies for handling decontamination shower wastewater. Management methods range from complete water retention in a storage unit to uncontrolled release (e.g., into parking lot or storm drain). The choice is usually based on the circumstances under which the individual decontamination system will be used. For example, these hospitals have generally arranged for some level of treatment or containment of wastewater generated by their primary decontamination systems (i.e., the systems that would be used most frequently). However, the same hospitals do not typically apply specific controls to wastewater from additional, open-air showerheads intended for use only as backup shower capacity (in the event that an unexpectedly large number of victims overwhelms the hospital's primary decontamination system).

Hospital B has a memorandum of understanding with the municipal wastewater treatment facility, which allows the hospital to drain water from its large, permanent, indoor decontamination system to the sanitary sewer. The agreement specifies that the hospital notify the treatment facility immediately when the shower is used to treat contaminated victims. Hospital B includes this notification in the EMP protocol for activating the shower.

Hospital A and Hospital C incorporate large (1,000 or more gallons) underground storage tanks into the design of their permanent, enclosed decontamination systems. When necessary, the water can be held until tested. After consultation with local environmental authorities, the hospital can either treat the wastewater, pump it out, or drain the water to the sanitary sewer or storm drain.

Among the hospitals interviewed, those that have obtained portable decontamination systems typically use a wastewater-containment device built into the base of the system enclosure. These containment devices usually include a low supportive wall (a few inches high) around the perimeter of the shower and a plastic lining to catch and hold wastewater. The hospitals often pump water from the shower base containment into a separate bladder to limit the volume in the shower base and to increase water storage capacity.

An important consideration for positioning wastewater storage receptacles is the eventual need to drain or transport them (once filled, these containers are heavy and can only be shifted using special equipment). Hospital D noted that its hazardous waste management contractor provided useful advice about locating the wastewater receptacle where it could be easily accessed by the contractor's equipment, or could be drained with little assistance if water treatment was not required. This advice influenced the ultimate decontamination area design.

MAINTAINING FUTURE READINESS

To sustain a functional level of emergency preparedness, hospitals need to maintain equipment, supplies, and employee training. They should devote time and attention to evaluating and updating the HVA and EMP and coordinating these activities with the community. These efforts all require resources that will not be available without support at all levels of management. Hospitals D and F note that emergency planners can take active steps to help hospital management recognize the need for continuing effort. These steps might include providing management with after-action reports following drills and updated information regarding the community's expectations of the hospital.

Administrators need to be aware that all aspects of the EMP should be maintained equally. Continued employee training alone will not provide adequate protection if protective equipment (including respirator cartridges) is not replaced after use or when its shelf life expires. Some equipment, such as PAPR batteries, requires routine maintenance (e.g., charging and battery-life evaluation) for the life of the equipment. In addition, a well-maintained decontamination facility will not function well if employees do not have the experience of active, recent drills.

Hospitals in more mature stages of emergency management planning might require less concentrated efforts than during start-up, but continue to dedicate full- or part-time staff to ensure the hospital retains a full level of preparation. Emergency managers use creative methods to obtain additional help when needed. Hospital D uses an energetic emergency manager to direct the activities of employees from other departments who temporarily require light-duty work due to medical restrictions (after an illness or injury). These individuals provide some of the labor needed to update and improve the already-mature HVA and EMP.

Appendix B

ACRONYMS AND DEFINITIONS

Atmosphere supplying respirator (ASR)

A respirator that provides clean air from an uncontaminated source to the facepiece. Examples include supplied-air (airline) respirators, SCBA, and combination supplied-air/SCBA.

Assigned protection factor (APF)

a rating assigned to a respirator style by OSHA or NIOSH. This rating indicates the level of protection most workers can expect from the properly worn, maintained, and fitted respirator used under actual workplace conditions. An APF of 1,000 indicates that the concentration of contaminant inside the facepiece would be 1,000 times lower than concentration in the surrounding air. A respirator with an APF of 1,000 will provide greater protection than a respirator with an APF of 100. (*Note*: The APF should not be confused with a similar measure, the "fit factor," obtained during quantitative fit testing. Fit factors, which tend to be higher numbers, provide a relative indication of how well a respirator fits an individual, but do not represent the level of protection the respirator would provide in the workplace.)

Awareness Level

See First Responder Awareness Level.

CBRN

Chemical, biological, radiological, or nuclear [agent or substance].

Clinicians

Physicians, nurses, nurse practitioners, physicians' assistants, and others.

Doff

To take-off or remove (e.g., PPE).

Don

To put on, in order to wear (e.g., PPE).

ED:

Emergency Department.

EMP

Emergency Management Plan.

First Receiver

Employees at a hospital engaged in decontamination and treatment of victims who have been contaminated by a hazardous substance(s) during an emergency incident. The incident occurs at a site other than the hospital. These employees are a subset of first responders.

First Responder

Personnel who have responsibility to initially respond to emergencies. Some examples are firefighters, HAZMAT team members, law enforcement officers, lifeguards, forestry personnel, ambulance attendants, and other public service personnel. In the case of hazardous materials incidents, these personnel typically respond at the site where the incident occurred.

First Responder Awareness Level

Individuals who might reasonably be anticipated to witness or discover a hazardous substance release and who have been trained to initiate an emergency response sequence by notifying the proper authorities of the release. They would take no further action beyond notifying the authorities.

First Responder Operations Level

Individuals who respond to releases or potential releases of hazardous substances as part of the initial response to the site for the purpose of protecting nearby persons, property, or the environment from the effects of the release. These individuals shall have received at least 8 hours of training or have sufficient experience to objectively demonstrate competency in specific critical areas.

HAZCOM

OSHA's Hazard Communication Standard.

HAZMAT

Hazardous Material.

HAZWOPER

OSHA's Standard on Hazardous Waste Operations and Emergency Response. In particular, paragraph (q) of this standard covers employers whose employees are engaged in emergency response to hazardous substance releases.

Hazard Vulnerability Analysis (HVA)

The identification of potential emergencies and direct and indirect effects these emergencies may have on the health care organisation's operations and the demand for its services.

Hazardous Substance

Any substance to which exposure may result in adverse effects on the health or safety of employees. This includes substances defined under Section 101(14) of CERCLA; biological or disease-causing agents that may reasonably be anticipated to cause death, disease, or other health problems; any substance listed by the U.S. Department of Transportation as hazardous material under 49 CFR 172.101 and appendices; and substances classified as hazardous waste.

Hospital Emergency Incident Command System (HEICS)

an example of an optional NIMS-based ICS tailored specifically for use by hospitals and designed to function in conjunction with other common ICSs used by emergency response organisations (e.g., Fire Service Incident Command System).

Hospital Decontamination Zone

This zone includes any areas where the type and quantity of hazardous substance is unknown and where contaminated victims, contaminated equipment, or contaminated waste may be present. It is reasonably anticipated that employees in this zone might have exposure to contaminated victims, their belongings, equipment, or waste. This zone includes, but is not limited to, places where initial triage and/or medical stabilization of possibly contaminated victims occur, pre-decontamination waiting (staging) areas for victims, the actual decontamination area, and the post-decontamination victim inspection area. This area will typically end at the emergency department door. In other documents, this zone is sometimes called the "Warm Zone," "contamination reduction zone," "yellow zone," or "limited access zone."

Hospital Post-decontamination Zone

The Hospital Post-decontamination Zone is an area considered uncontaminated. Equipment and personnel are not expected to become contaminated in this area. At a hospital receiving contaminated victims, the Hospital Post-decontamination Zone includes the emergency department (unless contaminated). This zone is sometimes called the "Cold Zone" or "Clean Area."

IDLH

Or Immediately dangerous to life or health, means an atmospheric concentration of any toxic, corrosive or asphyxiant substance that poses an immediate threat to life or would interfere with an individual's ability to escape from a dangerous atmosphere. Incident Command System (ICS): A flexible organisational structure which provides a basic expandable system developed by Fire Services to mitigate an emergency situation of any size. Incident Commander (IC): The individual who holds overall responsibility for incident response and management.

Incident Command System (ICS)

A flexible organisational structure which provides a basic expandable system developed by Fire Services to mitigate an emergency situation of any size.

Incident Commander (IC)

The individual who holds overall responsibility for incident response and management.

JCAHO

Joint Commission on Accreditation of Health Care Organisations.

LEPC

Local Emergency Planning Committee.

Mass Casualty

"A combination of patient numbers and patient care requirements that challenge or exceed a community's ability to provide adequate patient care using day-to-day operations" (Barbera and MacIntyre, 2003).

NIMS

The National Incident Management System, established by the US Department of Homeland Security as a standardized management approach to incident response that all responders will use to coordinate and conduct response actions.

NFPA

National Fire Protection Association.

Operations Level

See First Responder Operations Level.

Personal Protective Equipment (PPE)

Examples include protective suits, gloves, foot covering, respiratory protection, hoods, safety glasses, goggles, and face shields.

Powered Air-Purifying Respirator (PAPR)

A respirator that uses a battery-powered blower to force air through a filter or purifying cartridge before blowing the cleaned air into the respirator facepiece.

Release Zone

An area in and immediately surrounding a hazardous substance release. It is assumed to pose an immediate health risk to all persons, including first responders. For the purposes of this document the Release Zone is always REMOTE from the hospital. This zone is also referred to as the "exclusion zone", the "red zone", and the "restricted zone" in other documents.

Self-contained Breathing Apparatus (SCBA)

A respirator that provides fresh air to the facepiece from a compressed air tank (usually worn on the worker's back).

Supplied-air Respirator (SAR)

A respirator that provides breathing air through an airline hose from an uncontaminated compressed air source to the facepiece. The facepiece can be a hood, helmet, or tight fitting facepiece.

Triage

The process of screening and classifying sick, wounded, or injured persons to determine priority needs in order to ensure the efficient use of medical personnel, equipment, and hospitals.

WMD: Weapon of Mass Destruction.

Appendix C

ADVANTAGES AND DISADVANTAGES OF VARIOUS RESPIRATOR FACEPIECE STYLES

FACEPIECE STYLE	ADVANTAGES	DISADVANTAGES
Half face-piece	• Employee may wear any appropriate eyewear that does not interfere with the respirator seal	• If there is a break in the seal between the mask and the face, contaminated air can enter. Fit testing must be performed prior to use and user seal checks must be done by the user every time the respirator is used. • Does not provide eye protection.
Full face-piece	• When used with a powered air-purifying respirator (PAPR), a tight fitting facepiece might allow a worker to pull filtered air into the face piece if the battery fails.	• If there is a break in the seal between the mask and the face, contaminated air can enter. Fit testing must be performed prior to use and user seal checks must be done by the user every time the respirator is used. • Workers who wear glasses may require spectacle kits to be used inside the facepiece.
Loose fitting helmet/ hood	• Provides eye protection. • Provides eye protection. • Provides skin protection for the head and (certain models) neck. • Fit testing is not required. • Some workers find loose fitting respirators more comfortable than tight fitting models.	• When used with a PAPR, the hood will provide little or no protection if the battery fails.

- Can be worn by employees with facial hair and facial scars/deformities.
- Employees may wear their own glasses under the helmet/hood.

Adapted from Personal Protective Equipment Guide for Military Medical Treatment Facility Personnel Handling Casualties from Weapons of Mass Destruction and Terrorism Events (Technical Guide 275). U.S. Army Center for Health Promotion and Preventive Medicine (USACHPPM), August 2003.

Appendix D

KAISER PERMANENTE HAZARD VULNERABILITY ANALYSIS

This document is a sample Hazard Vulnerability Analysis tool. It is not a substitute for a comprehensive emergency preparedness programme. Individuals or organisations using this tool are solely responsible for any hazard assessment and compliance with applicable laws and regulations.

Instructions

Evaluate potential for event and response among the following categories using the hazard specific scale. Assume each event incident occurs at the worst possible time (e.g. during peak patient loads). Please note specific score criteria on each work sheet to ensure accurate recording.

Issues to consider for probability include, but are not limited to:

1. Known risk
2. Historical data
3. Manufacturer/vendor statistics

Issues to consider for response include, but are not limited to:

1. Time to marshal an on-scene response
2. Scope of response capability
3. Historical evaluation of response success

Issues to consider for human impact include, but are not limited to:

1. Potential for staff death or injury
2. Potential for patient death or injury

Issues to consider for property impact include, but are not limited to:

1. Cost to replace
2. Cost to set-up temporary replacement
3. Cost to repair
4. Time to recover

Issues to consider for business impact include, but are not limited to:

1. Business interruption
2. Employees unable to report to work
3. Customers unable to reach facility
4. Company in violation of contractual agreements
5. Imposition of fines and penalties or legal costs
6. Interruption of critical supplies

7. Interruption of product distribution
8. Reputation and public image
9. Financial impact/burden

Issues to consider for preparedness include, but are not limited to:

1. Status of current plans
2. Frequency of drills
3. Training status
4. Insurance
5. Availability of alternate sources for critical supplies/services

Issues to consider for internal resources include, but are not limited to:

1. Types of supplies on hand/will they meet need?
2. Volume of supplies on hand/will they meet need?
3. Staff availability
4. Coordination with any medical office buildings (e.g., doctors' offices and clinics) included in the EMP.
5. Availability of back-up systems
6. Internal resources ability to withstand disasters/survivability

Issues to consider for external resources include, but are not limited to:

1. Types of agreements with community agencies/drills
2. Coordination with local and state agencies
3. Coordination with proximal health care facilities
4. Coordination with treatment specific facilities
5. Community resources

Complete all worksheets including Natural, Technological, Human and Hazmat. The summary section will automatically provide your specific and overall relative threat.

APPENDIX E

HOSPITAL EMERGENCY INCIDENT COMMAND SYSTEM, JANUARY 1998

Confusion and chaos are commonly experienced by the hospital at the onset of a medical disaster. However, these negative effects can be minimized if management responds quickly with structure and a focused direction of activities. The Hospital Emergency Incident Command System (HEICS) is an emergency management system which employs a logical management structure, defined responsibilities, clear reporting channels, and a common nomenclature to help unify hospitals with other emergency responders. There are clear advantages to all hospitals using this particular emergency management system.

Based upon public safety's Incident Command System, HEICS has already proved valuable in helping hospitals serve the community during a crisis and resume normal operations as soon as possible. A survey of California hospitals in the Spring of 1997, reveals a significant number of hospitals have, or will be incorporating HEICS within their emergency plans. HEICS is fast becoming the standard for health care disaster response and offers the following features:

- predictable chain of management
- flexible organisational chart allows flexible response to specific emergencies
- prioritized response checklists
- accountability of position function
- improved documentation for improved accountability and cost recovery
- common language to promote communication and facilitate outside assistance
- cost effective emergency planning within health care organisations

ORGANISATIONAL CHART

- Positions may or may not be activated.
  Each emergency must be evaluated as to the specific positions which will need activation in order to address challenges of the emergency. The disaster's nature, proximity, and other factors may mandate all or very few of the positions to be staffed.
- Positions may be filled immediately or later based upon needs and staffing.
  A particular disaster may require that a certain number of positions need to be filled. However, if there are only a few managers available for the next 12 hours, then each manager

must take more than one position. If this is not acceptable, then the top priority positions must be identified and carried out in the best manner possible.

- More than one position may be assigned to an individual. Many managers are capable of carrying out more than one function at a time. Situations of a critical nature may require an individual to perform multiple tasks until additional support can be obtained. The use of checklists should facilitate the task of multiple position assignment.

APPENDIX F

U.S. COAST GUARD NATIONAL STRIKE FORCE

I. Medical Monitoring

a. Medical monitoring shall be conducted on all entry, backup, and decon personnel prior to Exclusion Zone entries. Follow-up medical monitoring shall also be conducted on all entry, backup, and decon personnel at the conclusion of each work shift. For workers wearing impermeable chemical protective clothing, workers shall also be monitored when the temperature in the work area exceeds 70°F (21°C). Medical monitoring shall be conducted during the rest period following each work cycle in accordance with chapter 8 of reference 1. If the work cycle specified in Table 8-10 of Reference 1 is less than 30 minutes, the supervisor may consult the Commanding Officer for authorization to extend the work cycle up to 30 minutes.

b. Recommended values from the American Heart Association are to be used as guidance for pre-entry medical monitoring:
Blood Pressure (Max): 140 bpm Systolic/100 Diastolic*
Pulse Rate (Max): 100 bpm
Temperature: 98.0°F (Min), 99.2°F (Max) (or +/- 0.6°F from normal)

c. When a medical value is found to be outside the accepted guidance, the supervisor should be informed immediately. Anomalous readings require medical advice prior to continued entries by an individual.

d. Use appropriate forms to record field medical monitoring.

e. When questions regarding medical monitoring arise, the unit Safety and Occupational Health Coordinator (SOHC) shall be contacted.

* *Note*: At the onset of an incident, fear and anxiety may cause employees' blood pressure to be elevated.

HEAT STROKE. Heat stroke is the most serious of health problems associated with working in hot environments. It occurs when the body's temperature regulatory system fails and sweating becomes inadequate. The body's only effective means of removing excess heat is compromised with little warning to the victim that a crisis stage has been reached.

A heat stroke victim's skin is hot, usually dry, red or spotted. Body temperature is usually 105°F or higher, and the victim is mentally confused, delirious, perhaps in convulsions, or unconscious. Unless the victim receives quick and appropriate treatment, death can occur.

Any person with signs of symptoms of heat stroke requires immediate hospitalization. However, first aid should be immediately administered.

This includes removing the victim to a cool area, thoroughly soaking the clothing with water, and vigorously fanning the body to increase cooling. Further treatment, at a medical facility, should be directed to the continuation of the cooling process and the monitoring of complications which often accompany the heat stroke. Early recognition and treatment of heat stroke is the only means of preventing permanent brain damage or death.

HEAT EXHAUSTION. Heat exhaustion includes several clinical disorders having symptoms which may resemble the early symptoms of heat stroke. Heat exhaustion is caused by the loss of large amounts of fluid by sweating, sometimes with excessive loss of salt. A worker suffering from heat exhaustion still sweats but experiences extreme weakness or fatigue, giddiness, nausea, or headache. In more serious cases, the victim may vomit or lose consciousness. The skin is clammy and moist, the complexion is pale or flushed, and the body temperature is normal or only slightly elevated. In most cases, treatment involves having the victim rest in a cool place and drink plenty of liquids. Victims with mild cases of heat exhaustion usually recover spontaneously with this treatment. Those with severe cases may require extended care for several days. There are no known permanent effects.

HEAT CRAMPS. Heat cramps are painful spasms of the muscles that occur among those who sweat profusely in heat, drink large quantities of water, but do not adequately replace the body's salt loss. The drinking of large quantities of water tends to dilute the body's fluids, while the body continues to lose salt. Shortly thereafter, the low salt level in the muscles causes painful cramps. The affected muscles may be part of the arms, legs, or abdomen; but tired muscles (those used in performing the work) are usually the ones most susceptible to cramps. Cramps may occur during or after work hours and may be relieved by taking salted liquids by mouth.

FAINTING. A worker who is not accustomed to hot environments and who stands erect and immobile in the heat may faint. With enlarged blood vessels in the skin and in the lower part of the body due to the body's attempts to control internal temperature, blood may pool there rather than return to the heart to be pumped to the brain. Upon lying down, the worker should soon recover. By moving around, and thereby preventing blood from pooling, the patient can prevent further fainting.

HEAT RASH. Heat rash, also known as prickly heat, is likely to occur in hot, humid environments where heat is not easily removed from the surface of the skin by evaporation and the skin remains wet most of the time. The sweat ducts become plugged, and a skin rash soon appears. When the rash is extensive or when it is complicated by infection, prickly heat can be very uncomfortable and may reduce a worker's performance. The worker can prevent this condition by resting in a cool place part of each day and by regularly bathing and drying the skin.

TRANSIENT HEAT FATIGUE. Transient heat fatigue refers to the temporary state of discomfort and mental or psychological strain arising from prolonged heat exposure. Workers unaccustomed to the heat are particularly susceptible and can suffer, to varying degrees, a decline in task performance, coordination, alertness, and vigilance. The severity of transient heat fatigue will be lessened by a period of gradual adjustment to the hot environment (heat acclimatization).

PREPARING FOR WORK IN THE HEAT

Adjustment to heat, under normal circumstances, takes about a week, during which time the body will undergo a series of changes that will make continued exposure to heat more endurable. With each succeeding daily exposure, hazardous physiological responses will gradually decrease, while the sweat rate will increase. When the body becomes acclimated to the heat, the worker will find it possible to perform work with less strain and distress.

Gradual exposure to heat gives the body time to become accustomed to higher environmental temperatures. Heat disorders in general are more likely to occur among workers who have not been given time to adjust to working in the heat or among workers who have been away from hot environments and who have gotten accustomed to lower temperatures. Hot weather conditions of the summer are likely to affect the worker who is not acclimatized to heat. Likewise, workers who return to work after a leisurely vacation or extended illness may be affected by the heat in the work environment. Whenever such circumstances occur, the worker should be gradually reacclimatized to the hot environment.

Heat stress depends, in part, on the amount of heat the worker's body produces while a job is being performed. The amount of heat produced during hard, steady work is much higher than that produced during intermittent or light work. Therefore, one way of reducing the potential for heat stress is to make the job easier or lessen its duration by providing adequate rest. Rather than be exposed to heat for extended periods of time during the course of a job, workers should, wherever possible, be permitted to distribute the workload evenly over the day and incorporate work-rest cycles. Work-rest cycles give the body an opportunity to get rid of excess heat, slow down the production of internal body heat, and provide greater blood flow to the skin.

REST AREAS. Providing cool rest areas in hot work environments considerably reduces the stress of working in those environments. There is no conclusive information available on the ideal temperature for a rest area. Rest areas should be as close to the work area as possible, and provide shade. Individual work periods should not be lengthened in favor of prolonged rest periods. Shorter but frequent work-rest cycles are the greatest benefit to the worker.

DRINKING WATER. In the course of a day's work in the heat, a worker may produce as much as 2 to 3 gallons of sweat. Because so many heat disorders involve excessive dehydration of the body, it is essential that water intake during the workday be about equal to the amount of sweat produced. Most workers exposed to hot conditions drink less fluids than needed because of an insufficient thirst drive. A worker, therefore, should not depend on thirst to signal when and how much to drink. Instead, the worker should drink 5 to 7 ounces of fluids every 15 to 20 minutes to replenish the necessary fluids in the body. There is no optimum temperature of drinking water, but most people tend not to drink warm or very cold fluids as readily as they will cool ones. Whatever the temperature of the water, it must be palatable and readily available. Individual drinking cups should be provided—never use a common drinking cup.

Heat acclimatized workers lose much less salt in their sweat than do workers who are not adjusted to the heat. The average American diet contains sufficient salt for acclimatized workers even when sweat production is high. If for some reason, salt replacement is required, the best way to compensate for the loss is to add a little extra salt to the food. Salt tablets SHOULD NOT be used.

PROTECTIVE CLOTHING. Clothing inhibits the transfer of heat between the body and the surrounding environment. Therefore, in hot jobs where the air temperature is lower than skin temperature, wearing clothing reduces the body's ability to lose heat into the air. When air temperature is higher than skin temperature, clothing helps to prevent the transfer of heat from the air to the body. The advantage of wearing additional clothes, however, may be nullified if the clothes interfere with the evaporation of sweat (such as rain slickers or chemical protective clothing).

APPENDIX G

PATIENT DECONTAMINATION PROCEDURE (NORTHERN VIRGINIA EMERGENCY RESPONSE COALITION)

Ambulatory Patients

1. Direct patient to Decon Sector.
2. Children should be kept with their parents if at all possible; if no parent or older sibling is available then a Decon Team member should provide needed assistance to a child.
3. Patient should be given Personal Decon set as soon as it is available and be given rapid instructions on its use—PLAY THE TAPE recorded set of instructions, if available.
   - The kit stays with you as you proceed through the process.
   - Open up the bag - it has three parts.
   - Take out the plastic bags now.
4. Patient should quickly remove all clothing, putting valuables into the clear plastic bag and clothing into the large bag, then put both bags into the 3rd bag and cinch tight w/tag number in pack. Patient should put numbered tag around their neck and wear it through decon and treatment.
5. The clothing bag should be set aside in a secure area.
6. If staff is available, patient's name and number should be recorded on the Patient Decon Record.
7. Patient should continue forward into the Decon Sector with remaining part of Personal Decon Kit.
8. Patient should quickly rinse themselves from head to toe with water using either the hand held sprayer, garden hose, or shower head.
9. Patient should next wash with soap and wash cloth or brush from the kit in a systematic fashion, cleaning open wounds first and then in a head-to-toe fashion for 5 minutes when the agent is non- persistent and 8 minutes when a persistent or unknown agent is involved. Discourage the patient from rubbing too vigorously while washing. Eye irritation may require the use of a topical anesthetic first before irrigating.
10. The Decon Team should closely observe each victim to ensure they are thorough in washing themselves. Particular attention should be made to ensure they wash the axilla, creases, folds, and hair. Help should be offered as necessary.
11. Once the washing is completed, each patient should thoroughly rinse themselves (this should require about a minute to complete).
12. Decon soap, wash cloths, brushes, and sponges should be put into a nearby trash can and NOT carried into the Cold Zone.

13. After the rinse/wash/rinse cycle is complete the patient should next proceed to the towel off area and complete drying off and leave the towel in the trash can.
14. Following drying off, the patient should put on the patient gown and proceed to the Triage Officer for rapid assessment and assignment to a Treatment Sector.
15. Additional treatment will be limited only to those interventions deemed life saving by the Decon Officer. Antidote administration should be done via the intramuscular (IM) route after cleaning the affected area first.
16. Decon Team members should be alert to the possibility that an ambulatory patient may clinically deteriorate and require immediate removal to the Non-Ambulatory Sector via backboard, stretcher, or wheelchair.

Non-Ambulatory Patients

1. Patient should be brought to the Decon Sector and tended to by a minimum of 4 decon personnel.
2. Each patient should be put onto a backboard or EMS stretcher w/the pad removed.
3. All patient clothing should be removed and valuables put into the clear plastic bag and clothing into the large bag, then put both bags into the 3rd bag and cinch tight w/tag number in pack. Clothing should be cut away where necessary.
4. Attention should be paid to minimizing the aerosolization spread of particulate matter by folding clothing inside out as removal is being done and dabbing the skin with sticky tape and or vacuuming.
5. Patient should have their clothing bag tag around their neck and wear it through decon and treatment.
6. The clothing bag should be set aside in a secure area. If staff is available, the patient's name and number should be recorded on the Patient Decon Record.
7. While resting the backboard on saw horses or other device or with the patient on an EMS stretcher, the patient should quickly be rinsed from head to toe with water using either the hand held sprayer, garden hose, or shower head; protection from aspiration of the rinse water should be ensured.
8. Next the patient should be washed with soap and either a brush or wash cloth in a systematic fashion, cleaning airway first followed by open wounds then in a head to toe fashion for 5 minutes when the agent is non persistent and 8 minutes when a persistent or unknown agent is involved. Avoid rubbing too vigorously.

9. The patient should be rolled on their side for washing of the posterior head, neck, back, buttocks and lower extremities by 2-4 personnel; attention to a possible neck injury should be given.
10. Careful attention should be given to washing the voids and creases such as the ears, eyes, axilla, and groin.
11. Topical eye anesthetic may be required for effective eye irrigation to be done.
12. The patient should then be rinsed in a head to toe fashion that minimizes contamination spread for about one minute. Overspray or holding the rinsing devise too close so as to irritate the skin should be avoided.
13. Decon Team members should be alert to the probability that the non-ambulatory patient may require ABC's support (airway positioning, suctioning, O_2 administration, spinal stabilization, etc.) and administration of life saving antidote administration by IM injection. If IV therapy is needed the extremity site for the IV should be deconned quickly before the IV is started. If IV therapy is needed the patient should be pulled out of line in the Decon Corridor but remain in the Decon Sector.
14. The patient should be dried off, put into a hospital gown, and transferred to a clean backboard (or clean off and dry the board they are on if additional boards are not available). Patients on an EMS stretcher should be transferred to a clean backboard.
15. Decon soap, brushes and sponges should be put into a trash can and not carried into the Cold Zone. O_2 material should remain in the Decon Sector.
16. The patient should be taken to the Triage Officer for rapid assessment and assignment to area in the Treatment Sector.

Patients with Special Needs

Glasses/Contact Lenses

1. Patients with glasses should keep them if they cannot see without them. They must be washed and rinsed thoroughly during the decon process before being worn. Otherwise, the glasses should be placed in the valuables portion of the clothing bag.
2. Contact lenses should be removed and placed in the valuables portion of the clothing bag.

Canes/Walkers

1. Patients who use walking assist devices may retain them, but the device must be washed with soap and water during the decon process before being allowed into the Treatment Sector.

2. Patients who are unsteady standing and/or walking should be given a walker upon entry into the Decon Corridor. The walker should be used to assist with ambulation until they get to the end of the line when it should be retrieved, deconned, and returned to the front of the Decon Corridor for the next patient who needs it.

Percutaneous Lines/Saline Locks

1. Unless contaminated, percutaneous lines and saline locks should be covered with Tegoderm or Saran wrap before the area is decontaminated.
2. Contaminated percutaneous lines or saline locks should be removed before being decontaminated. After the area is cleaned, a dressing should be applied until in the Treatment Sector where antibiotic ointment and a new bandage should be applied.

Hearing Aids

1. Hearing aids CANNOT be immersed or otherwise be soaked with water. Thus, they should either be removed and placed in the valuables portion of the patient's clothing bag or if they must be used by the patient because there is no hearing without them, they should be carefully wiped off with a slightly saline moistened 4x4 gauze, dried off, put into a clear plastic bag, and handed to the patient. The cleaned hearing aid is NOT to be worn until the patient has completed the decon process (including washing the ears) and is in the Treatment Sector.

Dentures

1. Unless the oral cavity is contaminated dentures should remain in place and no decontamination is necessary.
2. If the oral cavity is contaminated, then the dentures should be removed, placed in a clear plastic bag with the patient's name or clothing identification number placed on it. The dentures should later be decontaminated in accordance with instructions received from the Poison Center and/or a dentist. The patient's mouth should be decontaminated with mouthwash or saline that is gargled and safely spit out into a bio-hazard bag. Note that, depending on the contaminant, it may not be possible to decontaminate plastic items, such as dentures.

Law Enforcement Officers with Weapons

1. In most cases law enforcement personnel who have been injured on the scene will have had their gun(s) removed before arrival

and given to a fellow officer. However, if that is not the case, the weapon should be left in the holster and the gun belt removed by a Decon Team member and placed in a clear plastic bag labeled with the patient's name and/or clothing number. The bag should then be passed to the Treatment Sector where it should be given to a fellow officer or hospital Security Officer for safe keeping until it can be given to a representative of the injured officers department. THE GUN SHOULD BE LEFT IN THE HOLSTER IF AT ALL POSSIBLE. If the gun must be removed, it should be handled by a Decon Team member familiar with firearms, rendered safe, placed in a clear plastic bag marked with the patient's name and/or clothing identification number, and given to a fellow officer or hospital Security Officer in the Treatment Sector.

2. Decon Team personnel should be aware that oftentimes an officer may have a backup weapon usually found in a holster near the ankle, in their pocket, in a ballistic vest, or near an armpit. The holster with the weapon in place should be removed and secured as described above.
3. An officer's gun belt may also contain items that could prove dangerous if allowed to get in the wrong hands. Thus, the belt should be collected and separately bagged ASAP and passed to a fellow officer or hospital Security Officer in the Treatment Sector. Deconning of an officer's weapon and/or gun belt will be the responsibility of the police department.
4. If the officer is wearing a ballistic vest it must be removed prior to undergoing decon. The vest is usually easily removed by loosening the Velcro straps and then pulling the vest apart and off the patient. It should then be placed in a large plastic bag identified with the patient's name and/or clothing number on it and passed to a fellow officer or Hospital Security Officer in the Treatment Sector.

APPENDIX H

TECHNICAL DECONTAMINATION PROCESS FOR HOSPITAL PERSONNEL

Personnel should remove protective clothing in the following sequence.

1. Remove tape (if used), securing gloves and boots to suit.
2. Remove outer gloves, turning them inside out as they are removed.
3. Remove suit, turning it inside out and folding downward (first loosen and secure PAPR belt). Avoid shaking.
4. Remove boot/shoe cover from one foot and step over the clean line. Remove other boot/shoe cover and put that foot over the clean line.
5. Remove respirator. The last person removing his/her respirator may first wash all other respirator hoods or facepieces with soapy water and thoroughly wipe PAPR fan housing, then clean his/her own equipment before removing his/her suit and gloves. Place the masks in plastic bag and hand the bag over the clean line for placement in second bag held by another staff member. Send bag for decontamination. Discard items that cannot be effectively cleaned (e.g., it may not be possible to completely remove persistent contaminants from PAPR belts).
6. Remove inner gloves and discard them in a drum inside the dirty area.
7. Secure the dirty area until the level of contamination is established and the area is properly cleaned.
8. Personnel should then move to a shower area, remove undergarments and place them in a plastic bag. Double-bag all clothing and label bags appropriately.

Personnel should shower and redress in normal working attire and then report for medical surveillance.

3

Triage in Mass Casualty Disasters

A key component of the delivery of medical care to mass casualties is the process of *triage,* from the French word triagere, meaning "to sort". This concept was introduced in Napoleon's battlefield and has since become a cornerstone of military medical care. It involves matching the limited resources to the needs of casualties by assigning those who are most seriously injured to receiving priority care. This requires rapid identification of the severely injured in order to apply these resources most appropriately. The greater the casualty burden, the more difficult this becomes, and the more training and expertise are required.

THE CONCEPT AND IMPORTANCE OF TRIAGE

Physicians largely do not apply the principles of triage. All injured patients are brought to hospitals, and extensive resources are applied to every injury to maximize the benefit to each individual. However, triage must assume great importance in mass casualty scenarios in which the large numbers of casualties overwhelm existing medical resources.

The greater the number of casualties, the more difficult this becomes, the more time it may take to find those needing immediate care, and the greater the likelihood of preventable deaths caused by delay in treatment of the most severely injured. There are generally four accepted standard triage categories: 1. casualties requiring immediate treatment, such as hypotension, airway compromise, active external hemorrhage, open chest wounds, and intermediate burns; 2. injuries requiring treatment, but in whom delay is acceptable, such as open extremity fractures, extremity vascular injuries, and soft tissue wounds; 3. minimal injuries requiring no treatment (walking wounded); and 4. expectant injuries, or those that are so severe and require such time and resources that it is not possible to provide care without jeopardizing other more salvageable victims, and which therefore should not receive care, such as severe head injury, open skull fractures with extruding brain, cardiac arrest, and extensive and deep burns. This latter category most typifies the basic change in mindset necessary in mass casualty management from our normal management of trauma, from the greatest good for each individual to the greatest good for the greatest number. The decision as to what specifically constitutes an expectant injury must be individualized according to the numbers and types of casualties, and the available resources, and requires some advance planning and knowledge of mass casualty principles.

Over-triage, or the proportion of survivors assigned to immediate care, hospitalization, or evacuation who are not critically injured, is considered more an administrative, logistical, and economic problem under ordinary circumstances, since expensive and limited hospital resources and man-hours are applied unnecessarily.

Generally, an over-triage rate of 50% is considered necessary to reduce potentially life-threatening under-triage to zero, and this is accepted by trauma centers under normal circumstances as a necessary price to pay to avoid missing injuries that should be found.

However, in a mass casualty disaster, it is reasonable to postulate that overtriage could be as life-threatening as under-triage, because of the inundation of overwhelmed medical facilities with large numbers of non-critical casualties all at once, which may prevent the timely detection of that small minority with critical injuries who need immediate treatment, and jeopardize their survival.

The direct linear relationship between over-triage and critical mortality in these disasters confirms that over-triage can result in the loss of potentially salvageable lives in this setting.

The injuries themselves tend to be similar to those normally encountered in daily trauma practice, although they may be more severe and unique in certain settings (i.e. severe soft tissue disruption, shrapnel wounds or blast lung in victims of explosive disasters, cyanide poisoning in chemical events, and acute radiation syndrome in radiological events). However, the large number of casualties greatly impede the ability to fully evaluate and treat each injured individual in a conventional manner.

Medical evaluation and treatment must be rapid to allow for a continuing influx, and yet must remain accurate in identifying those critically injured victims who require immediate life-saving care. The standard goal of providing the greatest good for each individual patient must change in a mass casualty setting to the greatest good for the greatest number. These concepts are necessary to salvage the greatest number of lives in these circumstances.

The abundant medical resources in developed nations allow essentially unlimited application of care and expense to each patient, which makes rationing of care unnecessary. However, in the situation of developing and poor countries or in the event of true mass casualty disaster some kind of rationing is required to the quality of services and for that the principles of triage should also be known. This is why education and training assumes major importance in the care of mass casualties from any form of disaster, in view of how different the decision-making must be if the salvage of life is to be maximized.

THE CHALLENGE

Terrorist bombings can serve as a model for these patterns since they have historically been the most common agents of man-made violence, and thus provide abundant information on the resulting injury spectrum. Recent terror attack on Mumbai is a recent example. The incidence of immediate deaths following explosive events varies with the magnitude of the explosive force, how quickly surgical capability is available, whether the explosion occurs in open air or confined spaces, and whether structural collapse occurs. The great majority of initial survivors of these events are not critically injured, as the most lethal injuries kill immediately, and they typically have soft tissue and skeletal injuries from the blast. However, this predominance of non-critical injuries makes it difficult to rapidly identify that minority of casualties (10%–25%) with potentially life-threatening injuries who require immediate care to optimize their survival. This is where medical management can make the greatest impact, and where triage assumes its important role. The critical mortality rate, or the percentage of deaths only among the critically injured, is therefore the most appropriate measure of outcome, and the effectiveness and accuracy of triage is a major determinant of this rate.

Triage decisions depend on the severity of injury and how urgently the treatment is needed. Those who are most severely injured and require immediate life-saving care are typically the first priority for treatment. However, in a mass casualty event, the limited resources impose an additional factor to be considered, that of the potential salvageability of a casualty. It is impossible in this setting to devote the extensive time and resources necessary for the most severely injured with the lowest chance of survival without jeopardizing the lives of many more with less severe injuries and a better chance of surviving with less time and resources. The abandonment of those casualties who normally would undergo heroic and resource-intensive interventions, regardless of their chances of survival, is the hardest principle for medical providers to learn. Nonetheless, this principle must be applied in these circumstances if salvage of the population is to be maximized. This is the essence of the principle of the greatest good for the greatest number.

TRIAGE CATEGORIES

There are five standard triage categories. However, in the initial phases of casualty influx during the greatest period of chaos, when the ultimate number of casualties to be received cannot be known, when rapid assessment is essential, and when resources must be conserved, the only two categories that matter are those who need immediate care and those who do not. There is little role at this stage for laboratory testing or radiographic imaging. Once casualty influx subsides, and the nature and extent of injuries and available resources are known, more extensive evaluation may be carried out, and more triage categories can be defined. The immediate category includes those life-threatening injuries and conditions that require rapid but relatively simple intervention to keep a casualty alive long enough to reach definitive care. The most immediate threats to life of airway compromise, open chest wounds, tension pneumothorax, unconsciousness with focal signs, hypotension, active external hemorrhage, and intermediate burns are examples. These casualties should have first priority for transfer to the operating room. Endotracheal intubation, tube thoracostomy, burr holes, direct compression of external bleeding, and laparotomy for splenectomy are examples of rapid life-saving interventions that may be applied. After these interventions, a casualty may be downgraded to a less urgent category as they stabilize, making room for other immediate casualties.

The delayed category includes hemo-dynamically stable casualties with injuries and physiologic conditions that will require treatment, but which can be delayed without significantly affecting their outcome. Examples include open and closed extremity fractures, unconsciousness without airway compromise or lateralizing signs, pelvic fractures, spinal fractures with or without spinal cord injury, extremity vascular injuries, soft tissue wounds, and penetrating torso wounds. Generally treatment is not a part of the triage process. The concept of minimal acceptable care should be applied to these victims, involving only brief interventions to minimize morbidity and discomfort, such as immobilizing fractures, covering open wounds, starting intravenous lines, volume repletion, and administering antibiotics and analgesics. These casualties should be transported to a space away from the main triage and immediate treatment area to avoid crowding and confusion.

The minimal category is also referred to as the walking wounded. These casualties have relatively minor injuries and normal mental status, require no treatment beyond first aid, and do not require hospitalization. They are identified by their ability to walk under their own power. In many disasters, they are the first to reach the hospital, and may be the first indication to medical personnel that an event has occurred. These victims must also be monitored by medical personnel to identify any deterioration that may require urgent intervention.

It includes casualties who are alive, but with such severe injuries and low likelihood of survival that treatment would jeopardize the survival of many more victims by diverting the limited resources away from them. Severe head injury with open skull fractures and unconsciousness, extensive and deep burns, and imminent cardiac arrest with major torso trauma are examples of such victims, who should be denied care and segregated from those considered more salvageable, at least during the period of acute casualty influx and uncertain resource availability.

Generally, such maneuvers as closed chest compressions and ER thoracotomy are inappropriate in a mass casualty scenario. Expectant casualties should still be kept comfortable and monitored for any improvement in their condition that may warrant care later in the evolution of the disaster response.

The dead category is important to recognize in order to segregate them from all others to minimize inappropriate attempts at resuscitation and intervention, and to facilitate later identification and communication of their outcome to families. Any unresponsive victim who is rapidly determined to have no pulse or respirations should be considered dead, especially with evidence of major external trauma (i.e. traumatic extremity amputation, open torso or head wounds). No resuscitation or care should be initiated.

TRIAGE ERRORS

It should be evident that the accuracy of triage decisions could affect casualty outcomes and the overall success of the medical response to a disaster. There are two types of triage errors. Under-triage is the inappropriate assignment of critically injured victims with life threatening problems to a delayed category.

Even in the routine management of emergency patients, under-triage is considered a medical problem that could lead to adverse consequences or death from treatment delay. Certainly the potential for death is even greater in a mass casualty event, and must be minimized as much as possible. Over-triage is the assignment of non-critical casualties to immediate care. It is generally accepted in the routine care of injured patients in most developed countries with abundant resources, in order to minimize under-triage. With small numbers of patients at any given time, it represents an economic, logistical, financial, and administrative strain on hospitals, personnel and resources, but not a medical problem that could threaten lives. However, the essential difference in a mass casualty event is the inundation of hospitals with large numbers of casualties all at once. In this setting, overtriage could be as life-threatening as under-triage, because of the small minority of casualties who typically have critical injuries requiring urgent care. The large numbers of non-critical casualties make the rapid identification of the severely injured very difficult, increasing the chance of delaying their urgently needed care and of their preventable death. Thus, triage decisions in mass casualty scenarios must be both rapid and highly accurate to minimize both under-triage and over-triage, and to achieve the goal of the greatest good for the greatest number.

In the setting of a trauma system, studies have shown that over-triage can be reduced by focusing on physiologic and anatomic criteria rather than on mechanism in selecting patients for transport to trauma centers, and that over-triage can be minimized without increasing under-triage. Almogy *et al.* have shown from their experience with suicide bombings in Israel that a number of specific external signs of trauma are predictive of the risk of blast lung injury and the need for immediate care, including penetrating head and torso wounds, burns >10 % total body surface area, traumatic amputation, skull fracture, and closed space vs. open air explosions. A collective review of terrorist bombings reported similar markers of severity to aid in triage. Although trauma scoring correlates closely with survival of injured victims, it has been less useful in prioritizing care through triage.

In reality, it is impractical to expect high levels of triage accuracy during the initial chaos of a true mass casualty event. It is clear that the greater the casualty load, the poorer the quality of care and the more difficult the treatment decisions. Errors in both pre-hospital and in-hospital triage should be expected. The best approach is to minimize the adverse consequences of these errors through a number of steps that should be built into disaster plans to create an error-tolerant system. In pre-hospital triage, this can be accomplished with multiple sites of triage at areas between the disaster scene and the hospital, known as casualty collection points. By allowing secondary and tertiary triage to be carried out at multiple sites, non-critical casualties can effectively be filtered out with increasing discrimination, which would allow initial errors to be corrected at each successive echelon of care, so that only those who truly need hospitalization will finally be admitted. Under-triage may be mitigated by some mechanism for monitoring all casualties not triaged to immediate care for any deterioration, to the extent this is possible in the field.

In the hospital, over-triage is corrected by further triage in the emergency room to reassign those not requiring immediate care. Also, non-critical casualties are again monitored for any deterioration to mitigate the effects of under-triage. Certain innocent-appearing external injury patterns that may indicate severe visceral damage should be recognized by medical personnel, as another means of avoiding under-triage, such as multiple skin wounds following suicide bombings serving as markers of destructive internal shrapnel injuries. The greater the casualty load, the more important is such an error-tolerant system.

Triage accuracy is influenced by the location of a mass casualty disaster. Urban settings tend to be more tolerant of triage errors than more isolated and rural locales, because of the immediate availability of extensive medical resources for critical injuries. The adverse consequences of over-triage tend to be lessened by a large number of medical facilities and personnel, as this prevents large numbers of non-critical casualties from accumulating at one site, and from interfering with the identification of critical injuries. In more isolated locations, ovetriage is inevitable due to the scarcity of medical resources. The consequent delay in care resulting from this over-triage, and from casualty evacuation over long distances, further worsens casualty outcomes, explaining the generally higher critical mortality in these settings. The most severely injured casualties may be prone to over-triage in major mass casualty events. Inexperienced triage officers may assign to immediate care severely injured casualties with low salvageability who should be classified as expectant, reflecting a failure to change their approach to care in this setting. The resulting diversion of limited resources could lead to unnecessary mortality among more salvageable casualties, and should be recorded as over-triage. Deaths among expectant casualties should most properly be included among immediate deaths rather than among deaths in critically injured survivors, as they should never have received medical care and should not falsely skew the results of medical management. All cases of under-triage should be analyzed to learn how to avoid this in future events.

THE TRIAGE OFFICER

The two essential requirements of a triage officer are: (i) a thorough knowledge and clinical experience with the types of injuries anticipated for any specific disaster, and training and experience in the management of these injuries in the unique context of mass casualties. The ability to rapidly combine multiple sensory clues with physiologic and anatomic information to obtain an overall picture of a casualty is an important attribute. (ii) This person must know what resources are available and what the extent of the casualty load is at any given time (situational awareness), and understand the necessity for rationing of care so as to most efficiently apply the limited resources where they will do the most good for the whole population. In order to carry out this function, the officer must have absolute authority to make decisions as to casualty disposition if smooth and rapid casualty flow is to be achieved. This requires a person with good leadership and problem-solving capability, as well as the ability to work well under stress. Although physicians have been shown to improve triage accuracy as compared with non-physicians in the routine field evaluation of trauma victims, experienced nurses or pre-hospital medical professionals may perform this function as well in mass casualty events. In some unconventional disasters, such as from weapons of mass destruction (i.e. biological, chemical, radiological), other specialists may best direct triage, such as toxicologists, radiation biologists, infectious disease specialists or public health officials. However, acute care providers such as surgeons, emergency room nurses, or emergency medicine physicians are generally the best candidates for this role, because of their training and experience in the management of trauma. Computer simulation of mass casualty events has demonstrated that achieving the most stringent triage accuracy does not significantly improve casualty flow or outcome, suggesting that triage does not necessarily require the most experienced surgeons.

A number of factors will influence the process of triage, and must be considered in making these critical decisions. The extent and availability of resources, the nature of injuries, the mechanism of the disaster, and the number of casualties are examples. One of the most difficult, yet important, triage decisions in a mass casualty setting is determining which casualties should be classified as expectant and denied care. What exactly constitutes an expectant victim will necessarily differ with each specific disaster and location, and cannot be strictly defined in advance. In many mass casualty events it may not be necessary to have such a category. This determination should be made in the earliest phases of a disaster response through a consensus of those in charge of the major elements of that response. It is only at this time that a realistic assessment of the number and type of casualties and available resources is possible. For instance, a decision as to whether a casualty in respiratory failure should be in-tubated may be affected by the number of ventilators, auxiliary equipment and monitoring and support personnel available. A lack of electrical power could drastically alter necessary resources for many casualties and prevent some from receiving care. The need for major surgery must be adjusted according to the number of available operating rooms, anesthesiologists and surgeons. The potential salvageability of a casualty will be another major consideration in such decisions.

Triage in the field basically determines who will be transported to the hospital, and is determined by many of the same considerations. The location of this level of triage is in itself an important decision, as it should be situated away from the disaster scene due to the dangers this scene consistently poses to health care providers. Multiple successive pre-hospital triage sites are preferable to one, to improve triage accuracy through a progressive filtering process. It is equally important that initial triage of casualties not take place in the hospital, as this will tend to overwhelm the ability of hospital providers to carry out their essential function of care for those most in need. An additional essential component of field triage of mass casualties is an orderly distribution of victims from the scene among as many different hospitals as possible to avoid over-whelming any one facility, a process known as leap-frogging. Without this approach, the nearest hospital to the scene consistently becomes inundated with casualties, impairing effective casualty management.

Casualties assigned to a non-critical category must be monitored for any change in status. Those initially assigned to urgent care may stabilize and no longer merit priority over others. Once casualty influx has subsided, all triage assignments can be re-evaluated in accordance with available remaining resources. Those initially categorized as expectant may be reconsidered for initiation of treatment if still alive. As discussed earlier, such provisions enhance the error tolerance of triage and of the entire disaster medical response, and could maximize casualty survival.

Triage injuries tend to be either very different from those normally encountered in daily medical or surgical practice (i.e. acute radiation syndrome, toxic chemical exposure, blast lung injury, unusual infectious agents), or the extent and severity are much greater than typically seen (i.e. traumatic amputations, multiple shrapnel wounds, abdominal evisceration, decapitation).

There may be unusual combinations of injuries that make triage decisions especially difficult, such as a ruptured spleen with hemorrhagic shock in a casualty also contaminated with toxic chemicals. Medical personnel, especially triage officers, must be educated as to their recognition and approach to management, to avoid being caught off guard, and to maximize triage accuracy.

Documentation of triage decisions

Written documentation of triage decisions and casualty management is an essential tool for maintaining continuity of care during a mass casualty event. The chaotic environment can easily lead to losing track of casualties, and to critical omissions of treatment or redundant triage and management, as casualties move to successive echelons of care. This documentation also allows a post-event analysis of triage decisions, casualty management and casualty outcomes, from which important lessons can be derived to improve performance in future events. The results should be used to further train triage officers, and add to our body of knowledge of triage decision-making. This will allow us to strive toward the most effective triage in mass casualty disasters.

Lessons Learnt From Suicide Bombing Attacks in Israel

The last 2 decades have seen a dramatic increase in the number and extent of suicide attacks that target the civilian population. Although the concept of the suicide attacker is not new, we have recently evidenced the lethal effects of the ability of a suicide bomber to detonate a relatively large load of explosive material in proximity to his or her victims. The combination of military-grade explosive material, high-mass shrapnel, and precise control of the timing of detonation has transformed suicide bombing attacks into an ultimate tool in the hands of terrorists. Detonation of an explosive material causes injuries in 4 principal mechanisms. Primary blast injury is caused by the rapid outward spread of the shock wave, the energy of which is inversely proportional to the distance from the explosion's epicenter. Gas-containing organs such as the lung, tympanic membrane, and bowel are most often injured. Secondary blast injury is caused by penetrating missiles composed of bomb-based material (shrapnel) and debris that are propelled by the shock wave. Tertiary blast injuries result from a victim's body being displaced by expanding gases and high winds; trauma then occurs from tumbling and impacting objects. Burns and associated injuries from the collapse of buildings are defined as quaternary injuries and are also common among survivors of explosions. Blast lung injury (BLI) is caused by the rapid spread of the shock wave, a phenomenon that is exacerbated in confined spaces. Victims of suicide bombing attacks inside buses have been shown to suffer from diffuse alveolar injury, bilateral pneumothoraces, and broncho-pleural fistulas. Timely initiation of therapy, including unconventional methods such as high frequency jet ventilation, independent lung ventilation, and nitric oxide, may improve survival. Early recognition of BLI, a leading cause of in-hospital mortality, may improve outcome by directing patients to the appropriate level of care and initiating early treatment.

Following a suicide bombing attack, numerous victims are brought into the emergency department suffering from a combination of multi-organ injuries caused by the blast, penetrating injuries caused by shrapnel and other debris, and burns. In the initial phases, the signs and symptoms of BLI may be subtle and are often underestimated. The conditions of patients with BLI, however, quickly deteriorate and they often require sophisticated modes of mechanical ventilation such as high-frequency jet ventilation and 1-lung ventilation. By evaluating the degree of external trauma we can anticipate the risk of BLI, an important factor in patient survival after a suicide bombing attack.

Because of several mostly non-medical factors, the majority of severely injured casualties in Israel are currently being evacuated to the nearest medical facility and not to a level I trauma center. Following a suicide bombing attack, scores of victims suffering from a combination of blast injury, penetrating injury, and burns were brought to local hospitals from tie to time. Gidon Almogy et al conducted a study and retrospective analysis of all 15 suicide bombing attacks that occurred in Israel, to identify external signs of trauma that would assist medical crews in effectively triaging salvage-able and non-salvageable victims. They retrospectively collected data on all 15 suicide bombing attacks that took place in Israel between April 1994 and August 1997. Hospital records and trauma registry records were retrieved from the 13 different hospitals in which the victims were treated. Records were reviewed for demographic data such as age, sex, attack setting, and survival; the presence of BLI; the presence of tympanic membrane rupture; the presence and location of penetrating injuries; the presence and extent of burns; and the presence and location of fractures.

One hundred fifty-three victims died and 798 were injured in 15 suicide bombing attacks that took place in Israel. The targets were buses, semi-confined spaces (SCS) such as restaurants and covered open spaces, and open spaces (OS) such as bus stops and street cafés. The fatality-casualty ratios were 95:355 (26.7%), 25:304 (9.0%), and 33:292 (11.3%), respectively. The head was the most common site of penetrating injury among survivors who were inside a bus, the limbs were the most common site in SCS, and the torso was the most common site of penetrating injury in OS. The majority of patients with penetrating wounds to the torso also suffered from penetrating wounds to the head. Blast lung injury was significantly more common in survivors who had skull and facial fractures, burns covering more than 10% of the BSA, and penetrating wounds to the head or torso. Burns were common both in the dead and in survivors. The presence of amputations, open fractures, and burns was significantly greater in fatally injured victims than in survivors, regardless of the attack setting. These findings were even more prominent among casualties in buses. Only 2 of 41 victims who suffered from traumatic amputations inside a bus survived the blast; all 19 victims who suffered from burns covering more than 30% of the BSA inside a bus died of their wounds; and only 4 of 25 victims with open fractures who were injured inside a bus survived the blast.

The lessons learnt from the study were: Victims who died at the scene were more likely to suffer from burns, open fractures, and amputations in comparison with survivors. External signs of trauma should be used to triage victims to the appropriate level of care both at the scene and in the hospital.

References

Almogy G, Belzberg H, Mintz Y, Pikarsky AI, Zamir G, Rivkind AI. Suicide bombing attacks: update and modifications to the protocol. *Ann Surg*. 2004;239: 295-303.

Almogy G, Luria T, Richter E, Pizov R, Bdolah-Abram T, Mintz Y, Zamir G, Rivkind AI: Can external signs of trauma guide management? Lessons learned from suicide bombing attacks in Israel. *Arch Surg* 2005;140:390–393.

American College of Surgeons Committee on Trauma: Field categorization of trauma patients (field triage). *Bull Am Coll Surg* 1986;71:17–21.

Ammons MA, Moore EE, Pons PT, Moore FA, McCroskey BL, Cleveland HC: The role of a regional trauma system in the management of a mass disaster: an analysis of the Keystone Colorado chairlift accident. *J Trauma* 1988;28:1468.

Baxt WG, Berry C, Epperson M, Scalzitti V: Failure of pre-hospital trauma prediction rules to classify trauma patients accurately. *Ann Emerg Med* 1989;18:1–8.

Berry B: The medical management of mass casualties: the Scudder Oration in Trauma. *Bull Am Coll Surg* 1956;41:60–66.

Biancolini CA, DelBosco CG, Jorge MA: Argentine Jewish Community Institution bomb explosion. *J Trauma* 1999;47: 728–732.

Boffard KD, MacFarlane C: Urban bomb blast injuries: patterns of injury and treatment. *Surg Annu* 1993;25:29–47.

Brismar B, Bergenwald L. The terrorist bomb explosion in Bologna, Italy, 1980: an analysis of effects and injuries sustained. *J Trauma*. 1982;22:216-220.

Brismar B, Bergenwald L: The terrorist bomb explosion in Bologna, Italy, 1980: an analysis of the effects and injuries sustained. *J Trauma* 1982;22:216–220.

Burkle FM, Newland C, Orebaugh S, Blood CG: Emergency medicine in the Persian Gulf War—Part 2: triage methodology and lessons learned. *Ann Emerg Med* 1994;23:748–754.

Burris DG, Welling DR, Rich NM: Dominique Jean Larrey and the principles of humanity in warfare. *J Am Coll Surg* 2004; 198:831–835.

Caro D, Irving M: The Old Bailey bomb explosion. *Lancet* 1973;1:1433–1435

Champion HR, Sacco WJ, Gainer PS, Patow SM: The effect of medical direction on trauma triage. *J Trauma* 1988;28:235–239.

Cook CH, Muscarella P, Praba AC, Melvin WS, Martin LC: Reducing over-triage without compromising outcomes in trauma patients. *Arch Surg* 2001;136:752.

Cooper GJ, Maynard RL, Cross NL, Hill JF. Casualties from terrorist bombings. *J Trauma*. 1983;23:955-967.

Cooper GJ, Maynard RL, Cross NL, Hill JP: Casualties from terrorist bombings. *J Trauma* 1983;23:955–967.

Cushman JG, Pachter L, Beaton HL: Two New York City hospitals' surgical response to the September 11, 2001, terrorist attack in New York City. *J Trauma* 2003;54:147–155.

Einav S, Feigenberg Z, Weissman C, *et al*. Evacuation priorities in mass casualty terror-related events: implications for contingency planning. *Ann Surg*. 2004; 239:304-310.

Eiseman B. Combat casualty management for tomorrow's battlefield: urban terrorism. *J Trauma*. 2001;51:821-823.

Frykberg ER, Tepas JJ, Alexander RH: The 1983 Beirut airport terrorist bombing: injury patterns and implications for disaster management *Am Surg* 1989;55:134–141

Frykberg ER, Tepas JJ: Terrorist bombings: lessons learned from Belfast to Beirut. *Ann Surg* 1988;208:569–576.

Frykberg ER. Medical management of disasters and mass casualties from terrorist bombings: how can we cope? *J Trauma.* 2002;53:201-212.

Frykberg ER: Disaster and mass casualty management: a commentary on the American College of Surgeons position statement. *J Am Coll Surg* 2003; 197:857–859.

Frykberg ER: Medical management of disasters and mass casualties from terrorist bombings: how can we cope? *J Trauma* 2002;53:201–212.

Gagnon EB, Aboutanos MB, Malhotra AK, Dompkowski D, Duane TM, Ivatury RR: In the wake of Hurricane Isabel: a prospective study of post-event trauma and injury control strategies. *Am Surg* 2005;71:194–197.

Gutierrez de Ceballos JP, Turegano Fuentes FT, Perez-Diaz D,Sanz Sanchez M, Martin Llorente C, Guerrero Sanz JE: Casualties treated at the closest hospital in the Madrid, March 11, terrorist bombings. *Crit Care Med* 2005; 33 (Suppl):S107–S112.

Henderson JV: Anatomy of a terrorist attack: the Cu Chi mess hall incident. J World Assoc *Emerg Dis Med* 1986;2:69–73.

Hirshberg A, Scott BG, Granchi T, Wall MJ Jr, Mattox KL, Stein M: How does casualty load affect trauma care in urban bombing incidents? A quantitative analysis. *J Trauma* 2005;58:686–695.

Hirshberg A, Stein M, Walden R: Surgical resource utilization in urban terrorist bombing: a computer simulation. *J Trauma* 1999;47:545–550.

Hogan DE, Lairet J: Triage, in: Hogan DE, Burstein JL (eds), Disaster Medicine, Philadelphia, Lippincott Williams and Wilkins, 2002, pp. 10–15.

Iremonger MJ. Physics of detonations and blast-waves. In: Cooper GJ, Dudley HAF, Gann DS, *et al.*, eds. Scientific Foundations of Trauma. Oxford, England Butterworth-Heinemann; 1997:189-199.

Jacobs LM, Goody M, Sinclair A: The role of a trauma center in disaster management. *J Trauma* 1983;23:697–701.

Jacobs LM, Ramp JM, Breay JM: An emergency medical system approach to disaster planning. *J Trauma* 1979;19:157–162.

Karmy-Jones R, Kissinger D, Golocovsky M, Jordan M, Champion HR. Bomb related injuries. *Mil Med.* 1994;159:536-539.

Katz E, Ofek B, Adler J, Abramowitz HB, Krausz MM. Primary blast injury after a bomb explosion in a civilian bus. *Ann Surg.* 1989;209:484-488.

Kennedy K, Aghababian R, Gans L, Lewis CP: Triage: techniques and applications in decision-making. *Ann Emerg Med* 1996;28:136–144.

Kreis DJ, Fine EG, Gomez GA, Eckes J, Whitwell E, Byers PM: A prospective evaluation of field categorization of trauma patients. *J Trauma* 1988;28:995–1000.

Leibovici D, Gofrit ON, Shapira SC. Eardrum perforation in explosion survivors: is it a marker of pulmonary blast injury? *Ann Emerg Med.* 1999;34:168

Leibovici D, Gofrit ON, Stein M, *et al.* Blast injuries in a bus versus open air bombings: a comparative study of injuries in survivors of open air versus confined space explosions. *J Trauma.* 1996;41:1030-1035.

Leibovici D, Gofrit ON, Stein M, Shapira SC, Noga Y, Heruti RJ, Shemer J: Blast injuries: bus versus open air bombings—a comparative study of injuries in survivors of open air versus confined space explosions. *J Trauma* 1996;41:1030

Lengerich, Germany, Pabst Science Publishers, 2003, pp. 378–393.

Llewellyn CH: Triage: in austere environments and echeloned medical systems. *World J Surg* 192;16:904–909.

Mahoney EJ, Harrington DT, Biffl WL, Metzger J, Oka T, Cioffi WG: Lessons learned from a nightclub fire: institutional disaster preparedness. *J Trauma* 2005;58:487–491.

Mallonee S, Shariat S, Stennies G, Waxweiler R, Hogan D, Jordan F: Physical injuries and fatalities resulting from the Oklahoma City bombing. *JAMA* 1996;276:382–387.

Millie M, Senkowski C, Stuart L, Davis F, Ochsner G, Boyd C: Tornado disaster in rural Georgia: triage response, injury patterns, lessons learned. *Am Surg* 2000;66:223–228.

Peleg K, Aharonson-Daniel L, Stein M, Michaelson M, Kluger Y, Simon D, Noji EK, Israeli Trauma Group (ITG): Terror-related injuries: Gunshot and explosion injuries: characteristics, outcomes, and implications for care of terror-related injuries in Israel. *Ann Surg* 2004; 293:311–318.

Phillips YY. Primary blast injuries. *Ann Emerg Med.* 1986;15:1446-1450.

Pizov R, Oppenheim-Eden A, Matot I, *et al.* Blast lung injury from an explosion on a civilian bus. Chest. 1999;115:165-172.

Pyper PC, Graham WJH: Analysis of terrorist injuries treated at Craigavon Area Hospital, Northern Ireland, 1972–1980. Injury 1982;14:332–338.

Rignault DP: Recent progress in surgery for the victims of disaster, terrorism and war. *World J Surg* 1992;16:885–887.

Sklar DP: Casualty patterns in disasters. *J World Assoc Emerg Dis Med* 1987;3:49–51

Stein M, Hirshberg A. Limited mass casualties due to conventional weapons: the daily reality of a level I trauma center. In: Shemer J, Shoenfeld Y, eds. Terror and Medicine: Medical Aspects of Biological, Chemical and Radiological Terrorism. Lengerich, Germany: Pabst Science Publishers; 2003:378-393.

Stein M, Hirshberg A. Medical consequences of terrorism: the conventional weapon threat. *Surg Clin North Am.* 1999;79:1537-1552.

Stein M, Hirshberg A: Limited mass casualties due to conventional weapons: the daily reality of a level I trauma center. In: Shemer J, Shoenfeld Y (eds), Terror and Medicine: Medical aspects of biological, chemical and radiological terrorism.

Stein M, Hirshberg A: Medical consequences of terrorism: the conventional weapon threat. *Surg Clin North Am* 1999;79: 1537–1552.

Tekin A, Namias N, O'Keeffe T, Pizano L, Lynn M, Prater-Varas R, Quintana OD, Borges L, Ishii M, Lee S, Lopez P, Lessner-Eisenberg S, Alvarez A, Ellison T, Sapras K, Lefton J, Ward CG: A burn mass casualty event due to boiler room explosion on a cruise ship: preparedness and outcomes. *Am Surg* 2005; 71:210–215.

Tucker K, Lettin A: The Tower of London bomb explosion. *Br Med J* 1975;3:287.

Waeckerle JF: Disaster planning and response. *NEJM* 1991;324: 815–821

Waterworth TA, Carr MJT: Report on injuries sustained by patients treated at the Birmingham General Hospital following the recent bomb explosions. *Br Med J* 1975;2:25–27.

Wightman JM, Gladish SL. Explosions and blast injuries. *Ann Emerg Med.* 2001;37:664-678.

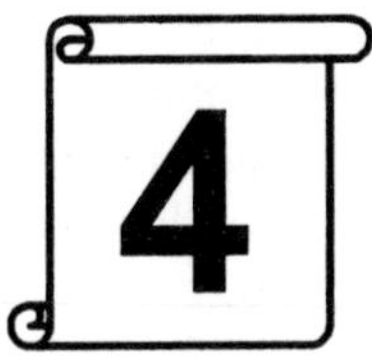

Role of Appropriate Medical Leadership and Technology during Disaster

Civilian populations increasingly constitute the front line in modern warfare as the prevalence of terrorist-related events and state-sponsored bombings rise worldwide. Any hospital adjacent to the location of the incident may be called on to function as an evacuation hospital, thus becoming pivotal in patient treatment during the event. Optimal trauma care of a patient requires multidisciplinary coordination. Treatment of multiple patients simultaneously demands excellent managerial decisions and teamwork, when hospital capacity may be overwhelmed despite full resource mobilization. Strategies for medical/surgical management of Disaster victims (DV) are currently undergoing rapid evolution. Major discrepancies may occur between estimated and actual resource requirements. Both the disaster plan and the key decision-makers must be flexible enough to make course corrections in real time to provide the optimal response. Surgeons have traditionally functioned as leaders in trauma care of the single patient, but the strategies for overall hospital organisation and the specific roles of the surgeon in hospital management and teamwork during Disasters are yet to be clarified. The panic, chaos, and emotional trauma of such disasters can magnify the loss of life, and are best combated by prompt and vigorous leadership, and a pre-existing plan for the immediate rescue, disposition, and treatment of casualties. Advanced Technologies like Disaster Emergency Logistics Telemedicine Advanced Satellites System (DELTASS), and Nanotechnology can help a great deal in locating the victims or their screening and assessment for a better triage and adequate management.

Indian leadership can be undoing to the management

After a disaster has struck, people all over the country become emotionally labile and want to help those affected or admitted in the hospitals with major or minor injuries. In Indian conditions as soon as any disaster strikes the people go in a state of panic, excitement, shock, disbelief, critical, spiritual, philosophical, emotional, philanthropic, and the like. Many others take it an opportunity to earn publicity, importance, money, goods, etc., aided by public ignorance and generosity. Many self styled smarty start collecting money and material for the welfare of the victims and often such donations do not reach the targets. Media plays its own role in spreading rumors and panic. Leaders of various hues descend on the scene in a apparent bid to manage the problems, often doing exactly opposite. A large number of self styled volunteers may throng the site of the disaster and thus effectively choke the areas excluding the essential manpower and life saving material. A state of chaos is created all over the country in general and the site of disaster and the adjoining hospitals in particular. This is exactly what should not be allowed in happen, given the quality of leadership in the managers at various levels.

Despite the best intentions of the donors, donated goods that are unsolicited or inappropriate frequently cause more harm than good. Unnecessary and unmanageable items can compete with essential relief goods for the limited capacity of personnel and operating facilities, and in turn, delay the delivery of necessary provisions to those most urgently in need. By following specified guidelines, timely donations will arrive at the scene of a disaster in an orderly way and will help rather than hinder the recovery and rebuilding process. Similarly, excited people of the area or others whose relatives are expected to be admitted to the hospital after an attack may create real hurdles in the way of relief and rescue team. Some take the happenings like another *Mela* like event. The political leadership should restrain them to get political mileage from the dead and disabled of disaster and only act in a non-publicized humanitarian manner. The hospitals can assume a specified type of leadership to organize the causalities in the space available and also use to the maximum the sources that are available or can be mobilized or that are offered by well meaning donors.

Before proceeding further let us take some frequently asked questions and their answers.

Q. I want to help the injured admitted to the hospitals. What should I do?

Find out the needs of the disaster victims and respond properly. Immediately following a disaster, local disaster relief officials will determine the needs of their community. These officials will then provide the media and various disaster relief organisations with a needs list. Look for reports from the media.

Volunteer agency experienced in disaster response such as your chapter of Red Cross, before you take any action. Don't rush yourself or any other material to the hospitals.

Q. What do disaster victims need most, when in hospitals?

Money. Financial contributions are the most useful form of disaster assistance. They help guarantee that relief workers have the funds necessary to provide disaster victims with needed supplies in a timely fashion. Donating money also eliminates many of the logistical concerns such as transportation, distribution and spoilage frequently associated with donations of unsolicited, unsized clothing and perishable mixed food items. Money also helps the local economy recover. Financial contributions should be made through a recognized volunteer agency to help insure that donations are put to their intended use. These organisations can accept checks or credit card donations earmarked for the disaster region. In addition, these organisations can provide telephone numbers of relief agencies in the disaster area. Prime minister's relief Fund is a safe bet.

Q. Do disaster victims need clothing in the hospitals?

For the most part, the answer is "no." Unless specifically asked for, donations of clothing are generally discouraged. Clothing and shoes are usually not needed after a disaster. Immediately after a disaster has occurred, there is neither the time nor distribution channels to ensure that donated items don't go to waste.

If clothing is requested, new clothes are preferred. Used clothing should be cleaned and in good condition. All articles should be sorted by category: age, gender and type. Donors should also consider the local climate when choosing what to send.

Q. Can I send food to the hospital in the disaster area?

Unless specifically asked for, donations of food are also discouraged. In most disasters, food scarcity is not an immediate problem. If food is requested, baby food is needed first, then ready-to-eat, non-perishable food items. It is also important that donated food be clearly labeled to facilitate distribution.

Q. What about medicine?

The arrival of unnecessary medicines at a hospital near disaster scene can be a burden rather than an asset. Medical supplies are highly specialized commodities that must have a distribution channel of qualified personnel. If medical supplies are called for, medicines sent must have a shelf life of at least six months after arriving at the disaster site, and they must also be clearly labeled. Old prescription medications should never be sent.

Q. Can I go directly to the disaster scene and volunteer to help?

Although well-intentioned, volunteers who have not been specifically requested at a disaster site frequently just add to the existing chaos. If you want to go to the disaster scene, first call either the Red Cross or the nodal officer of disaster relief. Local emergency services directors can also be contacted about volunteering for disaster relief efforts.

Q. How can businesses and organisations help?

Businesses and organisations wishing to make donations should first contact local officials to find out what is needed. Once the needs have been determined, it is helpful for the business or organisation to choose a single type of item to donate. This facilitates organisation and distribution at the disaster site. The donors should also be prepared to provide for the transportation of the goods and arrange for the delivery and unloading of the supplies at a specified location. Loading and unloading is much more efficient when shipments are transported on portable platforms that can be transferred using a standard forklift.

Also, businesses and organisations can conduct fund-raising efforts in their community with the proceeds going to the disaster area.

Q. What about donating blood?

Blood is always needed following a major disaster. Contact your local Red Cross chapter or a local hospital for information on how you can donate blood for disaster victims.

An Israeli study describes the shift in hospital leadership in MCE

This study describes the experience in hospital management during MCEs in Israel. These incidents all resulted from conventional terrorism. Differences in management concepts may be required for biological and/or chemical terror as well as for MCEs resulting from modes of operation that are different from those commonly experienced in Israel. For example, almost all physicians in Israel have extensive military training and experience (which has been shown to affect preparedness), which may not be true in other countries. Although these issues are pertinent, the results of this study can be extrapolated to hospitals outside Israel because of the large variety of experiences they represent.

It describes the shift in hospital leadership and management responsibilities and the pivotal roles of surgeons and anesthesiologists in this system. Surgeons are involved in hospital command and control and provide clinical care and should therefore be highly involved in hospital MCE planning and training. Anesthesiologists are vital for OR management and critical care and should be trained to participate in the clinical decision-making process during MCEs. (Sharon Einav, Israel).

It was designed to identify quality of leadership among key members for hospital organisation and to obtain information regarding the strategies that have been developed and implemented for efficient overall hospital management during MCEs. Investigated categories include: (1) overall organisation, (2) emergency department (ED) management, (3) operating room (OR) management and scheduling, (4) intensive care unit (ICU) management (e.g., admissions and transfers), and (5) use of post-anesthesia care unit (PACU) resources. The specific role of the surgeon as the team leader was studied within each of the investigated categories.

OVERALL ORGANISATION

Event Management

The clinical coordinator, usually an attending surgeon, is responsible for minute-by-minute decisions regarding priorities in distribution of resources for patient treatment. The administrative coordinator is responsible for recruitment of staff and resources. A representative of the hospital administration is responsible for communication with the media. Tight security measures were implemented by the on-duty hospital security officer. These included limitation of access of non-authorized vehicles/ persons to the hospital, closure of key hospital locations to the media and the general public, and searching the various hospital locations and the personal possessions of new arrivals for weapons.

Conventional communication systems have been known to collapse during MCEs, highlighting the importance of correct prioritization of staff recruitment from outside the hospital. In Israel, several attending surgeons and anesthesiologists regularly receive pages directly from the national emergency services. When a TMCE occurs, they are notified immediately. Almost half of the respondents noted that the collapse of conventional communication systems during MCEs impedes staff recruitment and emphasized that priority should be given to resolution of this issue.

When requested to define priorities for staff recruitment, respondents unanimously demanded the immediate presence of the chief of surgery, attending surgeons, and surgical residents. Respondents were also unanimous in their demand for attending anesthesiologists, the director of anesthesiology, and anesthesiology residents. Specialists in orthopedic surgery, emergency medicine, and critical care were called in immediately by more than 90% of respondents. All respondents considered in-hospital security staff crucial for event management and efficient crowd control. The proportion of respondents demanding immediate recruitment of the hospital chief of security (85%) was similar to the proportion of respondents demanding specialists in thoracic surgery, vascular surgery, and radiology.

Most respondents noted that the presence of too many staff members had interfered with their work in reception area (83%), ORs (7%), and PACU (10%). Surgeons felt that their work as team leaders was hampered by the presence of bystanders (93%) and OR (16%). Superfluous staff members were primarily physicians (78%), administrative staff (57%), and nurses (27%). Several respondents suggested that rather than turning away additional staff members, these individuals should be directed to a standby location from where their assistance may be requested later on.

THE EMERGENCY DEPARTMENT (ED)

Only 45% of the respondents felt that the quality of data provided to hospital staff regarding the situation in the field was satisfactory. Satisfaction with the quality of the information received from the field was more common among surgeons (57%) than among anesthesiologists (31%).

Most respondents concurred that primary triage should be performed by an attending general surgeon (73%) outside the entrance to the ED (82%). Eighty percent of the respondents who were attending surgeons concurred that ideally the triage officer should be a surgeon experienced in trauma. When a MCE occurs, the trauma specialist serves as the hospital incident commander who is in charge of hospital management. This surgeon often circulates among hospital locations to monitor events occurring at the multiple treatment sites and at the same time acts as supervisor/consultant to other physicians providing patient care in these locations.

Primary triage is usually performed in the first stage of the event by the most experienced surgeon present in the hospital at the time and later, by a senior surgeon with experience in trauma surgery.

Operating Rooms

Operating room (OR) administration hierarchy usually remained unchanged from the routine practiced in times of calm, and a large number of respondents noted the importance of maintaining this routine. The respondents concurred that elective surgery had been and should be suspended.

Post-anesthesia Care Unit

The PACU had been used for at least 1 of the following 3 functions in all but 1 hospital: as an extension of the ICU (12 of 14 hospitals), as an extension of the ED for severely injured patients (9 of 14 hospitals), and as a temporary location for patients waiting to enter the OR (13 of 14 hospitals). Surgeons participate in the selection of patients to be evacuated from the PACU in 4 of 14 hospitals. Most of the surgeon respondents considered it preferable that these decisions be made by the anesthesiologists.

ICU MANAGEMENT

In these unique circumstances, pressure is often placed on ICUs to evacuate patients already in the ICU at the time of the TMCE. Most respondents (75%) claimed that patients were routinely evacuated from the ICU in their hospitals (13 of 14 hospitals) to admit casualties. A quarter (25%) of the respondents knew of an ICU patient whose condition had deteriorated secondary to being transferred from the ICU. Surgeons spearhead not only the trauma care of individual patients but also function in most MCEs as clinical coordinators (attending surgeons) and supervisors/consultants and are responsible for primary triage (attending surgeons with trauma experience). Anesthesiologists are responsible for OR scheduling and intensive care regardless of location.

Hospital management during MCEs resembles a military hierarchy. Early and efficient implementation of security measures enables uninterrupted provision of professional medical treatment despite a potentially disruptive environment (e.g., ED inundation with patients and excess non-surgical staff). Division of authority between the clinical and administrative coordinators allows the clinical coordinator to focus on patient treatment and flow and the administrative coordinator to concentrate on recruitment of resources and personnel, both major issues in the chaotic environment. The decision-making process must be rapid and therefore depends on a few, select key decision-makers, often replacing normal managerial decision processes. The prerogatives of the clinical coordinator temporarily overrule those of the normal management hierarchy. As a commanding officer, the role of the physician is to use both clinical expertise and organisations skill to command the care of a large number of patients. Surgeons are the natural leaders in this scenario not only because of their traditional commitment to trauma care and their technical expertise but also because of their understanding of the management of the multiply injured patient and their training in rapid screening; selection of surgical options and decision-making are also crucial. Communication capabilities and skills are vital for management of MCEs.

Disaster Emergency Logistics Telemedicine Advanced Satellites System (DELTASS)

This advanced satellite system is a breakthrough in the technology and leadership during disasters. DELTASS uses both geostationary and low earth orbit communication satellites enabling 'top-down' management of emergency workers dispersed across a disaster zone, as well as letting medical experts located hundreds of miles away carry out on-the-spot diagnoses of casualties. Such a communication system for emergency telemedicine greatly multiplies the effectiveness of rescue workers within the affected area, especially as existing communications networks might not have survived. Apart from the damage to terrestrial communications infrastructure done by the likes of an earthquake or floods, the first thing that becomes unavailable is the cellular network, which quickly gets overloaded. First aid and ambulance teams are equipped with Portable Telemedicine Work-stations for two-way communication with medical experts at a nearby Medical Field Hospital. Patient data such as ECGs and vital signs can be transmitted along with still images of injuries.

It is from here that mobile teams' activities are coordinated, patients are gathered, treated and their data tracked, and decisions are made about evacuating them elsewhere. Broadband communication links enhances patient treatment, enabling videoconferencing with hospital staff in another country as well as tele-diagnosis techniques such as ultrasound. "Most of DELTASS allows us to 'follow' each patient from his first contact with the search and rescue team through the quite complex chain of events that characterizes the diagnostic and therapeutic intervention, distributed over time and space."

Nanotechnology can protect against bioterrorist attacks!

Medical leadership and professionalism may be activated by the enhanced surveillance, detection and data storage capacities offered by nanotechnology. It is a new weapon of leadership now available to the scientists and medical professionals. The targeting of hospitals by bioterrorist agents may be part of a tactic to disable disaster response plans. Nanotechnology allows medical professionals to effectively assess, warn and protect the public in relation to such bioterrorist threats (T.A. Faunce). Applications of nanotechnology are also likely to enhance forensic capabilities in almost every area, including enhanced surveillance capabilities and capacity to detect toxicological compounds and forensic evidence in tissue, materials and soil.

What the terrorists can do?

Bioterrorist threats could involve aerosol attacks on individuals or crowds, 'dirty' bombs and targeted contamination food sources (Alberts, 2005) such as Botulinum in milk (Wein and Liu, 2005), or release of pathogenic organisms or biotoxins in the water supply (Nuzzo, 2006). Such threats might also exploit unexpectedly virulent scientific discoveries such as mousepox IL-4 (Jackson *et al.*, 2001), or medical publication of the full genetic sequence of a highly lethal strain of influenza virus, such as caused the Spanish influenza pandemic in the winter of 1918-19 (Taubenberger *et al.*, 2005; Tumpey *et al.*, 2005).

Atlantic Storm was a simulated bioterrorism exercise based on the deliberate release of smallpox viruses in various European and North American cities. It revealed many nations had inadequate vaccine stockpiles and plans, while highlighting the need to develop innovative technologies (including nanotechnology) capable of allowing health workers to rapidly diagnose such an atypical infection and effectively communicate its details to public health authorities (Hamilton and Smith, 2006).

What is nanotechnology?

Nanotechnology involves the engineering design, fabrication, application and regulation of products at atomic, molecular or macromolecular levels of approximately 1 nanometer to 100 nanometers; a nanometer constituting one-billionth of a meter (United States FDA, 2006). Nanotechnology offers the prospect that bio-security in the future may be critically dependent on billions of widespread invisible sensors, integrated into clothing, buildings, vehicles and natural objects, collating unprecedented amounts of data for capacious nano-data storage units in a form of ambient intelligence. Skin-implanted nanosize radio frequency ID (RFID) tags, for instance, could control access to biosecure premises. Nano-fluidics may provide rapid analysis of biological samples (such as blood, semen and saliva) by forcing them through nano-sized channels etched onto a microchip (Thomas, 2006).

The Forensic Science Centre at Lawrence Livermore National

Laboratory in the United States is developing nano-structured materials for applications to forensics and homeland security. These include silica-based nano-materials, molecular imprinted polymers, and silicon platforms, for the collection, concentration and detection of chemical weapons or other related compounds (Reynolds and Hart, 2004) A major concern for physicians involved in such forensic use of nanotechnology for bio-security purposes is likely to be safety for themselves and their patients.

A glance at the type of injuries an MCE can cause

Before studying the role of nanotechnology let us look at various types of injuries that can occur in a terrorist attack. Analysis of casualties from terrorist bombings shows that the majority of survivors, generally those furthest from the blast and presenting earliest to hospital, suffer only minor, non-critical injuries; for example, minor penetrating trauma, tinnitus, psychological stress, and simple fractures (Leibovici, Gofrit, Stein, Shapira, Noga *et al.*, 1996). These injuries are often to the face, hands and arms; probably showing the protective effects of clothing (Brismar and Bergenwald, 1982; Golan, Golan, Alder, Sternberg, Zagher *et al.*, 1982). Only approximately 10% to 20% of survivors require admission to an intensive care unit (Frykberg, 2002). The traditional teaching about terrorist bomb injuries classifies as 'primary' those deriving from the blast wave itself (Freund, Kopolovic, and Durst, 1980). 'Secondary' injuries are described as arising relatively immediately from shrapnel, structural debris or heat propelled by the blast wave. 'Tertiary' injuries are caused by the patient's immediate displacement against solid objects or from building collapse or fire. Building collapse is a deliberate terrorist aim to maximize casualties from a bomb blast. Most mortality from bombing in World Trade Centre attack in 2001, for example, arose from tertiary injuries caused by building collapse and fire (Mallonee, Shariat, Stennies, Waxweiler, Hogan *et al.*, 1996). A fourth category of terrorist bomb injury, however, could arise from the terrorists' deliberate intention to create secondary hazards for victims, rescuers or medical staff. Techniques include a second bomb attached to a mock or pseudo-victim, or particularly relevant in this context, additional use of radiation or biologic vectors.

How nanotechnology works?

First, the patients would have been subjected to nanotechnology screening for bioterrorist chemical and viral vectors before being brought into the ICU.

Second, nanosize radio frequency ID (RFID) tags would have controlled and documented access of staff and relatives to these biosecure premises. Nanofluidics would have provided rapid analysis of biological samples from the patients. Nanotechnology diagnostics would more rapidly detect pleural effusions, rib fractures, ruptured organs and blood vessels and shrapnel. The resultant chest drains would be coated with nano-particles to reduce risk of infection. Split skin grafting and wound debridement would be facilitated by nanotechnology sensors able to detect and remove minute shrapnel and debris particles.

Nanotherapeutices

Nanotherapeutices e.g. nano-manufactured artificial red blood cells) may provide better treatments for septicemia and multi-organ failure. Nanofluidics would have facilitated rapid analysis of such biological samples. Nano-computing would have assisted rapid compilation of a large amount of information about the nature of the injuries, the associated risks and best responses thereto. This widespread use of nanotechnology in such a setting would raise significant issues for health professionals about balancing patient and staff confidentiality and privacy with the requirements of public health disaster plans and quarantine laws (Rubinson *et al.*, 2005). Use of nanotechnology in critical care bio-surveillance is likely to make staff and patients feel more secure and do their jobs better in such pressure, tense and often fear-filled situations.

The successful implementation of such plans may actually depend on how carefully they have been integrated with basic standards and principles of medical professionalism.

MCE from Terrorist Bombings; Time for medical leadership to rise

Explosions and bombings remain the most common deliberate cause of disasters involving large numbers of casualties, especially as instruments of terrorism, yet we still have not learned how to anticipate and manage the tragic carnage they cause with any degree of effectiveness. Our naiveté and inexperience in this area have been demonstrated by the predictably confused responses to recent terrorist disasters. Trauma physicians and trauma centers are uniquely qualified to play a leading role in the medical management of disaster victims and in the overall coordination of disaster response. They already are an integral part of the pre-hospital emergency medical system and public health efforts of many communities, and their infrastructure, training, and experience are specialized for the comprehensive evaluation and treatment of injury.

Predictably and logically, medical response to terrorist disasters tends to be most sophisticated and most effective in those countries that most commonly are exposed to them, or among those groups who regularly train for these contingencies, such as the military. Military medical forces are well prepared and well trained to cope with true mass casualty events, even though they actually deal with such events as infrequently as the civilian sector. This training and the systematic planning for orderly triage, stabilization, and evacuation of casualties through a chain of treatment stations and hospitals in times of war have allowed them to cope with massive casualty burdens that would overwhelm the ordinary civilian community.

The generally untrained and unprepared civilian sector must learn from this resource and from those who have handled mass casualties, because it is the civilian medical community that typically is confronted by terrorist acts.

Different types of disasters, such as fires, shootings, floods, infectious or chemical agents, radiation, or earthquakes, result in very different patterns of injury and medical needs.

The Explosive Injury

There are three forms of bodily injury induced by explosive blasts—primary, secondary, and tertiary blast injuries. Primary blast injury is caused by the shock wave that spreads radially outward from an explosion, at the speed of sound, and is transmitted more rapidly and powerfully, and over a longer distance, in water than in air. In air, this shock wave dissipates rapidly, in relation to the cube of the distance from the blast. The more powerful the blast, the greater the distance at which damage may occur. When the shock wave passes through the body, tissues are disrupted at air-liquid interfaces in a process called "spalling," and the ears and lungs are most commonly injured. The bowels are damaged only in the most powerful blasts, most typical of under-water blasts. The degree of tissue injury is directly related to the magnitude and the duration of the peak overpressure of the blast shock wave. After this is a longer phase of negative pressure, when implosion may occur, and then a major movement of air known as "blast wind." Most victims of primary blast lung injury from explosions are killed immediately, as the vital organs are likely to be fatally injured in anyone who is close enough to the blast to be hit by the shock wave before it dissipates. Death is often caused by massive cerebral and coronary air embolism, as well as the most powerful forms of secondary and tertiary injuries this close in to the explosion. Late deaths among the small number of survivors with primary blast lung injury are caused by progressive pulmonary insufficiency, which has all the radiographic and pathologic signs of parenchymal hemorrhage, similar to blunt contusions. Indoor detonations tend to cause more severe primary blast injuries than open-air bombings outdoors, because the blast wave is magnified, rather than dissipated, as it is reflected off walls, floors, and ceilings.

Secondary blast injury is caused by debris set in motion by the shock wave that impacts the body. Tertiary blast injury involves the actual displacement of the victim's body to crash into other objects. These two forms of explosive injury cause typical bodily trauma, and it is these injuries that predominate among survivors of bombings.

Collapse of the World Trade Center in New York

The collapse of the twin towers of the World Trade Center in New York City on September 11, 2001, was devastating in terms of how unexpected it was, and the realization of how vulnerable the United States is to such attacks. The jetliner crashes into these buildings, quite analogous to bombings, are estimated to have imparted the equivalent of 12,500 tons of force. The subsequent building collapse is estimated to have released the equivalent explosive force of 900 tons of TNT, resulting in approximately 3,000 deaths, and several hundred survivors with predominantly non-critical injuries (dead/wounded ratio of 5:1). With only a few survivors rescued from the collapsed buildings, the immediate death rate among those in the buildings was over 99%.

Patterns of Injury, Severity, and Mortality

It is important to distinguish the two goals of terrorist attacks: casualty generation, or the total number injured and killed from the single use of a weapon; and lethality or the proportion of casualties killed. The magnitude of an explosion, and the number of people in the vicinity, primarily determine casualty generation, whereas indoor location and building collapse maximize lethality.

Analysis of past bombing disasters reveals definite patterns of injury and mortality, which provide the opportunity to plan and prepare for future events. Immediate deaths, or those who die before reaching medical care, appear related to the magnitude of the explosion, the occurrence of building collapse, and an indoor location. A comparison of those bombings involving a major component of building collapse shows substantial rates of immediate deaths, and relatively constant critical mortality rates among survivors, with widely varying explosive forces. Those incidents involving an additional component of indoor location were associated with the highest immediate death rates. This suggests that building collapse is the most important determinant of outcome among these variables. Indoor blasts not only magnify the destructive power of the primary blast shock wave but also promote complete building collapse, which maximizes both casualty generation and lethality of a bombing.

The virtually 100% immediate death rate of casualties within the collapsed World Trade Center towers clearly showed the relative importance of building collapse, over and above explosive force, as a prognostic variable. The magnitude of explosive force has its greatest impact on lethality, rather than only casualty generation, when it is applied to building collapse, and when greater than a 1-ton TNT equivalent.

Another determinant of mortality among victims of bombings is the availability of medical resources at the disaster scene. Over 20 survivors of the World Trade Center disaster on September 11, 2001, were transported to a burn center with severe burns. The anatomic distribution of injuries among bombing victims tends to be out of proportion to the total body surface area. Head injuries occur more frequently than would be predicted on the basis of the 12% body surface area of the head and neck exposed to the environment, whereas torso and extremity trauma occur less frequently than their relative surface areas would suggest. This has been explained by clothing distribution, with covered areas of the body being less exposed to some of the forces of injury, such as flash burns.

Emotional shock is a common consequence of terrorist bombings, especially among female survivors. Although it is not as lethal as physical injury, there is significant potential for long-term psychological disability. This should be considered in the same category as other major injuries with respect to the need for treatment. Disaster planning should include provisions for emotional evaluation and rehabilitation of casualties. One of the most consistent injury patterns noted among survivors of terrorist bombings is the overwhelming predominance of relatively minor, non-critical injuries that are not life-threatening. The planning for medical management of casualties must revolve around this basic lesson learned from prior bombing disasters, as medical resources must be allocated accordingly.

Communication problems can retard the process of triage and smooth flow

Klein and Weigelt reported their experience with three sequential aircraft crash disasters in Dallas, Texas, over a period of 3 years. As a result of analyzing the problems they encountered, they were able to modify the community and hospital disaster plans to more effectively manage the logistics and medical management of large casualty loads. The major problems they encountered were communications between the disaster scene and hospital, the authority and command structure, security considerations for scene and medical personnel safety, and the organisation of medical management, all also typical of most reported disasters. Communications were secured through protected phone lines controlled by the administrative post, and the use of walkie-talkies, to circumvent the completely overwhelmed hospital phone lines by unrestricted incoming calls. They emphasized the importance of restricting laboratory and radiology testing in this setting, which is largely overused even in ordinary circumstances, but may significantly hamper casualty flow, and jeopardize lives, in disasters.

The time of greatest danger to orderly casualty handling, and of risk of hospital overload, is in the immediate aftermath of a bombing, a period of chaos. A rapid institution of strong authority and leadership over the care of victims is necessary to avoid loss of life in this initial phase of disaster management, and this is only possible with preplanning and rehearsal. If there is any biologic, chemical, or radiation contamination involved in the disaster, this period could lead to the hospital itself being shut down if prompt control is not established. Triage sites must be established in large open areas, and must be located outside of the hospital. It is recommended that a second triage site be established to further screen initially evaluated casualties to enhance triage accuracy, and to ensure that only those needing hospitalization are admitted. It is also important that the triage sites be located away from the bombing scene, to avoid the risk of a second bomb blast, which terrorists have used commonly to take out initial survivors, rescue personnel, and unwitting on lookers. Protection of medical assets must be a major priority of disaster management.

Medical Management and Casualty Flow

After rescue, treatment of bombing casualties begins at the triage site with rapid stabilization, control of hemorrhage, splinting of fractures, and cleaning and covering wounds. Immediate determination of concomitant radiation, chemical, or biologic contamination must be made and a decontamination process instituted before victims reach the hospital. Extensive or definitive treatment should not be performed at this stage. Many interventions can be applied on the basis of clinical findings alone, such as tube thoracostomy and laparotomy. Only when the casualty influx subsides should physicians reassess all evaluated casualties more completely, and begin considering treatment or evacuation of those in the delayed and expectant categories. At this time there will be a better understanding of available resources. Primary blast lung injury poses a major challenge in treatment, and fortunately occurs in only a small minority of bombing survivors. It presents as acute respiratory failure, and its radiographic findings are similar to pulmonary edema. Oxygenation must be supported, but positive pressure should be avoided if possible because of the tendency to induce air embolism. Noninvasive ventilatory support should be tried initially. If intubation is necessary, high-frequency jet ventilation, independent lung ventilation, or volume-controlled ventilation should be considered to reduce ventilation pressures. The classic presenting triad of apnea, bradycardia, and hypotension must be treated, and resuscitative fluids should be judiciously restricted.

A liberal approach is warranted to early abdominal, head, and thoracic operations in those with critical injuries to these anatomic areas in view of their high specific mortality. This emphasizes the importance of immediate availability of surgeons and surgical support personnel and facilities to minimize morbidity and mortality of bombing survivors. All deaths among survivors should be analyzed to determine the quality of medical care, especially among cases of under-triage or deaths among non-critically injured victims. Any immediate care provided to expectant injuries should be considered overtriage, and the inevitable death of these patients will result in raising the critical mortality rate as a result. Such mis-triage could result in unnecessary loss of life among more salvageable patients.

Mortality among properly triaged expectant injuries should be categorized as immediate deaths, as they never received medical care, and therefore should not skew the critical mortality rate as a measure of medical care.

Looking at the future leadership of medical personnel

The advance formulation of a disaster plan is essential for the successful management of mass casualties, because these incidents are unpredictable in their timing and location. In order that the plan be relevant and workable, it must be based on the published experience to the extent possible. Surgical capability must be a central feature of these plans. An effective disaster plan must incorporate all community and hospital assets that will be required for the proper handling of mass casualties. These plans should be rehearsed regularly through simulation drills, and a critique of these drills should lead to appropriate revision of the plans. A post-event briefing of involved personnel is important soon after a disaster, so as to revise the disaster plans according to the problems encountered. Above all, flexibility must be built into these plans to allow adaptation to the unique circumstances characteristic of every disaster, but still within the context of the broad principles reviewed above. We must all have the "imagination" to be prepared for the most unexpected forms of attack to provide the best care for the victims. Another necessity for future preparations for bombing disasters is that physicians, and especially surgeons, become more involved in the planning process than they have been historically. Trauma surgeons, trauma centers, and trauma organisations are uniquely suited to leadership roles in the planning, organisation, and implementation of disaster care.

References

Adler J, Golan E, Golan J, *et al.* Terrorist bombing experience during 1975–79: casualties admitted to the Shaare Zedeck Medical Center. *Isr J Med Sci.* 1983;19:189–193.

American College of Surgeons, Committee on Trauma. Field categorization of trauma patients (field triage). *Bull Am Coll Surg.* 1986;71:17–21.

American College of Surgeons, Committee on Trauma. Resources for Optimal Care of the Injured Patient. Chicago, IL: American College of Surgeons; 1998.

Ammons MA, Moore EE, Pons PT, *et al.* The role of a regional trauma system in the management of a mass disaster: an analysis of the Keystone Colorado chairlift accident. *J Trauma.* 1988;28:1468–1471.

Bellamy RF. The medical effects of conventional weapons. *World J Surg.* 1992;16:888–892.

Berry FB. The medical management of mass casualties: the Scudder Oration on Trauma. *Bull Am Coll Surg.* 1956;41:60–66.

Biancolini CA, DelBosco CG, Jorge MA. Argentine Jewish Community Institution bomb explosion. *J Trauma.* 1999;47:728–732.

Brismar B, Bergenwald L, The terrorist bomb explosion in Bologna, Italy, 1980: an analysis of the effects and injuries sustained. *J Trauma.* 1982;22:216–220.

Candole CA. Blast injury. *Can Med Assoc J.* 1967;96:207–214.

Caro D, Irving M. The Old Bailey Bomb explosion. *Lancet.* 1973;1:1433–1435.

Caro D. Major disasters. *Lancet.* 1974;2:1309–1310.

Champion HR, Sacco WJ, Gainer PS, *et al.* The effect of medical direction on trauma triage. *J Trauma.* 1988;28:235–239.

Champion HR, Sacco WJ. Trauma severity scales. In: Maull KI, ed. Advances in Trauma. Vol 1. Chicago: Yearbook Medical Publishers; 1986:1–20.

Chan TC, Killeen J, Griswold W, Lenert L. Information technology and emergency medical care during disasters. Acad Emerg Med. 2004;11:1229-1236. FULL TEXT | ISI | 69. Centers for Disease Control and Prevention (CDC). Hurricane Katrina response and guidance for health care providers, relief workers, and shelter operators. *MMWR Morb Mortal Wkly Rep.* 2005;54:877.

Ciraulo DL, Frykberg ER, Feliciano DV, *et al.* A survey assessment of the level of preparedness for domestic terrorism and mass casualty incidents among Eastern Association for the Surgery of Trauma members. *J Trauma.* 2004;56:1033-1039.

Clemedsson CJ. Blast injury. Physiol Rev. 1956;36:336–354.

Cook CH, Muscarella P, Praba AC, *et al.* Reducing overtriage without compromising outcomes in trauma patients. *Arch Surg.* 2001;136:752–756.

Cooper GJ, Maynard RL, Cross NL, *et al.* Casualties from terrorist bombings. *J Trauma.* 1983;23:955–967.

Einav S, Aharonson-Daniel L, Weissman C, Freund HR, Peleg K, Israel Trauma Group. In-hospital resource utilization during multiple casualty incidents. *Ann Surg.* 2006;243:533-540.

Einav S, Feigenberg Z, Weissman C, *et al.* Evacuation priorities in mass casualty terror-related events: implications for contingency planning. *Ann Surg.* 2004; 239:304-310.

Eiseman B. Combat casualty management for tomorrow's battlefield: urban terrorism. *J Trauma.* 2001;51:821–823.

Feliciano DV, Anderson GV, Rozycki GS, *et al.* Management of casualties from the bombing at the Centennial Olympics. *Am J Surg.* 1998;176:538–543.

Frykberg ER, Hutton PMJ, Balzer RH. Disaster in Beirut: an application of mass casualty principles. *Mil Med.* 1987;11:563–566.

Frykberg ER, Tepas JJ, Alexander RH. The 1983 Beirut airport terrorist bombing: injury patterns and implications for disaster management. *Am Surg.* 1989;55:134–141.

Frykberg ER, Tepas JJ. Terrorist bombings: lessons learned from Belfast to Beirut. *Ann Surg.* 1988;208:569–576.

Frykberg ER. Medical management of disasters and mass casualties from terrorist bombings: how can we cope? *J Trauma.* 2002;53:201-212. ISI | PUBMED

Frykberg, E.R. (2002). Medical management of disasters and mass casualties from terrorist bombings: how can we cope? *Journal of Trauma,* 53, 201-212.

Frykberg, E.R., Tepas, J.J., and Alexander, R.H. (1989). The 1983 Beirut airport terrorist bombing: Injury patterns and implications for disaster management. *The American Surgeon,* 55, 134-141.

Gidron, Y. (2002). Posttraumatic stress disorder after terrorist attacks: A review. *Journal of Nervous and Mental Disease,* 190, 118-121.

Glanz J. In collapsing towers, a cascade of failures. *New York Times.* November 11, 2001:B1, B11.

Glaser B, Stauss AL. The Constant Comparative Methods of Qualitative Analysis: Discovery of Grounded Theory. New York, NY: Aldine de Gruyter; 1967:101-116.

Golan J, Golan E, Adler J, *et al.* Plastic surgery and civilian casualties due to "terrorist" activities. *Ann Plast Surg.* 1982;8:359–362.

Golan, J., Golan, E., Alder, J., Sternberg, N., Zagher, U., Rosenberg, B. *et al.* (1982). Plastic surgery and civilian casualties due to 'terrorist' activities. *Annals of Plastic Surgery,* 8,359-362.

Grossman, L.K. (1995). The electronic republic: Reshaping democracy in the information age. New York: Viking.

Gunn, J., Yang, A., Palmbach, T., Dongguang, W., and Sinha, S. (2006). Nano-forensics-nanoparticles in gun-shot-residues emerging technologies. Nanoelectronics, 2006 IEEE Conference, 269-272.

Gutierrez de Ceballos JP, Turegano Fuentes F, Perez Diaz D, Sanz Sanchez M, Martin Llorente C, Guerrero Sanz JE. Casualties treated at the closest hospital in the Madrid, March 11, terrorist bombings. *Crit Care Med.* 2005;33(1 suppl):S107-S112.

Guy RJ, Kirkman E, Watkins PE, *et al.* Physiologic responses to primary blast. *J Trauma.* 1998;45:983–987.

Hadden WA, Rutherford WH, Merrett JD. The injuries of terrorist bombing: a study of 1532 consecutive patients. *Br J Surg.* 1978; 65:525–531.

Hadden, W.A., Rutherford, W.H., and Merrett, J.D. (1978). The injuries of terrorist bombing: A study of 1532 consecutive patients. *British Journal of Surgery,* 655, 25-531.

Hamilton, D.S., and Smith, B.T. (2006). Atlantic storm. EMBO Reports, 7, 4-9. Jackson, R.J., Ramsay, A.J., Christensen, CD., Beaton, S., Hall, D.F., and Ramshaw, I.A.. (2001). Expression of mouse interleukin-4 by a recombinant ectromelia virus suppresses cytolytic lymphocyte responses and overcomes genetic resistance to mousepox. *Journal of Virology*, 75,1205-1210.

Henderson JV. Anatomy of a terrorist attack: the Cu Chi mess hall incident. *J World Assoc Emerg Disaster Med.* 1986;2:69–73.

Hill JF. Blast injury with particular reference to recent terrorist bombing incidents. *Ann R Coll Surg Engl.* 1979;61:4–11.

Hirshberg A, Stein M, Walden R. Surgical resource utilization in urban terrorist bombing: a computer simulation. *J Trauma.* 1999;47:545–550.

Hsieh HF, Shannon SE. Three approaches to qualitative content analysis. *Qual Health Res.* 2005;15:1277-1288.

Huller J, Bazini Y. Blast injuries of the chest and abdomen. *Arch Surg.* 1970;100:24–30.

Jacobs LM, Goody M, Sinclair A. The role of a trauma center in disaster management. *J Trauma.* 1983;23:697–701.

Jacobs LM, Ramp JM, Breay JM. An emergency medical system approach to disaster planning. *J Trauma.* 1979;19:157–162.

Karmy-Jones R, Kissinger D, Golocovsky M, *et al.* Bomb-related injuries. *Mil Med.* 1994;159:536–539.

Kennedy TL, Johnston GW. Civilian bomb injuries. *BMJ.* 1975;1:382–383.

Kernaghan L. Halifax explosion. Available at: http://tceplus.com/halifax.htm. Accessed December 20, 2001.

Kirschenbaum L, Keene A, O'Neill P, Westfal R, Astiz ME. The experience at St Vincent's Hospital, Manhattan, on September 11, 2001: preparedness, response, and lessons learned. *Crit Care Med.* 2005;33(1 suppl):S48-S52.

Klein JS, Weigelt JA. Disaster management: lessons learned. *Surg Clin North Am.* 1991;71:257–266.

Kluger Y, Mayo A, Soffer D, Aladgem D, Halperin P. Functions and principles in the management of bombing mass casualty incidents: lessons learned at the Tel-Aviv Souraski Medical Center. *Eur J Emerg Med.* 2004;11:329-334.

Kluger Y, Peleg K, Daniel-Aharonson L, Mayo A, Israeli Trauma Group. The special injury pattern in terrorist bombings. *J Am Coll Surg.* 2004;199:875-879.

Lee, A., Isaac, M., and Janca, A. (2002). Post-traumatic stress disorder and terrorism. Current opinion in psychiatry, 15, 633-637.

Leibovici D, Gofrit ON, Stein M, *et al.* Blast injuries: bus versus open- air-bombings—a comparative study of injuries in survivors of open-air *versus* confined-space explosions. *J Trauma.* 1996;41:1030–1035.

Leibovici, D., Gofrit, O.N., Stein, M., Shapira, S.C., Noga, Y., Heruti, R.J. *et al.* (1996). Blast injuries: Bus versus open-air bombings. A comparative study of injuries in survivors of open-air versus confined space explosions. *Journal of Trauma*, 41, 1030-1035.

Lowe, V. (1988-1989). The role of equity in international law. Australian Yearbook of International Law, 2, 54-81.

MacPherson WG. History of the Great War, Medical Services, General History. Vol 3. London: His Majesty's Stationery Office; 1924.

Mallonee S, Shariat S, Stennies G, *et al.* Physical injuries and fatalities resulting from the Oklahoma City bombing. *JAMA.* 1996;276:382–387.

Mallonee, S., Shariat, S., Stennies, G., Waxweiler, R., Hogan, D., and Jordan, F. (1996). Physical injuries and fatalities resulting from the Oklahoma City bombing. *Journal of the American Medical Association*, 276, 382-387.

Mann NC, MacKenzie E, Anderson C. Public health preparedness for mass-casualty events: a 2002 state-by-state assessment. *Prehospital Disaster Med.* 2004;19:245-255.

Marshall TK. Forensic aspects of terrorism. *Ann Acad Med Singapore.* 1984;13:32–36.

Martinez C, Gonzalez D. The World Trade Center attack: doctors in the fire and police services. Crit Care. 2001;5:304-306. FULL TEXT | ISI | PUBMED

Niezgoda, J.A., Cianci, P., Folden, B.W., Ortega, R.L., Slade, J.B., and Storrow, A.B. (1997). The effect of hyperbaric oxygen therapy on a burn wound model in human volunteers. *Plastic and Reconstructive Surgery,* 99, 1620-1625.

Nuzzo, J.B. (2006). The biological threat to US water supplies: Toward a national watersecurity policy. *Biosecurity and Bioterrorism,* 4, 147-159.

Phillips YY. Primary blast injuries. *Ann Emerg Med.* 1986;15:1446–1450.

Pyper PC, Graham WJH. Analysis of terrorist injuries treated at Craigavon Area Hospital, Northern Ireland, 1972–1980. *Injury.* 1982;14:332–338.

Rawlins JSP. Physical and pathophysiological effects of blast. Injury. 1977; 9:313–320.

Reynolds, J.G., and Hart, B.R. (2004). Nanomateriais and their application to defense andhomeland security. *Journal of Metals,* 56, 36-39.

Rignault DP, Deligny MC. The 1986 terrorist bombing experience in Paris. *Ann Surg.* 1989;209:368–373.

Rignault DP. Recent progress in surgery for the victims of disaster, terrorism and war. *World J Surg.* 1992;16:885–887.

Roco, M.C. (2006). National nanotechnology investment in the FT2003 Budget Request by the President. National Science and Technology Council's subcommittee on Nanoscale Science, Engineering and Technology (NSET). Retrieved August 28, 2006, from http://www. nano.gov/2003budget.html

Rosenberg B, Sternberg N, Zagher V, *et al.* Burns due to terroristic attacks on civilian populations from 1975–1979. *Burns.* 1982;9:21–23.

Royal Society. (2004). The individual and collective roles scientists can play in strengthening international treaties. London: The Royal Society.

Rubinson, L., Nuzzo, J.B., Talmor, D.S., O'Toole, T., Kramer, B.R., and Inglesby, .T.V. (2005). Augmentation of hospital critical care capacity after bioterrosist attacks or epidemics: Recommendations of the Working Group on Emergency Mass Critical Care. *Journal of the American Medical Association,* 33, El-El 3.

Rutherford WH. Experience in the accident and emergency department of the Royal Victoria Hospital with patients from civil disturbances in Belfast, 1969–1972, with a review of disasters in the United Kingdom, 1951–1971. *Injury.* 1972;4:189–199.

Sarkisian AE, Khondkarian RA, Amirbekian NM, *et al.* Sonographic screening of mass casualties for abdominal and renal injuries following the 1988 Armenian earthquake. *J Trauma.* 1991;31:247–250.

Schneider SM, Gallery. ME, Schafermeyer R, Zwemer FL. Emergency department crowding: a point in time. *Ann Emerg Med.* 2003;42:167-172.

Scott BA, Fletcher JR, Pulliam MW, *et al.* The Beirut terrorist bombing. *Neurosurgery.* 1986;18:107–110.

Shamir MY, Weiss YG, Willner D, *et al.* Multiple casualty terror events: the anesthesiologist's perspective. *Anesth Analg.* 2004;98:1746-1752.

Sklar DP. Casualty patterns in disasters. *J World Assoc Emerg Disaster Med.* 1987;3:49–51.

Slater MS, Trunkey DD. Terrorism in America: an evolving threat. *Arch Surg.* 1997;132:1059–1066.

Smallwood, R.A., Merianos, A., and Matthews, J.D. (2002). Bioterrorism in Australia. *Medical Journal of Australia,* 176, 251-253.

Sone, J., Fujita, J., Ochiai, Y., Manako, S., Matsui, S., Nomura, E. *et al.* (1999). Nanofabrication toward sub-10 ran and its application to novel nanodevices. *Nanotechnology,* 10, 135-141.

Stapczynski JS. Blast injuries. *Ann Emerg Med.* 1982;3:287–293.

Stein M, Hirshberg A. Medical consequences of terrorism: the conventional weapon threat. *Surg Clin North Am.* 1999;79:1537–1552.

Stephens HW. The Texas City Disaster, 1947. Austin, TX: University of Texas Press; 1947.

Taubenberger, J.K., Reid, A.H., Lourens, R.M., Wang, R., Jin, G., and Fanning, T.G. (2005). Characterization of the 1918 influenza virus polymerase genes. *Nature,* 437, 889-893

Thomas. I. (2006). Nanotechnology and surveillance. Little Brother is watching you. *Chain Reaction,* 97, 29.

Tucker K, Lettin A. The Tower of London bomb explosion. *BMJ.* 1975;3:287–290.

Tumpey, T.M., Basier, CF., Aguilar, P.V., Zeng, H., Solorzano, A., Swayne, D.E. *et al.* (2005). Characterization of the reconstructed 1918 Spanish influenza pandemic virus. *Science,* 310, 77-80.

U.S. Department of Defense. Emergency War Surgery. Washington, DC: U.S. Government Printing Office; 1975.

U.S. Department of State. International Terrorism. Selected documents, No. 24. Washington, DC: U.S. Government Printing Office; 1986.

United Nations. (1948). Universal declaration of human rights. Adopted 10 Dec. 1948. (GA Res 217A (III). UN Doc A/810 (1948) 71)"

United Nations. (1949). Convention for the amelioration of the condition of the wounded and sick in armed forces in the field (UNTS 1949; 75: 31). Convention for the amelioration of the condition of the wounded, sick and shipwrecked members of armed forces at sea (UNTS 1949, 75, 85). Convention relative to the treatment of prisoners of war (UNTS 1949; 75: 135). Convention relative to the protection of civilian persons in time flow (UNTS 1949, 75, 287). Additional protocol I, 1977.

United Nations. (1966a). International covenant on civil and political rights. Adopted 16 Dec 1966, entry into force 23 March 1976. (GA Res 2200A (XXI). UN GAOR Sttpp (No 16) 52. UN Doc A/6316 (1966). 999 UNTS 17), reprinted in International Legal Materials, 2:967, 368.

Waterworth TA, Carr MJT. Report on injuries sustained by patients treated at the Birmingham General Hospital following the recent bomb explosions. *BMJ.* 1975;2:25–27.

Zuckerman S. Experimental study of blast injuries to the lungs. *Lancet.* 1940;2:219–238.

5

Preparedness and Emergency Communication Systems

We are now living in an era of unprecedented medical advances in patient care and quality of life, but at the same time face some of the most daunting challenges in the management of mass casualties from terrorist violence. Various man made disasters illustrate one of the most prominent and timely of these challenges to our skills, our adaptability to adversity, and to our commitment to the care of the injured. The massive numbers of casualties that exceed the resources of most hospitals, the victimization of innocent civilians, including children, and the especially severe and extensive patterns of injury that characterize current terrorist attacks, go so far beyond the standard surgical training and experience of most of the doctors, that a basic change in mindset is necessary in the approach to medical care of these victims to maximize the salvage of life. Physician participation in Metropolitan Medical Response System (MMRS) drills is valuable, since the use of unfamiliar medical jargon is a common problem, many health care workers are needed in the front lines of a medical response. Awareness of the National Response Plan is vital to understanding how the system will be working at the state or central level during a disaster. With a little forethought and preparation, we can all be safer and better able to help those around us. (James Harper)

LACK OF PREPAREDNESS IS UNIVERSAL

Although Indians have suffered several terrorist attacks and substantial loss of life from these causes over the past 20 years, and the threats of more attacks rise, we tend to have a short memory. The same mistakes continue to occur in our preparedness, response, and approach to casualty disposition and management following each of these events, including, among many others. After the World Trade Center destruction in

2001 in USA, recent terrorist attack on Mumbai India is a major event. It is past time that we begin taking to heart the critical need to learn the basic principles of mass casualty management from terrorist disasters which have been so well established from decades of experiences (Eric R. Frykberg).

War between countries or between the army of a nation and its insurgents can be a tricky disaster to deal. The on going fight between the LTTE and the Sri Lankan army is one such challenge for the red cross and others involved in mitigating the disaster. "We talk about approximately a quarter of a million persons who are fundamentally trapped in a very small restricted perimeter—250 sq km [96 sq m]—which is the theatre of very intense combat," he said.

"They find themselves simply under fire and highly vulnerable. Access to medical care is almost non-existent at this point. They are in need of food, they are in need of shelter and most of all they are in need of security."

The ICRC based its figure of hundreds dead on body counts by its staff in local hospitals.

Access for aid workers was so limited, it said, that the ICRC's own presence in the region was virtually meaningless. The ICRC wanted to evacuate 200 critically wounded people on Tuesday but did not receive security clearance. Those patients, it says, now face death. The UN secretary general and the European Union have also expressed deep concern for civilians caught in the fighting.

The military did take a group of journalists, including the BBC's Chris Morris, to the region on Tuesday. Brig Nandana Udawatte, who led the capture of Mullaitivu, said that "mortar fire, indirect fire and close-quarter battles" were going on 1.5 km from the town of Puthukkudiyiruppu. Pro-rebel sources have previously accused the army of killing hundreds of civilians with shellfire—allegations the military denies. A correspondent says that apart from soldiers on every corner in Mullaitivu, it is a ghost town. Most of the buildings, houses and shops are damaged or destroyed. He says its capture is a big victory for the army but that the Tigers also appear on the surface undaunted, with the sound of artillery fire not that far away echoing down the empty streets.

Let us look at certain experiences and the lessons learnt in preparedness for the same.

1. Bombings and shooting massacres are, historically, by far the most common form of terrorist violence. These means continue to be used, and therefore are most likely to be used in the future. These mechanisms are the easiest and least costly methods of achieving the terrorist goals of large-scale casualties. This explains why surgeons, along with other acute care trauma specialists, must be integrally involved as leaders in the field of disaster management, and in local hospital and community disaster planning. We must resist our current tendency to

become overly enamored with the "weapons of mass destruction" of biologic, chemical and radiological attacks, in terms of funding priorities and resource allocations that are wholly disproportionate to the clear reality of the terrorist bombing threat.

2. Importance of triage to the proper management of mass casualties from terrorist bombings and shootings, due to the fact that these disasters typically result in large numbers of casualties who are not critically injured, cannot be over-emphasised. Einav *et al.* report only 20% of casualties with critical injuries requiring urgent care. This leads to an inundation of scarce medical resources with hundreds of victims who do not require immediate attention (overtriage), which then threatens to delay the recognition and care of that small minority with urgent and salvageable life threatening injuries at immediate risk of death (undertriage). Almogy *et al.* stress the need to avoid providing care to those "expectant" survivors so severely injured that their ultimate salvage is unlikely. For this reason, Peleg *et al.* emphasize that injuries of moderate severity, rather than greatest severity, should take priority.

   Triage should be performed outside of the hospital as an aggressive screening process, to prevent all except those in most need of urgent attention from overwhelming this critical medical resource. sheer numbers of potentially urgent injuries require that initial assessment be rapidly performed by small medical teams, and that only minimal acceptable care be applied just to keep patients alive long enough to reach definitive care. The length of time influx continues is unpredictable in any given disaster, and usually not known because of breakdown in communications between the scene and hospital. Therefore, a plan for relief of medical teams after several hours, and for evacuation of treated casualties elsewhere to make room for more becomes necessary.

3. Surgeons must be prepared for especially complex and difficult wounding patterns that are not typically seen in routine practice, and that greatly increase morbidity and mortality, such as blast lung, and multiple penetrating injuries from both destructive shrapnel increasingly used in bombs and from automatic firearms.

Our emergency care system is in critical condition. The signs are unmistakable:

- Emergency room (ER) crowding
- Ambulance diversion

- Unpaid care
- Fewer "on-call" specialists
- The rising costs of care and fear of legal liability have led more specialists to opt out of taking ER call.
- If ERs and trauma centers are already jammed with patients, how could they respond to a disaster or a terrorist strike?
- Public hospitals are overcrowded and private hospitals do not find the emergency work lucrative.

Survival kit: Stock up on essentials for a disaster

In a disaster, keep in mind that neighborhood grocery stores and gas stations may run out of supplies. Essential services such as electricity, telephone and health care may be disrupted or shut down. Be prepared by assembling a survival kit to get you through these tough times.

You should have supplies to last everyone in your household—including pets—at least two weeks. Store supplies in a cool, dry place in easy-to-carry containers in case there's a need to evacuate. Check and replace any supplies past their expiration dates. Adapt this supply list to suit your specific needs.

SURVIVAL KIT CHECKLIST

Water

Plan on 1 gallon per person per day, for drinking and for sanitation.

Food

Select foods that require no refrigeration, have a long shelf life, and require little or no water to prepare. This may include ready-to-eat canned goods, protein bars, dried fruit and crackers.

Hygiene and sanitation

Respiratory masks or comparable make

Moist towelettes

Alcohol-based, waterless hand sanitizer

Toothpaste and toothbrush

Toilet paper and paper towels

Garbage bags, heavy duty, and ties

Prescribed medications

Store at least a one-month supply.

First-aid kit

Rubber gloves
Cleansing agent (soap or towelettes)
Antibiotic ointment and burn ointment
Cold packs
Adhesive bandages, cotton balls and swabs
Sterile dressing, tape and elastic wrap
Thermometer
Tweezers, sharp scissors, spoon
Eyewash solution
Medication for fever and pain relief, such as acetaminophen or ibuprofen
Anti-diarrheal medication
Antihistamines

Tools

Manual can opener
Eating utensils
Flashlight
Light sticks
Radio, battery powered
Batteries
Matches, in waterproof container
Duct tape
Knife
Wrench or pliers

Additional items

Cash and coins
Special needs such as inhalers, contact lenses, extra eyeglasses and hearing aid batteries
Copies of credit cards, bank numbers, important documents, medical prescriptions, driver's licenses and passports
Keys, extra sets
Feminine hygiene supplies
Infant supplies
Recreational materials
Food and supplies for pets

Items for evacuation

Blankets or sleeping bags
Change of clothing and footwear
Bathing supplies
Raincoat

Let not an Epidemic create pandemonium

To avoid chaos and help maintain a sense of order in your life during an epidemic, plan for a change in routine.

- *Food.* Plan for food shortages at supermarkets. Store enough food and water for two weeks.
- *Power.* Expect electrical and water service disruption. Keep batteries and candles on hand. Consider buying a generator.
- *Health Care.* Plan for overwhelmed medical services. Expect possible delays in medical treatment for all but the most serious problems. Keep enough medicine and first-aid supplies on hand. Know how to manage your chronic illness when you can't access medical services.
- *Money.* Anticipate bank, government, postal and telephone service disruptions. Stash some cash, sign up for online bill pay and keep your cell phone charged.
- *Work.* Expect work and school closures. Find out emergency plans for schools and work sites.
- *Entertainment.* Check for cancellation of worship services and entertainment events. Stock books and games to pass the time.
- *Travel.* Count on travel restrictions and lack of access to transportation networks. Have backup plans for conducting business from home.

Stay informed

Identify reliable sources that you can count on for information about the disease and its spread.

- *News.* Know how you'll keep up-to-date on developments. Stay abreast of the news through local radio or television broadcasts or Internet sites.
- *Work.* Find out how your business will operate during the emergency. Get set-up to work from home if possible. Establish a call tree to pass along important information. Consider plans for an extended leave of absence.
- *School.* If you have children, be aware of plans for school closings.

Stay in touch

Designate a friend or relative to be an emergency contact. No matter where family members are—that includes the extended family—everyone should know how to stay in touch during emergencies.

- *Make contact.* When there are major disruptions, it's often easier to contact someone far away than nearby.
- *Plan a meeting location.* Designate a primary and backup meeting location.

Plan for quarantine

To limit spread of disease in a pandemic, there may be restrictions on travel. Don't flee—you may spread the disease. Instead, be prepared for an extended stay at home.

But stay flexible. In another kind of crisis, you may need to evacuate. Know recommended routes and the location of emergency shelters. Designate where your family can meet, within and outside the community. In addition:

- Know how to turn off household utilities—water, electricity, gas.
- Be prepared to take pets with you. Have ID tags on collars.
- Keep your gas tanks at least half-full.

Recognize flu symptoms

Bird flu symptoms are similar to those of seasonal flu but may be more severe. Be suspicious if anyone shows signs of infection. Regularly monitor your health during a pandemic. Take your temperature often, and treat symptoms early.

By planning, not panicking, you can be confident during a crisis

The more you plan for an extreme event, such as a flu pandemic, the more in control of your situation you're likely to feel. In addition to making plans for water, food and medical supplies, it's a good idea to plan how you want to respond emotionally.

Before a crisis

Imagine that you've just heard on the news that bird flu has reached pandemic proportions. What would you need to do? Start doing those things now. As a guide, ask yourself these three questions:

1. *Am I prepared*? Do you have a stockpile of food and medical supplies in case these become unavailable? Do you know what to do if your workplace closes?
2. *Is my family prepared*? Have you reviewed disaster plans with your family? Plan how you will help young children understand what's going on or how you'll transport college students home in the event schools close.
3. *What key local resources can I draw on*? Local and state public health and law enforcement agencies will likely be important sources of information on what's happening in your immediate area and what you should do. Find out how to get that information, whether on the radio, television or through a Web site.

Focusing on these priorities now will help you stay organised and make your planning more efficient. Then if you hear that a pandemic—or any crisis—is developing, stay calm and fall back on your preparations. Prioritize what you need to do, and begin addressing the most important matters first.

During a crisis: Stay balanced

A pandemic flu outbreak or other disaster in your area is likely to take its toll for a few weeks, perhaps longer. It's normal to feel concerned and anxious about safety. Use these tips to help manage stress during a crisis:

- *Continue to focus on the facts.* Stay informed. Follow official directions to protect yourself and your loved ones.
- *Keep your strength up.* That means eating right, exercising regularly and getting enough sleep. Avoid drugs and alcohol.
- *Stay connected.* It's possible that a flu outbreak will require that you and your family be quarantined for a time. But even if that's the case, you don't need to disconnect from the world. You can stay in contact with family, co-workers, friends and neighbors with e-mail, phone calls and text messaging.
- *Consider limiting news exposure.* If a family member—especially a child—is overwhelmed by the news and feeling anxious, limit access to TV or radio. Use it on a "need-to-know" basis.
- *Distract yourself.* Continue to enjoy pleasurable activities, such as listening to music, cooking a favorite meal, reading a good book or playing board games with your family.
- *Take time for relaxation.* Find a quiet place to collect your thoughts and feelings. Try some relaxation exercises, such as yoga, tai chi, deep breathing or progressive muscle relaxation. Encourage others to do the same.
- *Limit caffeine intake.* Caffeine can add to feelings of anxiety and agitation.

During a crisis: Help your child cope

Children may feel confused and frightened by what's happening. Help them through a crisis with these activities.

- *Encourage the child to ask questions.* Find out what, specifically, he or she is afraid of, and address those issues. Be ready to answer the same question several times, because once may not be enough. If you can't answer a question, it's OK to say so.
- *Talk at a level he or she can understand.* Don't overwhelm your child with details. Keep your answers short and simple for young children.
- *Spend time with your child.* Be physically affectionate. Reassure your child that you care and that you understand his or her concerns.

- *Keep regular schedules as much as possible.* Regular playtimes, mealtimes and bedtimes can help a young child feel secure.

Vaccine to prevent bird flu

There's no vaccine to prevent bird flu, there are things you can do to reduce your risk of becoming ill.

1. Stay healthy

It's impossible to know how a flu pandemic might take shape, but being in good health can help protect you. A healthy body means a strong immune system that fights off infection. Eating a balanced diet, exercising regularly and getting adequate sleep are all things you can do to maintain good health.

2. Get a seasonal flu shot

Although your yearly flu shot won't protect you from the bird flu, it's still protective against the more common seasonal flu viruses. It's also a precaution against the possibility of getting simultaneous infections with both the common flu and bird flu. This is important because simultaneous infections are the main way that viruses swap genes and create new strains that potentially can cause flu pandemics.

3. Wash your hands frequently

Use soap and water. When traveling or when water is scarce, an alcohol-based (60 percent to 95 percent) hand sanitizer can be used to help prevent the spread of infection. It's especially important to wash your hands after likely exposure, and before handling food or touching your nose, mouth or eyelids. When you wash, use warm water and soap and scrub for at least 15 seconds. Alcohol-based hand sanitizers are actually better than soap and water at killing bacteria and viruses. Even after washing, avoid touching your mouth or eyes with your fingers.

4. Use proper respiratory hygiene

Cover your mouth and nose with tissue when you cough or sneeze. Discard used tissues immediately. If no tissue is available, cough or sneeze into your upper sleeve.

5. Consider wearing a mask

A respiratory mask may prevent you from inhaling airborne particles from an infected person's coughs or sneezes. The snug-fitting N95 face mask is the gold standard for infection protection.

6. Wear gloves

Consider wearing latex gloves when caring for someone with flu, as gloves may reduce the risk of direct contact with influenza viruses (but still wash your hands). Use latex-free gloves if you have a latex allergy.

7. Keep your home and work areas clean

Use disinfecting wipes or cleanser to clean such common surfaces as door handles, phones, computer keyboards, countertops and tools.

8. Be careful about the food you eat

Don't eat undercooked poultry or raw eggs. Thoroughly cooking poultry and eggs—and other types of meat—kills bacteria and viruses within these products.

9. Avoid contact

Avoid contact with birds and bird-related material in areas where bird flu is occurring; whether feeding ducks at a park or walking through an open-air market, touching or being close to birds or bird droppings can lead to bird flu transmission, if birds in that area are infected.

10. Keep distance

In the event of a epidemic, avoid public areas, work from home, avoid unnecessary travel, stay three to six feet away from people who are coughing or sneezing, and avoid shaking hands, hugging or kissing.

If you are a diabetic; make special preparation.

An earthquake or blizzard or flu pandemic may disrupt life for days, weeks or months on end. When Hurricane Katrina struck the Gulf Coast in August 2005, more than 200,000 people with diabetes were affected. Some lost medical services and found themselves in shelters without access to lifesaving insulin injections. But even minor emergencies—such as a temporary power outage in your neighborhood—can present challenges when it comes to managing diabetes. Your safety depends on planning your responses now. Use the following strategies to guide your actions for any type of emergency.

1. Emergency kit

Begin by gathering enough supplies to last for at least a week. In case of emergency, you'll need:

- *Medical supplies.* Pack tissues, alcohol swabs, syringes, cotton balls, testing strips, blood glucose meters and any other items key to managing diabetes. Also include a pencil and pad of paper for recording blood sugar levels.
- *Medications.* Be prepared to store insulin, glucagon and other drugs in a cooler. Keep ice or freezer packs handy in case refrigeration fails. Remember that your needs for medication may change if your weight or stress levels change during the emergency period.
- *Non-perishable drinks and snacks.* Set aside bottled water, granola bars, peanut butter, crackers, cereal, orange juice, or any other snacks recommended for controlling your blood sugar.

Remember that you may need to eat more at times when your activity level increases—for example, when walking long distances or lifting heavy objects.

- *Routine emergency items*. Include a first-aid kit, whistle, candles, matches, gloves, flashlight and radio with spare batteries.
- *Medical records*. Pack copies of your insurance card and prescriptions in a waterproof plastic bag. Also keep a list of your health care providers and emergency contacts. If your child has diabetes, include a copy of the health care records you've shared with your child's school.

Store your emergency kit in a place where you can easily find it. Make sure that relatives, friends and neighbors know where you keep the emergency kit. Inspect the kit at least once a year, updating medical records and replacing expired items as needed.

2. Tell others about your diabetes

If you're evacuated to a shelter or other location, identify yourself as a person who has diabetes. If you have diabetes-related complications, mention those as well. Sharing this information immediately means that you're more likely to get appropriate attention from relief workers. It's also important to wear appropriate medical identification at all times.

3. Protect your medications

Keep insulin as cool as possible without freezing it. Also protect it from direct heat and direct sunlight. Remember that extremes of temperature and humidity can affect medications, blood glucose monitors and test strips. Keep the package inserts for these items and check for information on how to use them in unusual conditions. Keep your medication containers, too. As long as you have the original containers, you might be able to get medications in case of emergency without a prescription.

Discard any medications that come in contact with flood water or other contaminated water. Make a possible exception for lifesaving drugs. If pills are still dry and clean, use them until you can find replacements.

4. Avoid dehydration

High blood sugar can lead to dehydration. If you're exposed to high temperatures, you can lose body fluids through sweating—which only compounds the risk. During a disaster, clean drinking water may be in short supply. Ask relief workers if you can boil water for drinking. If not, turn to the water in your emergency kit. Supplement this with bottled drinks that don't include sugar or other carbohydrates.

5. Prevent wounds and infections

Diabetes can cause problems with blood circulation and make it harder for you to recover from wounds and infections. During a disaster, do everything you can to avoid injuries. Check your feet daily for sores, cuts and blisters. Also look for signs of infection, such as swelling, redness or discharge from a cut. If you're injured or notice signs of infection, seek treatment right away. Treating open wounds immediately can help prevent potentially life-threatening infections.

6. Wash your hands

Washing your hands is one of the most important ways to prevent illness and infection. This simple strategy is especially important in emergency conditions. Soap and clean, fresh water work best. If these aren't available, look for alcohol-based hand wipes or gels. The steps you take to keep your hands clean can go a long way toward promoting good health during an emergency.

Be sure to wash your hands:

- Before preparing or eating food
- After using the toilet, changing a diaper or helping a child use the toilet
- After coughing or blowing your nose
- After caring for someone who's sick
- After handling uncooked foods, especially meat and fish
- After handling animals or animal waste
- After handling garbage or storm debris

Humanitarian volunteer worker!

It is usually greeted with a smile and curiosity. "But what do you do?" High-profile philanthropists have recently brought renewed attention to world poverty and disease. Fund-raising and consciousness-raising are worthwhile, but there simply aren't enough qualified humanitarian workers in the world to put those funds and good intentions to work.

It is necessary to focus efforts on displaced persons, driven from their homes by disasters, natural or human-made—or a combination of both. To support displaced people takes more than money; it requires skilled workers. A humanitarian professional would need to help in crisis situations, but also know what to do in post-conflict reintegration and longer-term phases of development.

As a humanitarian professional, these are the core values:

- He cares about people outside his group.
- He sees himself as part of a larger effort.
- He is a citizen of the world, not only a country or a state.

What can he do? Here are 4 ideas:

(1) Sponsor a child, (2) volunteer to help resettlement of refugees, (3) learn about disaster preparedness, or (4) take courses in global health.

Health communication system; a study in the d.m. in east java W., H.D., TEGUHS.; M.D.

A Communication System is a subsystem in a disaster management (D.M.).

Briefly a disaster entails: (i) there are many victims many of them are in serious condition, (ii) it happens in a relatively short time, (iii) they need medical help in the shortest time possible, (iv) the existing facility and the routine mode of operation is not adequate to provide the needed help (Kaejadi *et al*).

There must be an effective Disaster Management Organisation that is able to do the following functions:

(i) It is capable to organize all available resources to respond in an effective and efficient way at any time when disaster happen, (ii) it is capable to obtain the earliest information about the occurance of disaster, (iii) it is capable to mobilize appropriate and adequate resource to respond effectively and efficiently to disaster, (iv) it is capable to coordinate the mobilized resource, (v) it acts in the shortest possible time, (vi) provides the support system viz. the communication system, the transportation system, the funding system. The Communication System that functions routinely day-to-day as a support system in the referral system is used more intensively and extensively when disaster happens. It is used to activate, mobilize and coordinate all resources involved in the disaster management.

The participating components include the hospital, the "Red Cross", the regional health officers, the armed forces, the police, the civil defense, etc.

The organisation will do all activities that are considered necessary for a successful disaster management, such as: (i) Standardization, registration and development of manpower, equipment, drugs and health facilities, (ii) Standardization, registration and development of communication and transportation system, and (iii) training and education for medical, para-medical personnel and laymen.

The role of the communication system is to activate, mobilize and Co-ordinate all the activities of the Disaster management team as given below.

The disaster management operation is done in 5 stages:

(a) The alert phase
(b) The initial phase
(c) The planning phase
(d) The operation phase
(e) The post operation/evaluation phase

The role of the communication system at those phases is:

(i) At the initial phase, to report, and give a true and correct description of the disaster such as, the location, the estimate of number of the victims, the prediction of the further development of the disaster. (ii) At the planning phase the communication system is used to inform health-units that are going to be involved at the operation stage, (iii) At the operation stage the communication system is used to coordinate the activities of the different components of the team, and (iv) At the post-operation stage the communication system is used to make a fine report that include the identification the number and the distribution of the victims in different hospitals.

The public must have access to the health unit to report the occurrence of a disaster. The health unit must have access to the public to ask for and to direct their participation.

The role of the Health Communication System

There are 2 basic role of the Health Communication System: (a) In time of no disaster it is used to support the referral system especially the referral system in Emergency Medical Service System. (b) In time of disaster it is used by the disaster team to activate, mobilize and coordinate all the activities of the different components of the team.

References

Amateur Radio Disaster Services (ARDS). American Radio Relay League. Available at: www.ares.org Accessed June 20, 2006.

American Academy of Pediatrics, American College of Emergency Physicians. Emergency information form for children with special needs. American Academy of Pediatrics, American College of Emergency Physicians. Available at: www.aap.org/advocacy/blankform.pdf Accessed June 20, 2006.

American Academy of Pediatrics. Family readiness kit. Elk Grove Village, Ill: American Academy of Pediatrics. Available at: www.aap.org/family/frk/frkit.htm Accessed June 20, 2006.

American Medical Association. Available at: http://www.ama-assn.org/ama/pub/category/6206.html Accessed January 18, 2007.

Children on the Brink 2004: A Joint Report of New Orphan Estimates and a Framework for Action. Available at: www.unicef.org Accessed January 18, 2007.

Christian Children's Fund. Available at: www.ccfusa.org Accessed January 18, 2007.

Federal Emergency Management Agency (FEMA). Are you ready? An in-depth guide to citizen preparedness. Washington, DC: FEMA. August 2004. Available at: www.fema.gov/areyouready/Accessed June 20, 2006.

Federal Emergency Management Agency (FEMA). FEMA Independent Study Programme: IS-100 Introduction to Incident Command System, I-100. Washington, DC: FEMA. Available at: www.training.fema.gov/EMIWeb/IS/is100.asp Accessed June 20, 2006.

Federal Emergency Management Agency (FEMA). FEMA Independent Study Programme: IS-700 National Incident Management System (NIMS), An Introduction. Washington, DC: FEMA. Available at: www.training.fema.gov/EMIWEB/IS/is700.asp Accessed June 20, 2006.

Federal Emergency Management Agency (FEMA). FEMA Independent Study Programme: IS-800 National Response Plan (NRP), an Introduction. Washington, DC: FEMA. Available at: http://www.training.fema.gov/EMIWEB/IS/is800.asp Accessed June 20, 2006.

Feliciano DV, Anderson GV, Rozycki GS, *et al.* Management of casualties from the bombing at the Centennial Olympics. *Am J Surg.* 1998;176:538–543.

Frykberg ER. Medical management of disasters and mass casualties from terrorist bombings: how can we cope? *J Trauma*. 2002;53:201–212. [PubMed].

Hein K. Just call us children: the impact of tsunamis, AIDS and conflict on children. American Osler Society, Inc. John P. McGovern Award Lectureship. April 2005.

Hirshberg A, Stein M, Walden R. Surgical resource utilization in urban terrorist bombing: a computer simulation. *J Trauma*. 1999;47:545–550.

Horton R. The trinity papers. *Lancet*. 2004;364:1069.

Human resources for health: overcoming the crisis. Joint Learning Initiative. *Lancet*. 2004;364:1984-1990.

International Rescue Committee. Available at: www.theIRC.org Accessed January 18, 2007.

Jacobs LM, Goody M, Sinclair A. The role of a trauma center in disaster management. *J Trauma*. 1983;23:697–701.

Johnston C, Redlener I. Critical concepts for children in disasters identified by hands-on professionals: summary of issues demanding solutions before the next one. *Pediatrics*. 2006;117:458-460.

Joint Commission on the Accreditation of Health Care Organisations. Comprehensive Accreditation Manual for Hospitals. Standard EC.1.4. Washington, DC: Joint Commission on the Accreditation of Health Care Organisations; 2006.

Mullan F, Panosian C, Cuff P, eds. Healers Abroad: Americans Responding to the Human Resource Crisis in HIV/AIDS. Washington, DC: The National Academies Press; 2005;1-125.

Slater MS, Trunkey DD. Terrorism in America: an evolving threat. Arch Surg. 1997;79:1537–1552.

Stein M, Hirshberg A. Medical consequences of terrorism: the conventional weapon threat. *Surg Clin North Am*. 1999;79:1537–1552.

US Centers for Disease Control and Prevention and the American Red Cross. Preparedness today: what you need to know. US Centers for Disease Control and Prevention and the American Red Cross. February 23, 2006. Available at: http://www.redcross.org/preparedness/cdc_english/CDC.asp Accessed June 20, 2006.

US Department of Homeland Security. Metropolitan Medical Response System (MMRS), Federal Emergency Management Agency (FEMA). Available at: www.mmrs.fema.gov/default.aspx Accessed June 20, 2006.

US Department of Homeland Security. National Disaster Medical System. US Washington, DC: Department of Homeland Security. Available at: www.ndms.dhhs.gov Accessed June 20, 2006.

World Health Organisation. Guide to Health Workforce Development in Post-Conflict Environments. NLM Classification: W 21. World Health Organisation; 2005. Available at: http://whqlibdoc.who.int/publications/2005/9241593288_eng.pdf Accessed January 19, 2007.

World Health Organisation. WHO (World Health Organisation) Humanitarian Charter and Minimum Standards: The Importance of Health Services. World Health Organisation; 2005:254-297. Available at: www.who.org Accessed January 18, 2007.

6

Management of Blast and Burn Injuries during Disaster

Let alone India, most countries of the world including USA, have insufficient critical care staff, medical equipment, burn beds and ICU space to provide timely, usual critical care to a surge of critically ill victims due to blast and burn injuries. If a mass casualty critical care event were to occur tomorrow, many people with clinical conditions that are survivable under usual health care system conditions may have to forgo life-sustaining interventions owing to deficiencies in supply or staffing. This is true of not only India, but also western countries.

INTRODUCTION

Mass Burn injuries are common among victims of terrorism and war. Since bombs are the most common weapons used by terrorists all over the world, the inevitable results are a combination of blast injuries, penetrating injuries, and burns. The main difference between war and terrorist attacks is in the targeted population—soldiers in the former, civilians in the latter. Civilians are less protected compared to soldiers and therefore are more susceptible. The fact that acts of terrorism harm the very old and the very young confronts the medical system with a case-mix that is utterly different from the one expected in war. The extreme age groups are special populations in terms of morbidity and mortality from burns, and this adds a new dimension to the treatment of burns caused by terrorist attacks, compared to war injuries. Terrorist attacks may take the form of letter bombs, suitcase bombs, car bombs or truck bombs, and suicide bombers that result in blast and burn injuries on a large scale. Blast injuries in civilian populations can also occur as a result of fireworks, household explosions, or industrial accidents. Injuries occur from the effects of the blast itself, propelled foreign bodies, or, in large blasts, from falling objects. Military blast injuries may also involve personnel submerged in water. Water increases energy transmission and the possibility of injury to the viscera of the thorax or abdomen. Crush injury results from rapid displacement of the body wall and may result in laceration and contusion of underlying structures. Minor displacements may produce serious injury if the body wall velocity is high. In addition, the motion of the body wall generates waves that propagate within the body and transfer energy to internal sites. Large explosions cause multiple foreign body impregnations, bruises, abrasions, etc. Bali terrorist bombings in October 2002 caused several such injuries. A surviving patient suffered lacerations and displacement injuries in a smaller initial blast. The two cases, closer to a larger blast in the vicinity minutes later, suffered severe immediate and ultimately fatal internal and external injuries. All three experienced significant full thickness burns and complex wound infections (Thomas Faunce).

War injuries generally involve fire and blast

In the military environment burn injury is a ubiquitous threat, and war burns have been described for more than 5,000 years of written history. Fire was probably utilized as a weapon long before that. With the ever-increasing destructive power and efficiency of modern weapons, casualties, both fatal and non-fatal, are reaching new highs, particularly among civilians who are becoming the major wartime targets in recent wars, accounting for most of the killed and wounded. Even though medical personnel usually believe that a knowledge of weaponry has little relevance to their ability to effectively treat injuries and that it may in some way be in conflict with their status, accorded under the Geneva and Hague treaties, it is imperative that they know how weapons are used and understand their effects on the human body. Burns and injuries from shrapnel fragments or small arms are the most common wounds to be expected in modern conventional conflicts. Over the last hundred years, the burn threat has ranged from small shoulder-launched missiles to nuclear weapons. Materials such as napalm and white phosphorus plainly present a risk of burn, but the threat extends to encompass also personnel in vehicles attacked by anti-armor weapons, large missiles, fuel-air explosives, and detonations/conflagrations on weapons platforms such as ships. While advances in protective gear, not available for protection of civilians, such as helmets and body armor combined with faster, more efficient battlefield medical care and even better appreciation of resuscitation and life-support measures are saving lives and getting heightened attention from both the military and the medical profession, these protective measures cannot keep soldiers from being injured or killed. The new armored Kevlar vests composed of a multiple-layer mesh of woven fabrics that soldiers are wearing in the present war in Iraq, for example, stop projectiles and bullet rounds, efficiently protecting the human torso, and have definitely saved countless lives. Unfortunately the surviving victims are often paying a terrible price and are left with serious mutilations and handicaps from burns and shrapnel wounds over body areas not protected by the vest.

Mortality is falling, morbidity is rising

Though the firepower utilized in modern-day conflicts has increased, lethality has been decreasing gradually owing to changes in the strategies and systems of battle care. In World War II, 30% of the Americans injured in combat died. In Vietnam, the proportion dropped to 24%. In the war in Iraq and Afghanistan, about 10% of those injured have died. Though burn injuries that were fatal just a few years ago no longer are so, with rapid and proper response, burns are still complicated injuries that require lengthy therapy and treatment, particularly when they are complicated by other serious injuries. As the technology of weaponry advances, the number and severity of burn injuries will certainly increase. Good management of burn injuries during armed conflicts starts with a good understanding of the mechanisms of injury and the properties and characteristics of the offending agents. Various weapons may result in a higher incidence of killed in action than others that may produce a greater incidence of burns and penetrating wounds. Kamikaze attacks for example have yielded significantly more burns than incidents involving bombs, gunfire, torpedoes, mines, and multiple other weapons, whereas mine explosions were responsible for more strains, sprains, and dislocations than the other weapon types. Even though medical personnel usually believe that a knowledge of weaponry has little relevance to their ability to effectively treat injuries and, in some way, may be in conflict with their status accorded under the Geneva and Hague treaties, it is imperative for them to understand the forces at work when casualties are sustained and how weapons are used and to understand their effects on the human body. This knowledge will allow the soldier and civil rescue worker to accurately assess the nature and extent of injuries. It also enables them to predict more accurately the number and type of casualties that may result from a combat action so that adequate medical support can be arranged and more effective treatment and evacuation decisions may be taken. The end result will certainly be a reduced death rate and morbidity; moreover, countermeasures and protective equipment can be more adequately designed.

War-related chemicals and nuclear burn injuries can be massive

The atomic detonation at Hiroshima in 1945 instantaneously generated 59,500 burn casualties. That massive number and a comparable number of burns at Nagasaki alerted the Army to burn injury as being a major problem in future conflicts, refocusing the Army's Surgical Research Unit on the problem of burns and their management. Materials such as napalm and white phosphorus plainly present a risk of burn, but the threat extends to encompass personnel in vehicles attacked by anti-armor weapons, large missiles, fuel-air explosives, and detonations/conflagrations on weapons platforms such as ships. Sulphur mustard, a vesicant blistering agent producing chemical burns, has been used extensively in the past. The potential use of mustard gas in present-day conflicts remains a significant threat that would result in a large number of casualties with severely incapacitating partial-thickness burns characterized by considerably slower wound healing.

War-related burn injuries, even among civilians, are unlikely to be the only trauma and are generally more extensive, deeper, more complicated, associated with inhalation injuries, and under-treated, compared with the "normal" case mix of accidental burns in our everyday life.

Severe burns in a battlefield setting historically had a very low salvage rate. A recent American survey of military burn casualties among personnel involved in ongoing conflicts demonstrated, however, an improved mortality rate of 5% in combat and 2% in non-combat patients. The same optimistic outcome was demonstrated in a study of the treatment of servicemen with combined burn injuries in the Chechen Republic, where the development of medical treatment systems made it possible to reduce lethality from 13.5% to 7.5%. Despite the severity of combat burns, mortality at present is low and outcomes generally good. Nevertheless, the burden on military medical services in handling burn casualties is daunting, as all the physiological systems become affected.

Unfortunately, the field of combined injury is relatively unfamiliar to burn surgeons. On the whole, the mortality and morbidity of combined injuries is higher than that of injuries separately, and awareness of the possible injury associations is critical. As an example, cervical spine injury—uncommon in burn patients, except in those injured in explosions, high-speed vehicular accidents, and falls, or by contact with high-voltage electricity—if unrecognized may result in serious morbidity, if not mortality. Moreover, burns are a "distracting injury". Treatment with narcotics of pain secondary to burns may make the clinical diagnosis of associated injuries such as spinal injury rather difficult. It is evident that special medical care practices are required to manage armed conflict burns, whether affecting civilians or military personnel, that are different from practices usually applied to treat civilian-type burns.

Burn and trauma management in warfare situations

War wounds, whether inflicted during conventional war or asymmetric warfare, as well as mass casualties, produce in general significant additional burdens and impose a heavy load on existing medical facilities and emergency, trauma, and critical care systems. Within the military institution, management of battlefield casualties constitutes the climax of any military medical activity. However, as armed conflicts are spreading and terrorist threats are not subsiding, and owing to new enhanced-blast munitions and some tactical considerations, military physicians, in addition to managing injuries of military personnel, are also required more and more to diagnose and treat mainly civilian primary blast injury casualties. Most clinicians have considered caring for victims of explosions and bombings a remote possibility unless the provider is a member of the military or an overseas aid group. That is no longer the case. Clinicians should be aware of the types of potential injury and of the appropriate management in these mass casualty situations so that definitive care can be provided to victims while utilizing hospital resources effectively.

Although there are many similarities between civilian and military trauma care, multiple additional logistic challenges unique to the combat environment cause increased difficulty in effectively managing multiply traumatized war casualties requiring a continuous chain of activities, starting with the first aid given by other servicemen and continuing with the measures taken by the medical corps men, the battalion (regimental) first-aid station, the medical company ('field ambulance'), etc. The management of civilian casualties is no different. Needless to say, in peacetime it is rare to see the wide spectrum of injury encountered during armed conflicts; hence surgeons can be unaware of optimal management protocols to be followed. The majority of military war injuries are inflicted on the battlefield, far away from advanced medical services, where evacuation to a rear hospital or even a basic medical echelon may be significantly delayed due to battle conditions, while medical teams work in life-threatening surroundings and under the emotional stress of the fighting zone. Moreover, proper medical preparedness for mass burn casualties in military conflicts requires an active commitment to the full sharing of data on burns in the multi-trauma patient.

Civil v/s Army

The circumstances of any given war and the available medical resources dictate the medical care delivered to war casualties. The sheer magnitude of casualties often requires extensive infrastructure to support the surgeons on the battlefield and to care for the wounded. In civilian practice, with optimum resources available, every burn patient receives emergency care and the seriously injured are transferred to a burn unit facility with optimum resources. In the combat setting, the tactical situation, logistical limitations, or limited availability of health care personnel may necessitate reduction in the upper limits of what is considered optimal care. Medical care also depends on the importance that cultures or circumstances place on it: on the one hand, the "precious" casualty of western armies whose medical support is organised in a concept (forward medical and surgical care, ultra-rapid medical evacuation) tailored to each case, and as close as possible to the medical care of a civilian trauma patient whose models remain the North American ballistic wound managed in trauma centers; on the other, civilian victims in large numbers in poor, disorganised countries, often abandoned to their own fate or sorted by "epidemiological" triage which guarantees as efficient as possible a distribution of limited medical care. In war, advanced medical care and precarious medicine may work side by side according to two logics which do not exclude one another. Moreover, as wars are changing in nature, military medical skills, training, and available resources must reflect these fundamental changes in preparation for future conflicts.

The treatment of local burns in the field consists of bandaging, alleviation of pain, and treatment of shock by intravenous administration of fluids. However, in mass casualty situations such as war, the fluid resuscitation of burn patients presents a formidable challenge. The possibility of overwhelming numbers of patients to be treated by inexperienced personnel dictates the adoption of a safe, simple and effective regimen that is computed in advance and displayed in simple tabular form. Smoke inhalation, with subsequent respiratory difficulties, remains frequent major problem in the initial field management of burn victims. Patients with small burns can be treated and returned to duty. Patients with a moderate burn that is all partial-thickness can be treated and then evacuated to the hospital closest to his or her home. Patients with more extensive burns associated with full-thickness skin loss can be further resuscitated and, when stable, safely evacuated. The first-aid treatment of casualties with chemical burns and imbedded phosphorus particles requires immediate care of the burn wound. The offending agent must be washed from the body surface as soon as possible with copious water lavage and removal of the identifiable particles, following which the involved areas are covered with a saline-soaked dressing and kept moistened until the patient reaches a definitive treatment installation. If the transfer is going to require more than 12 h, the involved areas should be covered with a liberal application of topical antimicrobial agent to prevent microbial proliferation and the re-ignition of retained phosphorus particles.

It has been mentioned that, in the best of circumstances, optimum treatment of war-related burn injuries results in salvage of approximately 50% of patients whose burns involve 60-70% of the total body surface in contradistinction to a salvage rate of approximately 50% of young adults with civilian-type burn injuries whose burns involve 80% of the total body surface area (TBSA) or more. With limited resources, available burn care resources should be applied to the group of patients in whom the greatest benefit will be realized, with less attention being paid to those with minor or more extensive burns. In a battlefield triage scenario with resource restrictions or large numbers of casualties, expectant care should be considered for patients with burns that exceed 80%. Care can be delayed for patients with burns of 20% or less who are otherwise stable. Available care facilities and resources must be applied to those with burns in 20-70% TBSA. With even greater restriction of health care availability, the upper limit of the maximum treatment group should be reduced by stepwise decrements of 10% until the surgical workload matches available resources. Triage modifiers include significant coexisting inhalation injury and associated mechanical injury, each of which lowers the upper limit of the maximum treatment group by 10%. Conversely, burns in the hands, face, feet, and perineum in patients with lesser TBSA burns will increase the medical care necessary for such patients.

Evacuation of battle casualties is a complex operation

Subsequently, an optimal medical-evacuation system during local armed conflicts and wars is essential. Evacuation of battle casualties is a complex operation and should be performed under medical supervision to ensure that appropriate care is given.38 Western military surgeons have at their disposal a highly sophisticated, complex transportation system for rapid patient evacuation. All medical personnel must understand this system's advantages, limits, and potential. Undoubtedly, the judicious use of aero-medical evacuation markedly reduces the time lapse from injury to definitive care. Evacuation is in two stages: initially to a first medical aid and resuscitation centre, and then to specialized medical care services (Phase Two). The decision to evacuate a patient by air to the next echelon should be made with the full knowledge of flight schedules, lag times, and the care available at each stage in the chain of evacuation. Every effort should be made to reduce the workload within the system to the essentials required for good patient care. The flight attendants should not be burdened with unnecessary dressing changes, topical medications, special diets, or other procedures that would distract them from caring for more seriously injured patients. Physicians at the originating hospital should ensure that the patient is ready to withstand the complications of the trip. Although the patient will be monitored by other physicians, it should not be assumed that they will have the opportunity to fully evaluate the patient en route. Physicians are reminded that patients with oxygenation or pulmonary-function problems at sea level may be expected to have increased difficulty at higher altitudes. For routine aero-medical evacuation the patient should have stable vital signs, no active bleeding, and adequate hydration. The importance of the inclusion of a surgeon in the aero-medical evacuation team and the usefulness of cling film as an initial burns dressing during evacuation were demonstrated by Operation Bali Assist following the Bali bomb explosions in 2002.

In combat, the tactical situation can however prevent rapid evacuation towards definitive care, or a casualty overload can tie up the surgical teams. All medical personnel and their supporting cadre should therefore be able to manage wounds and burns. Controlling bleeding and airways, cleaning and debriding wounds, and dressing or splinting injuries are essential knowledge as well as training for enlisted and officer personnel in all medical departments. Experience of a UK reserve field surgical hospital during military operations in Iraq in March/April 2003 demonstrated the importance of the integration of surgical specialties and of consultant-led and multidisciplinary team-working in the treatment of military and civilian casualties from all sources and of all causes. The close integration of general, orthopedic, plastic-reconstructive, maxillofacial, ophthalmic, and neurological surgeons and general and intensive treatment unit and anesthetists allowed the delivery of a range of specialist treatment to a heterogeneous patient population, including children as young as 6 months and a lady in the advanced stages of pregnancy. The range of casualties treated by the Defence Medical Services in the recent Gulf conflict reaffirmed the important role of plastic and reconstructive surgery within the military.

Mass burn injuries, psychological health, and the treating team

Psychological problems are a frequent component of burn injury. Burn victims often display symptoms that can impede recovery, causing severe long-term impairment, both physical and psychological.68 Psychiatric problems frequently seen in burn patients are depression and post-traumatic stress disorder (PTSD), characterized by a fear reaction during the trauma and subsequent intrusions, avoidance, and hyper-arousal. The rate of PTSD among burn victims varies between 9 and 35% at 2 to 4 months after the burn injury. Unfortunately, the extent to which psychological factors such as coping style predict the psychological outcome for burn patients is not well understood. The true incidence of post-traumatic stress disorder after combat burn injury also remain important unresolved question. Nevertheless, a variety of services must be provided at any burns centre. It is important to provide families with free lodgings near the burns care facility. Soldiers should be supported by events such as award ceremonies and visits by military leaders and dignitaries. It is generally believed that having the burns service members grouped in one location facilitates this type of support and probably has intangible benefits from a morale standpoint.

Although physicians, nurses, and paramedical personnel routinely deal with crises, the rapid influx of patients with multiple burns, particularly in the context of conventional or asymmetric warfare, tests the adaptability of any medical facility as well as the physical and psychological stamina of the treating team. During the crisis, the emergency team usually encounters a surreal treatment environment and has little time to understand the magnitude of the unfolding disaster. Despite frequently uncomfortably hot conditions in a crowded emergency facility or department and pungent odors of burned flesh and toxic residue, the staff usually remains focused on the basics and clinical aspects of patient trauma care. It is only after the acute crisis has passed that the full-blown emotional impact on the emergency staff becomes manifest. Usually nurses repeatedly speak about the overwhelming psychological effects of seeing so many severely burned patients. Nevertheless, the psychological trauma of the emergency treating team is unfortunately not really appreciated.

The status of trauma ICU or burns unit staff is not very different. Doctors, nurses, and various members of the health care team, all of whom spend a considerable amount of their time in intense interactions with patients, are vulnerable to various visual and psychological stressors. However, the majority of staff working in the stressful environment of a burns unit associated with chronic occupational stressors do not experience emotional exhaustion and do not seem to have a high incidence of burnout syndrome, which is characterized by emotional exhaustion, depersonalization, and reduced personal accomplishment. Nevertheless, promotion of staff morale and emotional support to frontline clinicians and nurses are of utmost importance. Trauma ICU nurses usually find patient care to be physically demanding, particularly with time-consuming burn dressings. Patients' rooms are generally kept warm and nurses are required to wear gowns, gloves, and face masks when providing care, which makes staying in the patients' rooms rather laborious. Despite this, nurses find it difficult to leave the burns unit at the end of their shifts. Many have guilt feelings about not being available longer to assist colleagues and some prefer to keep busy rather than think about the experience. Nurses may be emotionally resilient because they care for trauma patients every day, which helps to contain the emotional distress of witnessing mass suffering; however, young staff usually identifies with young burn victims, and may require emotional support from colleagues. As patients start to recover, the treating team is faced also with providing them with psychological support, which is emotionally draining. Although some staff members suffer no overt psychiatric consequences, most suffer transient acute stress symptoms, including irritability, restlessness, sleep disturbance, mood lability, fatigue, and intrusive imagery. These symptoms generally resolve rapidly and do not require psychiatric intervention, but a few staff that are directly involved in caring for the burn patients do suffer an acute exacerbation of past trauma symptoms or unresolved grief. All these symptoms and manifestations are naturally amplified in an armed conflict situation, which carries its inherent stressor factors.

Prevention of war injuries and burns

In wartime, all possible strategies need to be undertaken to minimize and prevent injuries. Perhaps the only true benefit of war is the higher standards of trauma care it forces us to develop and pass on to succeeding generations. Unfortunately, the threat from war burns is unlikely to diminish; indeed, new developments in weapons seek to exploit the vulnerability of the serviceman and servicewoman to burns. Clothing can be a barrier to some types of burns, not only inherently in the properties of the material but also by trapping air between clothing layers. Conversely, ignition of the clothing may exacerbate a burn. Even light-weight combat clothing can offer significant protection to skin from short-duration flash burns; the most vulnerable areas are the parts of the body that are not covered,, i.e. the face and hands. In one study, 98% of tank crewmen who sustained burn injuries were wearing fireproof suits at the time. Only 12% of them sustained abdominal burns whereas 77% had facial burns, as none of them were wearing fireproof masks. Only 9% of the burned soldiers who wore fireproof gloves sustained hand burns, compared with 75% who did not wear the gloves. Wearing protective suits increased the percentage of minor burns from 21 to 51% and reduced the percentage of burns greater than 40%, TBSA from 29 to 18%. Multilayered combat clothing can offer significant protection for short periods from engulfment by flames, whereas lightweight tropical wear with few layers offers little protection. However, under high heat loads in the laboratory, combat clothing can ignite, even though there is little evidence that clothing ignition is a common occurrence in military burn casualties. Thermoplastic materials, however, have many benefits in civil and military clothing. There is little objective evidence that they exacerbate burns or complicate burns management. Their use in military clothing must be based on objective evidence, not hearsay.

An unprecedented burden of what orthopedists term "mangled extremities", with severe limb soft-tissue, bone, and often vascular injuries, have also been noticed in association with wearing the standard Kevlar cloth ballistic vest. This, however, must not be construed as a reason for not using the vest; on any conceivable battlefield, the risk of being wounded by fragments far outweighs the threat of primary blast injury. Rather, the triaging physician must use this information to recognize that soldiers near an explosion may have had their lives saved by the vest but that primary blast injury to the lungs and abdomen may complicate their condition.

New approaches are needed to minimize trauma to civilians. Lessons learned from Bosnia and Lebanon show that the most effective way to achieve successful surveillance and injury prevention is to enhance local skills and resources. Both political advocacy and local efforts are needed. The use of incendiary weapons such as white phosphorus shells and napalm against civilian targets is banned by international treaties. Article 2, protocol III, of the 1980 UN Convention on Certain Conventional Weapons states: "It is prohibited in all circumstances to make the civilian population as such, individual civilians or civilian objects, the object of attack by incendiary weapons". Moreover, as chemical warfare has been widely condemned since it was first used on a massive scale during the First World War, some have claimed that the use of white phosphorus contravenes the 1993 Chemical Weapons Convention, which bans the use of any "toxic chemical" weapons which causes "death, harm or temporary incapacitation to humans or animals through their chemical action on life processes". Surprisingly, this opinion is not widely shared. A spokesman for the Organisation for the Prohibition of Chemical Weapons, which enforces the Convention, stated recently that the Convention permitted the use of such weapons for "military purposes not connected with the use of chemical weapons and not dependent on the use of the toxic properties of chemicals as a method of warfare", claiming that the burns caused by white phosphorus shells were thermal in nature rather than chemical and as such are not prohibited by the treaty.

Children bear disproportionate consequences of armed conflict

The twenty-first century continues to see patterns of children enmeshed in international violence between opposing combatant forces, as victims of terrorist warfare, and, perhaps most tragically of all, as victims of civil wars. Innocent children so often are the victims of high-energy wounding from military ordinance. They sustain high-energy tissue damage and massive burns. Children have also been deliberately targeted victims in genocidal civil wars in Africa in the past decade, and hundreds of thousands have been killed and maimed in the context of close-quarter, hand-to-hand assaults of great ferocity. One chronic legacy of contemporary warfare is blast injury to children from landmines. In many parts of the world, un-detonated military incendiary devices such as land mines and hand grenades contaminate the sites of abandoned battlefields. Such devices cause significant numbers of civilian casualties years and even decades after local hostilities cease. On the other hand, PTSD remains an under-treated legacy of children who have been trapped in the shot and shell of battle in addition to those displaced as refugees. The increase in, and plight of, child soldiers themselves has also been an urgent, unfocused, and unmet challenge. A new class of combatant comprises these children, who also become enmeshed in the triad of anarchic civil war, light-weight weaponry, and drug or alcohol addiction. The International Criminal Court has outlawed as a War Crime the conscription of children less than 15 years of age. Nevertheless, there remain more than 300,000 child soldiers active and enmeshed in psychopathic violence as part of both civil and international warfare. Only by vigorous and maintained advocacy of the rights and welfare of children in the context of the evolving 'Laws of War' can the world's children be better protected from the scourge of future wars.

In an effort to determine whether new medical technologies or enhanced training might contribute to a reduction in armed-conflict-related deaths, the causes of possible death viewed as most likely to be salvageable today include, among a few other conditions, severe burns, while the areas of training most often mentioned as having a potential impact on salvageability include burns management. Military medicine personnel must be aware that more time, energy, and material need to be spent on burn treatment as we enter the next millennium. The magnitude of the improvement in prognosis of burn casualties, and the velocity with which it has occurred, document the effectiveness of integrated clinical/laboratory research.

Types of injuries caused by an explosion

Overall, blast injuries result in mortality ranging between 7.8 percent in open air to 49 percent in a confined space. A majority of victims (70 percent) will sustain soft tissue injury, and traumatic amputations will occur in approximately 11 percent of cases. There are four general types of injuries caused by an explosion: (1) direct blast injuries—primary injuries, (2) injuries caused by flying objects accelerated by the explosion—secondary injuries, (3) injuries sustained by the victim's movement—tertiary injuries, and (4) miscellaneous injuries caused by the explosion or the explosives.

Injury patterns following an explosion are random and are affected by a number of factors including the nature of the explosive, its container, barriers between the explosive and the victim, and distance from the explosion.

There are two general types of explosives—high-order and low-order. Each type of explosive will create slightly different injury patterns. High-order explosives are chemicals with a very high rate of reaction. These chemicals include nitroglycerin, dynamite, C-4, and a mixture of ammonium nitrate and fuel oil. On detonation, the chemical is converted into a gas at a very high temperature and pressure. For example, an explosion of one-quarter pound block of C4 can generate an initial pressure of four million pounds per square inch (psi), a blast wave that expands outward in all directions. Low order injuries would be less deadly.

Several types of injuries can result from an explosion. These injuries include immediate death, primary injuries, secondary injuries, tertiary injuries, and miscellaneous injuries.

Immediate death

Death from an explosion can be instantaneous and result from massive pulmonary hemorrhage accompanied by rapid suffocation. Other causes of immediate death from an explosion include pulmonary air embolism, significant head injury, exsanquination from a traumatic injury, crush injury, and impalement. Because of the blast wave and its damage, the patient dies in spite of immediate and high-quality care. EMTs and paramedics should consider death in any victim of an explosion under the following conditions:

- Traumatic amputation along with absent vital signs.
- Absence of effective ventilation or pulse.
- Severe respiratory insufficiency cause by a blast effect.

Primary blast injuries

Primary blast injuries result from the blast wave created by high-order explosions and have an overall incidence of 20 percent. The extent of the injuries will depend on several factors, including—

- Peak pressure of the initial blast wave.
- Duration of over-pressurization.
- Medium in which the explosion occurs.
- Distance from the source of the explosion.

Primary blast injuries commonly affect the ear, respiratory system, and gastrointestinal system. The brain and cardiovascular system may also be affected. In the ear, the eardrum typically ruptures, especially when the overpressure exceeds 5 psi. With extremely high overpressures, the eardrum may be destroyed and the ossicles (bony structures) can be dislocated or fractured. At lower pressures, the eardrum may bleed without rupture. Signs and symptoms of eardrum rupture include pain, loss of hearing, and tinnitus. Blood may be present in the ear canal. The respiratory system can sustain significant injury typically as a result of supersonic pressure caused by the blast wave. Over-pressurization at 40 psi will cause pulmonary injury such as pneumo-thorax, air embolism, interstitial emphysema, pneuo-mediastinum, and subcutaneous emphysema. Pulmonary contusion is most common and generally found on the side of the body that was closest to the explosion. A patient who survives the initial explosion may develop "blast lung" immediately, but signs and symptoms can be delayed up to 48 hours after the event.

Blast injury to the gastrointestinal tract should be suspected in anyone exposed to an explosion with signs and symptoms that include abdominal pain, nausea, vomiting, hematemesis, rectal pain, testicular pain, unexplained hypo-volemia, and any finding suggesting an acute abdomen. The colon is the most common site of hemorrhage and perforation. The perforated bowel may be immediately evident or may perforate after a delay of up to 48 hours. Solid organ laceration and testicular rupture are also seen with primary blast injury, but are less frequent and often associated with large blast loads.

Primary blast injury can cause concussion or traumatic brain injury, although this finding is difficult to differentiate from a concussion because of impact with another object. Myocardial contusion accompanied by signs of dys-rhythmia or hypotension may develop.

Secondary blast injuries

These are caused by debris propelled by the blast wind of the explosion, resulting in both penetrating and blunt trauma. Individuals far from the scene of an explosion can be struck and injured by this debris. For example, after the 1998 terrorist bombing of the U.S. Embassy in Nairobi, flying glass wounded victims up to 2 kilometers away. Terrorist devices often have additional objects such as nails, nuts, and bolts added to the explosive mixture to increase the effects of secondary blast injury. Military devices such as shells and grenades may be designed in such a way as to

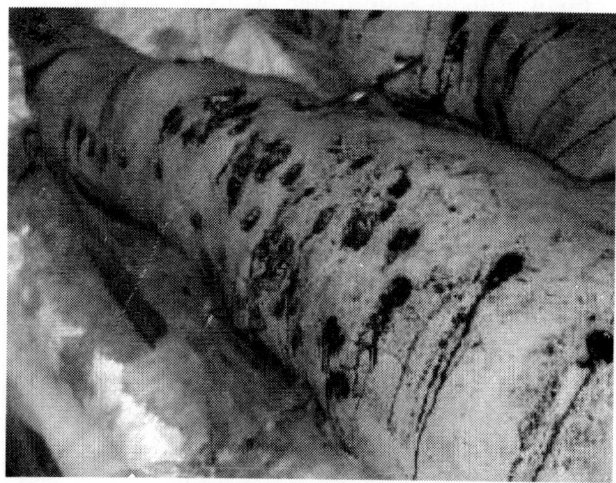

increase the number of fragments flung by the explosion. Secondary blast injuries are much more common than primary blast injuries and are the most common causes of death in blast victims. The penetrating injuries occur most often in the exposed areas of the body such as the head, neck, and extremities.

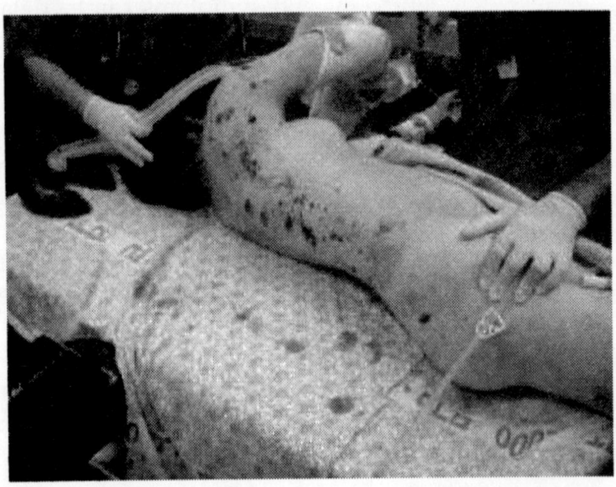

Secondary blast injuries may not be initially obvious. A seemingly small abrasion or wound may mask the entrance wound for a large fragment.

Tertiary blast injuries

These are caused when the victim's body is propelled into another object by the blast winds. Tertiary effects result from the bulk flow of gas away from the explosion and often occur when the victim is in close proximity to the explosion. However, these injuries can take place relatively far from the point of detonation if the victim is located in the path of gases venting from a structure, such as a doorway, window, or hatch. Likewise, if the patient is in an alley, magnification of the blast wind may occur because of the configuration of the buildings.

Injuries from this mechanism depend on what the victim strikes and can range from simple contusions to impalement. Victims may tumble along the ground sustaining abrasions, contusions, and "road-rash."

Miscellaneous injuries

These include burns from fire or radiation, crush injury associated with structural collapse, poisoning from carbon monoxide or other toxic products of the explosion, and inhalation of dust or chemicals from the explosion. The unprotected human body can survive a blast with a peak overpressure of 30 psi, but buildings and other structures collapse with stress of only a few pounds per square inch. This means that persons can survive the effects of the blast only to be injured by collapsing buildings. Finally, the blast may be a vector for chemical warfare agents and biological warfare agents and result in a myriad of medical complaints.

Pre-hospital Considerations

The predominant injuries found after an explosion will be penetrating and blunt trauma. Because the initial signs and symptoms of significant blast injury can be subtle, the early presentation of victims can be deceiving. Blast lung injury is the most common fatal injury among initial survivors of the blast. Pre-hospital medical care can follow some simple guidelines:

- Initial care is similar to regular trauma care.
- Ear and GI injuries do not need special care in the field.
- Rapid evacuation increases the chance of survival.
- Follow the principles of disaster management—do not treat during triage.
- Resuscitation efforts in the field should be minimal—CPR at the scene of a mass-casualty event is not indicated.

An explosion that occurs in a confined space (vehicles, mines, buildings, and subways) is associated with greater morbidity and mortality. If the structure collapses, this markedly increases the mortality. Experience has shown that terrorists will often set a second device timed to explode 30 to 100 minutes after the first device has detonated. This second device is designed to injure EMS, fire, and police personnel who may be at the scene. In some cases, the perpetrator of the explosion may be watching over the area of the explosion and either remotely detonate the second explosive or employ high-powered rifle fire to injure or kill responders. It is also important to check all victims for weapons, booby traps, and explosives. It is quite common for a bomber to become a victim of his own device.

Evaluation and Management

The most important step of management is assessment of life support needs and ensuring that the patient has an adequate airway, ventilation, and circulation. A thorough physical examination should be performed if time and resources permit. Unfortunately, when the EMS provider is faced with dramatic injuries such as amputations, fragment injuries, and multiple critically ill patients, it is easy to miss the subtle signs of blast injury. For each patient, attempt to determine the distance from the explosion and whether they were in open air, in an enclosed space, or in water is made. If the patient was wearing body armor, this should also be noted. Body armor increases the chance and severity of primary blast injury but provides significant protection against fragment injuries. Distance obviously decreases the risk of primary blast injury. If the patient was in water, this should be noted; the suspicion for intra-abdominal blast injury is heightened.

After ensuring the initial Assessment, supplemental oxygen and IV fluids should be administered. Additionally, the EMS provider should be prepared to treat pneumothorax, hypotension, and air embolism until the patient is turned over to the emergency department.

Experiences of bomb attack on trains in Madrid, Spain

On Thursday, 11 March 2004, terrorist bombs attacked Spain, which led to one of the most calamitous mass injury situations of its kind in Europe during recent decades. Ten bags containing charges of TNT were detonated in four commuter trains at rush hour. The explosions took place between 07:39 and 07:42, and all emergency services were immediately alerted. Most critical body system injuries are found among those who are killed immediately, and these are the same body system injuries that most commonly cause death in all other forms of trauma. The most important means of preparing for the large casualty loads caused by bombing disasters is to understand the patterns of injuries and logistical problems that result. A retrospective analysis of implemented organisation and clinical management can identify helpful decisions and errors.

They defined as 'critical' any casualty presenting with an acute airway, or breathing, circulatory or neurological problems that required immediate surgical intervention and/or admission to an intensive care unit (ICU), and all patients admitted with endo-tracheal intubation. Blast lung injury (BLI) was diagnosed on the basis of hypoxaemia and characteristic radiographic lung opacities, with or without pneumothorax, and absence of rib fractures or chest wall injury.

Initial emergency treatment and triage was carried out by emergency medical services near the scenes of the blasts, and the victims were subsequently transferred to hospitals. The vast majority of survivors were evacuated by ambulance and many others by private vehicles.The explosions resulted in 2062 casualties, 177 (8.6%) of whom were killed immediately. There were 14 subsequent deaths (in-hospital deaths), which occurred either on the same day or later on, among 82 victims who were reported to be in a critical condition at 21:00 on that day, bringing the total death toll to 191 and the overall 'critical mortality' rate to 17%.

With over 70,000 health personnel involved, 291 ambulances for transport, 200 firemen, 13 groups of psychologists, 500 volunteers, thousands of donations of blood at hospitals and in 10 mobile units, and 1725 blood donors from other regions of the country. The 112 emergency communication centers received more than 20,000 phone calls during the morning of the blasts. By 31 March 2004, only 30 patients remained hospitalized, five of whom were in a critical condition.

GMUGH, a 1800-bed teaching public hospital, serving a population of more than 650,000 people, and located in the centre of Madrid, received the first victim, who walked into the emergency department (ED) suffering from an ear blast injury.

Immediate action was taken to cancel all scheduled surgical

interventions in the 22 available rooms, and 161 hospitalized patients were discharged home from the various wards in under 2 hours. A number of patients in the ICU and surgical

ICU, with 28 beds in total, were evacuated to intermediate care units, as deemed appropriate. The recovery room, with a maximum capacity of 10–12 beds and adjacent to the surgical ICU, was also made available to receive critically ill patients. The 123 patients who were kept under observation at the ED at 07.30, before the blasts occurred, were either discharged home when appropriate or transferred to the wards, and only 10 of them remained in the ED at 09.30. All elective diagnostic procedures were deferred. At the same time, the Teaching Pavillion, adjacent to the ED, was used as an information center for the families, authorities and the media.

Triage was performed by senior faculty members at the entrance to the ED and continued until around 10.30. Two patients were directly taken for surgery, and most intubated patients and those who looked to be critically ill were immediately taken to the adjacent 'shock room' and other nearby rooms for primary survey and resuscitation, in accordance with Advanced Trauma Life Support protocols.

Teams of general surgeons and anesthesiologists examined all of the critically ill patients initially, and the need for further examination by sub-specialty teams such as orthopedic, neurosurgical, cardiovascular, thoracic, maxillofacial and plastic surgical teams was determined. All patients were examined, at some time during the day or later, by ear, nose and throat teams to rule out injury to the tympanic membrane.

Out of more than 27 victims assessed in the shock rooms, seven haemodynamically unstable patients were immediately taken for surgery and the others were triaged to radiology departments or ICUs. In these units, further assessment was undertaken and additional patients sent for surgery. Minor casualties were triaged to different areas of the ED for assessment, wound dressing and suturing. Focused abdominal sonography for trauma was performed in 37 patients during the first 3 hours, at different rooms and units, and 40 spiral computed tomography scans had been done by the end of the day, as well as 270 plain radiographs and three vascular interventional radiology procedures. The blood bank delivered 145 units of type-specific blood during the day (90 of them in the first 4 hours), 60 units of fresh frozen plasma and 75 units of platelets. The absence of previous experience with a mass casualty event of that proportion was probably counterbalanced by the commitment of every person directly or indirectly involved in the treatment of victims and by spontaneous leadership assumed in different areas. All in all, common sense, diligence in triage of patients and serenity seemed to prevail after the initial chaos and emotional trauma, which are unavoidable and common to such situations. There was in fact an abundance of medical teams, nursing staff and resources to treat the critically injured, and no critically injured patient experienced a delay in treatment.

Injuries sustained, mortality and surgical interventions

Many of the 243 assessed casualties were walking wounded and their injuries were minor-to-moderate, requiring only simple dressing or sutures, but some wounds were grossly contaminated and with much tissue loss. The most frequent injuries found in the 243 victims were tympanic membrane perforations, chest injuries, shrapnel wounds and fractures.

No patients were dead on arrival, but five died subsequently, two of them shortly after admission. One of the latter was a moribund patient who died at the ED within minutes of her arrival, probably from severe head trauma. Another died with an open cranial wound while being readied for surgical intervention. A third patient died in the ICU at 10:30 from bilateral lung contusion and a thoracic aorta tear. A fourth victim died on that morning while undergoing damage control.

laparotomy. The only death in a patient who had survived for more than 24 hours was due to multiple organ failure, and this death occurred on the day 7 after admission. She was 22 years old, and had with bilateral hemo-pneumothorax and lung contusion, maxillofacial fractures and avulsion of the left ear, apart from first-degree and second-degree burns. The five fatalities are included in the critical care group of 29 patients, and so the critical mortality rate was 17.2%.

Many procedures required collaboration among different surgical specialties, and soft tissue and musculoskeletal injuries accounted for almost 50% of all operations performed. Twenty-seven critically ill patients survived initially to be admitted to ICUs; as mentioned above, three of these patients died. Of all critically ill patients 67% presented with ear blast injuries, and in eight patients the damage to the tympanic membrane was combined with burns and avulsions of the ear. Twenty-four critical patients had lung lesions; 17 of them had BLI and seven had lung damage associated with injury to the chest wall. These lung injuries were bilateral in 71% of all cases. Of all critically ill patients 80% required mechanical ventilation for respiratory failure or coma, and 37% were mechanically ventilated for more than 7 days.

According to computed tomography scans, the severity of head injuries was assessed as severe in 60%, moderate in 13% and mild in 27% of the critically ill patients. Fractures to the base of the skull and brain contusions were the most common findings, whereas subarachnoid haemorrhage and brain swelling were also frequent. Ten critically ill patients had abdominal injuries, and half of them underwent surgical treatment. One-third of this critically ill population suffered fractures to extremities. Of these 60% were open and often associated with gross soft tissue damage. They were evenly distributed in the upper and lower limbs. Almost as many patients had maxillofacial fractures. Traumatic amputation of one ear proved to be a marker of severity, and only one critically ill patient arrived with a major traumatic amputation of the left lower limb. Four patients (15%), all of them severely wounded, presented with eye lesions. Three of them were very severe, with one traumatic unilateral enucleation, two blast eyes with intraocular haemorrhage, and two perforations with an intraocular foreign body, each resulting in partial or total loss of sight.

Major causes of injuries

The three major causes of injuries in such incidents include the blast effect or shock wave, flash burns from the heat of the explosion, and penetrating wounds from the ballistic effects of the shrapnel. Among survivors at GMUGH, soft tissue, musculoskeletal and ear blast injuries predominated in up to 80% of cases, but mostly they were noncritical in severity and contributed virtually nothing to mortality. There were multiple contaminated wounds containing various debris and fragments. Wound debridement in these patients was necessary to prevent infection and accounted for more than a third of all operations performed in the first 24 hours. The incidence of critical injuries among survivors varies between 9% and 22%. Chest and abdominal injuries, including BLI, and traumatic amputations occur very infrequently among survivors of bombings, because the most critical cases are selected out by the initial blast, succumbing to immediate death. However, the few surviving patients with these injuries have a substantial specific mortality, and these injuries should be recognized as prognostic markers of severity. Most victims of primary BLI from explosions are killed immediately, and late deaths among the small number of survivors with this injury are caused by progressive pulmonary insufficiency, which has all the radiographic and pathologic signs of parenchymal haemorrhage, similar to blunt contusions. The 63% incidence (17 cases) of BLI seen in our critically ill patients, which is higher than previously reported, probably reflects a bias in triage of many severely wounded patients, which was closest to the blasts. In a similar way, the ear—an organ that is very sensitive to blast injury—was damaged at a percentage similar to that for lung. Emotional shock is a common consequence of terrorist bombings. Although is not as lethal as physical injury, there is significant potential for long-term psychological disability.

An analysis of the patterns of injury and death from this event corroborates some important principles regarding disaster management. Most survivors had no critical injuries. The high immediate death rate, and the high dead/critically wounded ratio of >2:1 was probably because of the extreme magnitude of the explosive force at an indoor location, as observed by others. In Madrid the bombings occurred shortly before the start of a midweek work day when most clinicians and medical personnel were on their way to work or already at the hospital, and night shifts were still on duty. This, together with empty operating rooms and personnel waiting for the first scheduled cases, proved decisive as regards the adequacy of the medical and surgical response at GMUGH and other hospitals. Had the blasts occurred just 1 hour later, then the whole situation would have been much worse and very difficult to cope with.

Burn Trauma Disaster; West Pharmaceutical Plant Explosion

On January 29, 2003, an explosion occurred at the West Pharmaceutical chemical plant in Kinston, North Carolina. A volunteer fire fighter working at the plant immediately notified the explosion and requested assistance via his VHF radio because phone lines were lost in the explosion. Local emergency medical services (EMS) were immediately dispatched, and North Carolina Emergency Management was notified of the event and told of a potential for more than 200 victims. The initial cause was thought to be a plane crash because of radio communications reporting an employee had noticed a plane flying over the plant just minutes before the explosion. Preliminary findings indicate that the explosion was caused by the accumulation and dispersion of fine polyethylene powder that collected above a suspended ceiling. Initial attempts to decontaminate victims were cumbersome and difficult, and given reports that hazardous exposure was not expected, further attempts at decontamination were not pursued.

The explosion killed three people at the scene and resulted in more than 30 admissions to area hospitals. The disaster resulted in 10 critically ill burn patients, who were all intubated with inhalation injuries, many with combined burn and trauma injuries. All 10 critically injured patients were admitted to a tertiary care facility 100 miles away with both a Level I trauma center and a verified burn center. Ultimately, 7 of 10 patients survived (a mortality rate of 30%), and none were transferred to another trauma or burn center (Bruce, A. *et al.*). Burns occurred in only a small number of survivors, yet burns were a major determinant of late deaths and had the highest specific mortality (40% mortality) among all types of injury. Most combined burn and trauma patients required intensive care unit admission (55%). Furthermore, patients with combined burn and trauma had the longest hospital stay. One of the greatest challenges in caring for a combined burn trauma patient occurs at the scene where triage decisions are made. Is this primarily a burn patient or a trauma patient? Should they be taken care of in a burn center or in a trauma center or only in a combined burn–trauma center? Who makes the decision?

A review of the national trauma center inventory suggests that there is a substantial geographic disparity of trauma centers across the United States, with the greatest concern being in rural and medically underserved areas. Given that burns are frequently a component of traumatic disasters, it follows that RACs would also be responsible for the triage and care of combined burn trauma patients within their own region.

Lenoir Memorial hospital set-up an external triage area outside their emergency department and received the bulk of the walking wounded. Although many patients were treated only at the outside triage area and were not seen inside the Emergency Department, a significant number of patients were triaged into the Emergency Department (approximately 27), resulting in 16 admissions, 2 of whom were intubated for critical burn injuries while awaiting transfer to UNC Hospitals' North Carolina Jaycee

Burn Center. There were four critically injured patients transferred to the Level I trauma center at Pitt County Memorial Hospital and four critically injured burn patients transferred directly from the scene to UNC Hospitals using helicopter transport. There appeared to be little knowledge of how to activate the regional disaster response. Overall, the communication among the scene, transport systems, and UNC Hospitals has to be characterized as poor.

By 2:50 PM (1 hour after the explosion), the UNC Hospitals' Incident Command Center had been set-up so that by the time the first patient arrived, the hospital was at disaster level operations. This included canceling elective operations; holding and recalling staff; organizing disaster teams; notifying security, pharmacy, and the blood bank; triaging patients from the Emergency Room; and planning for contingent intensive care unit admissions. The medical director of the burn center called surrounding Region IV burn centers, as well as the American Burn Association Central Office, to arrange for additional burn beds should it appear that our burn center would become overwhelmed. These beds were arranged and ready when the first patient arrived from the scene at 4:12 PM (2 hours and 35 minutes after the explosion), followed by five additional patients by 5:15 PM

Hospital Course

A total of 10 patients were received at UNC Hospitals: 6 patients were directly admitted to the Burn Center, 2 were admitted to the surgical intensive care unit and, using intensive care unit (ICU) bed contingency plans, 1 was admitted to the cardiothoracic intensive care unit and 1 was admitted to the neurosurgical intensive care unit. All patients were critically injured, intubated with inhalation injuries, and had burn injuries ranging from 16% to 62% TBSA. Two patients had associated orthopedic injuries; two patients had associated abdominal injuries, one requiring exploratory laparotomy and splenectomy; and one had an associated closed head injury with a non-operative intracranial hematoma. Patients underwent an average of 3.5 to 2.4 operations. Seven patients survived to discharge, with an average length of stay of 48 days (range, 15–136 days), whereas three patients died, all with combined burn trauma, resulting in a critical mortality rate of 30%. A total of six patients developed deep venous thromboses, two patients developed cholecystitis requiring tube placement, and two patients developed adrenal failure requiring treatment with corticosteroids, one of whom died.

During the first 24 hours, regrouping, communication, and coordination of care, especially in non-Burn Center hospital ICU units that had received patients, was the first priority of the physicians responsible for their care. One issue that was discussed was whether the hospitals had overwhelmed their resources in keeping all 10 of the critically injured burn patients. The burn center was now exceeding its 11-bed ICU census by an additional 4 patients, and the surgical team caring for all 25 burn patients was involved in the management of the entire disaster the night before. In addressing this, one concern was which patient would be an optimal candidate for transfer. Several patients were clearly too unstable for transfer, whereas a number appeared to have fairly minimal injuries (for a critically injured burn patient) and would be expected to be extubated soon. In the end, the physicians responsible decided they could care for all the patients they had accepted, although clearly the system was stressed.

Overall burn center staff resources and hospital staffing pool (especially nursing) were taxed; however, a willing stream of staff volunteers worked to alleviate care delivery concerns. Coordination to assist the families through Family Support Services was established, with food and accommodations a priority. Families were able to stay close by and for the most part many commuted the 2-hour drive from Kinston to Chapel Hill while their loved one was in the hospital. Although the needs of these 10 critical patients were met, the resources at our institution were clearly and almost entirely maximized. Despite this, during the next 30 days, we were still able to accommodate an additional 28 admissions to the burn center: 12 to the ICU and 16 to the floor. This sustained effort resulted in a staffing increase from 7 to 8 caregivers per shift to 13 to 14 per shift. The increase was covered by 360 hours overtime at a cost of $22,177; 47 additional 12-hour shifts; additional agency and traveler nursing support at a cost of $48,011; conversion of nursing administration to patient care; 660 12-hour registered nurse shifts; and two nurses who postponed vacations. Morale during this time remained extremely high and was associated with only 9 missed shifts for the month, a remarkable 0.01% call out rate. Although the institution's response to the increased workload was impressive, it also was unsustainable over a long period of time.

"Witness after witness testified that despite 9/11, the private sector remains largely unprepared for a terrorist attack." Although North Carolina has one of the most advanced regional trauma systems in the United States, a lack of education, communication, and coordination continue to hamper their ability to efficiently and optimally respond to mass casualty events and, as the 9/11 Commission's report attests, it seems they are not alone in this critical assessment. As the experience with the West Pharmaceutical chemical plant explosion demonstrates, North Carolina and, as an extension, the entire United States, still has a number of issues to resolve before it can claim that it is prepared for a disaster. However, progress is being made. The state regional trauma system continues to expand and is becoming more organised. Members of the burn community are now active participants on the American College of Surgeons Committee on Trauma for North Carolina. Improved management of combined burn trauma patients after an explosion will depend on a number of factors. First, there must be a concerted effort to continue to identify, integrate, and improve burn and trauma-related resources on a state, regional, and national scale.

References

Aboutanos M.B., Baker S.P.: Wartime civilian injuries: Epidemiology and intervention strategies. *J. Trauma*, 43: 719-26, 1997.

Almogy G, Belzberg H, Mintz Y, *et al.* Suicide bombing attacks: update and modifications to the protocol. *Ann Surg* 2004;239:295–303.

American Psychiatric Association: "Diagnostic and Statistical Manual of Mental Disorders", 4th ed., Pilgrim Press, Washington, DC, 1994.

Armenian H.K.: Perceptions from epidemiologic research in an endemic war. Soc. Sci. Med., 28: 643-7, 1989.

Arnold J., Halpern P., Ming-Che T., Smithline H.: Mass casualty bombings: A comparison of outcomes by bombing type. *Ann. Emerg. Med.*, 43: 263-73, 2004.

Atiyeh B.S., Gunn S.W.A., Hayek S.N.: Armed conflicts and burn injuries. *Ann. Burns and Fire Disasters*, 18: 45-6, 2005.

Badger J.M.: A nurse's perspective on a nightclub fire: Fostering resilience during a disaster response. *Am. J. Nursing*, 104: 72AA-72FF, 2004.

Baker M.S.: Management of soft-tissue wounds, burns, and hand injuries in the field setting. *Mil. Med.*, 161: 469-71, 1996.

Barillo D.J., Cancio L.C., Hutton B.G., Mittelsteadt P.J. *et al.*: Combat burn life support: A military burn-education programme. *J. Burn Care Rehabil.*, 26: 162-5, 2005.

Bellamy R.F., Zajtchuk R.: The weapons of conventional land warfare. In: "Textbook of Military Medicine", Vol. 5, 1-52, Office of the Surgeon General, Department of the Army, Washington, DC, 1990.

Bhatnagar M.K., Curtis M.J., Smith G.S.: Musculoskeletal injuries in the Afghan war. *Injury*, 23: 545-8, 1992.

Biancolini CA, Del Bosco CG, Jorge MA: Argentine Jewish com- munity institution bomb explosion. *J Trauma* 1999, 47:728-732

Blood C.G., Puyana J.C., Pitlyk P.J., Hoyt D.B. *et al.*: An assessment of the potential for reducing future combat deaths through medical technologies and training. *J. Trauma*, 53: 1160-5, 2002.

Blood C.G.: Analyses of battle casualties by weapon type aboard U.S. Navy warships. *Mil. Med.*, 157: 124-30, 1992.

Borden Institute—The Textbooks of Military Medicine. Available at www.bordeninstitute.army.mil/cmbtcsltycare/surgeryguidelines.htm. Accessed 2 May 2007.

Brandt CP, Yowler CJ, Fratianne RB. Burns with multiple trauma. Am Surg 2002;68:240–3; discussion 243–4.

Brismar B, Bergenwald L: The terrorist bomb in Bologna, Italy, 1980: an analysis of the effects and injuries sustained. *J Trauma* 1982, 22:216-220.

Cancio L.C., Horvath E.E., Barillo D.J., David J. *et al.*: Burn support for Operation Iraqi Freedom and related operations, 2003 to 2004. *J. Burn Care Rehabil.*, 26: 151-61, 2005.

Cancio L.C., Horvath E.E., Barillo D.J., Kopchinski B.J. *et al.*: Burn support for Operation Iraqi Freedom and related operations, 2003 to 2004. *J. Burn Care Rehabil.*, 26: 151-61, 2005.

Carini L., Grippaudo F.R., Bartolini A.: Epidemiology of burns at the Italian Red Cross Hospital in Baghdad. *Burns*, 31: 687- 91, 2005.

Carsin H., Dutertre G., Le Bever H., Ainaud P., Le Reveille R., Rives J.M.: Multiple trauma and burns. *Cah. Anesthesiol.*, 43: 209-14, 1995.

Centers for disease control and prevention. Explosions and blast injuries: A primer for physicians. Available at www.bt.cdc.gov/masstrauma/explosions.asp. Accessed 2 May 2007.

Chambers L.W, Green D.J., Gillingham B.L. *et al.*: The experience of the US marine corps' surgical shock trauma platoon with 417 operative combat casualties during a 12-month period of Operation Iraqi Freedom. *J. Trauma*, 60: 1155-64, 2006.

Champion H.R., Bellamy R.F., Roderts P., Leppaniemi A.: A profile of combat injury. *J. Trauma*, 54: S13-19, 2003.

Ciraulo DL, Frykberg ER, Feliciano DV, Knuth TE, Richart CM,Westmoreland CD, Williams KA: A survey assessment of the level of preparedness for domestic terrorism and mass casualty incidents among eastern association for the surgery of trauma members. *J Trauma* 2004, 56:1033-1041

Colombia University. Emergency explosive incidents. Available at www.columbia.edu/cu/ccnmtl/projects/eprep/exp/print.html. Accessed 2 May 2007.

Committee on Trauma American College of Surgeons. Statement on disaster and mass casualty management. *J Am Coll Surg* 2003;197:855–6.

Comprint Military Publications. Burn specialist visits. J. National Naval Medical Center. Available at www.dcmilitary.com/navy/journal/archives/dec16/j_e121699.html. Accessed 5 May 2007.

Cooper GJ, Maynard RL, Cross NL, Hill JF: Casualties from ter- rorist bombings. *J Trauma* 1983, 23:955-967.

Covey DC. Blast and Fragment Injuries of the Musculoskeletal System. *J Bone and Joint Surgery* 2002; 84A: 1221-1234.

Cushman JG, Pachter HL, Beaton HL. Two New York City hospitals' surgical response to the September 11, 2001, terrorist attack in New York City. *J Trauma* 2003;54:147–54; discussion 154–5.

Cushman JG, Pachter HL, Beaton HL: Two New York city hospi- tals' surgical response to the September 11, 2001, terrorist attack in New York city. *J Trauma* 2003, 54:147-155.

Department of Defense, United States of America. Triage. In: "Emergency War Surgery NATO Handbook", part I, Types of wounds and injuries, chapter III, Burn injury, Borden Institute, US, 2004.

Department of Defense, United States of America. Weapons effects and parachute injuries. In: "Emergency War Surgery", 3rd revision, chapter 1, 1-14, Borden Institute, US, 2004.

Dillingham T.R., Spellman N.T., Braverman S.E., Zeigler D.N. *et al.*: Analysis of casualties referred to Army physical medicine services during the Persian Gulf conflict. *Am. J. Phys. Med. Rehabil.*, 72: 214-8, 1993.

Dougherty P.J.: Armored vehicle new casualties. Mil. Med., 155: 417-20, 1990.

Dreyfuss U.Y.: Burn injuries to military personnel during the Six Day War. *Harefuah*, 138: 737- 41, 2000.

Ehde D.M., Patterson D.R., Wiechman S.A., Wilson L.G.: Post-traumatic stress symptoms and distress one year after burn injury. *J. Burn Care Rehabil.*, 21: 105-11, 2000.

Einav S, Feigenberg Z, Weissman C, *et al.* Evacuation priorities in mass casualty terror-related events: implications for contingency planning. *Ann Surg* 2004;239:304–10.

Einav S, Feigenberg Z, Weissman C, Zaichik D, Caspi G, Kotler D, Freund HR: Evacuation priorities in mass casualty terror-related events. Implications for contingency planning. *Ann Surg* 2004, 239:304-310.

Eldad A.: War burns: The blow and the cure. *Clin. Dermatol.*, 20: 388-95, 2002.

Emile H, Hashmonai D: Victims of the Palestinian uprising (intifada): a retrospective review of 220 cases. *J Emerg Med* 1998, 16:389-394.

Evison D., Hinsley D., Rice P.: Chemical weapons. *BMJ*, 324: 332-5, 2002.

Fauerbach J.A., Heinberg L.J., Lawrence J.W., Munster A.M. *et al.*: Effect of early body image dissatisfaction on subsequent psychological and physical adjustment after disfiguring injury. *Psychosom. Med.*, 62: 576-82, 2000.

Feliciano DV, Anderson GV Jr, Rozycki GS, Ingram WL, Ansley JP, Namias N, Salomone JP, Cantwell JD: Management of casualties from the bombing at the

Centennial Olympics. *Am J Surg* 1998, 176:538-543.

Frykberg ER. Disaster and mass casualty management: a commentary on the American College of Surgeons position statement. *J Am Coll Surg* 2003;197:857–9.

Frykberg ER. Medical management of disasters and mass casualties from terrorist bombings: how can we cope? *J Trauma* 2002; 53:201-212

Frykberg ER. Principles of mass casualty management following terrorist disasters. *Ann Surg* 2004;239:319–21.

Frykberg ER: Medical management of disasters and mass casualties from terrorist bombings: how can we cope? *J Trauma* 2002, 53:201-212.

Garfield R.M., Neugut A.I.: Epidemiologic analysis of warfare: A historical review. *JAMA,* 266: 688-92, 1991.

Gosselin R.A.: War injuries, trauma, and disaster relief. Techniques in Orthopaedics, 20: 97-108, 2005.

Hart A.J., Mannion S., Earnshaw P., Ward A.: The London nail bombings: The St. Thomas' Hospital experience. *Injury,* 34: 830-3, 2003.

Harvey A.G., Bryant R.A.: The relationship between acute stress disorder and post-traumatic stress disorder: A prospective evaluation of motor vehicle accident survivors. *J. Consult. Clin. Psychol.,* 66: 507-12, 1998.

Hinsley D.E., Rosell P.A., Rowlands T.K., Clasper J.C.: Penetrating missile injuries during asymmetric warfare in the 2003 Gulf conflict. *Br. J. Surg.,* 92: 637-42, 2005.

Hirshberg A. Multiple casualty incidents: lessons from the front line. *Ann Surg* 2004;239:322–4.

Houdelette P.: Current aspects of war surgery. From the trauma center to precarious medical care. *Chirurgie,* 122: 187-91, 1997.

Independent News and Media (UK) Ltd, Buncombe A., Hughes S.: The fog of war: White phosphorus, Fallujah and some burning questions. Available at: www.commondreams.org/headlines05/1115-03.htm. Accessed 5 May 2007.

Ivantsov V.A., Sidel'nikov V.O., Pogodin I.U.I., Shchekochikhin S.A. *et al.*: Combined and multifactorial burn injuries in military conflicts: Tactical approaches to diagnosis and treatment. *Voen. Med. Zh.,* 326: 4-8, 2005.

Jacobs LM, Burns KJ, Gross RI. Terrorism: a public health threat with a trauma system response. *J Trauma* 2003;55: 1014–21.

JordanMH.The2003ABApresidentialaddress:9/11. . .this is not a drill! J Burn Care Rehabil 2004;25:15–24.

Journal of Burn Care and Rehabilitation 150 Cairns *et al.* March/April 2005.

Kauvar D.S., Cancio L.C., Wolf S.E., Wade C.E., Holcomb J.B.: Comparison of combat and non-combat burns from ongoing U.S. military operations. *J. Surg. Res.,* 132: 195-200, 2006.

Kluger Y.: Bomb explosions in acts of terrorism - detonation, wound ballistics, triage and medical concerns. Isr. Med. Assoc. J., 5: 235-40, 2003.

Kumar P., Jagetia G.C.: A review of triage and management of burn victims following a nuclear disaster. *Burns,* 20: 397-402, 1994.

Kuzman M., Tomic B., Stevanovic R., Ljubicic M. *et al.*: Fatalities in the war in Croatia, 1991 and 1992. Underlying and external causes of death. *JAMA,* 270: 626-8, 1993.

La Borde P.: Burn epidemiology: The patient, the nation, the statistics, and the data resources. *Crit. Care Nurs. Clin. North Am.,* 16: 13-25, 2004.

Lavonas E.: Blast injuries. Available at www.emedicine.com/emerg/topic63.htm. Accessed 5 May 2007.

Leibovici D, Gofrit ON, Stein M, Shapira SC, Noga Y, Heruti RJ, Shemer J: Blast injuries: bus versus open-air bombings: a comparative study of injuries in survivors of open-air versus confined-space explosions. *J Trauma* 1996, 41:1030-1035.

Mabrouk R.: Civilian and military burn injuries: A comparative study. *Ann. Burns and Fire Disasters,* 7: 11-12, 1994.

Mabrouk R.: The management of burn injuries in mass casualties. *Ann. Burns and Fire Disasters,* 3: 112-3, 1990.

Mabry R.L., Holcomb J.B., Baker A.M., Cloonan C.C. *et al.*: United States Army Rangers in Somalia: An analysis of combat casualties on an urban battlefield. *J. Trauma,* 49: 515-28, 2000.

MacKenzie EJ, Hoyt DB, Sacra JC, *et al.* National inventory of hospital trauma centers. *JAMA* 2003;289: 1515–22.

March JS, Amaya-Jackson L, Terry R, Costanzo P. Posttrau- matic symptomatology in children and adolescents after an industrial fire. *J Am Acad Child Adolesc Psychiatry* 1997;36:1080–8.

Marcikic M., Kraus Z., Dmitrovic B., Zibar L. *et al.*: View of a war from a pathology department: Croatian experience. *Med. War.,* 9: 33-9, 1993.

McLean A.D.: Burns and military clothing. *J.R. Army Med. Corps,* 147: 97-106, 2001.

Medtrng.com. Introduction to Ballistic, Blast and Burn Injuries. Available at www.medtrng.com/blackboard/ballistic_blast_burn.htm. Accessed 2 May 2007.

Meleney F.L.: A plan for the study of war wounds. *Ann. Surg.,* 114: 283-92, 1941.

Michaeli D.: Medicine on the battlefield: A review. *J. Royal Society Med.,* 72: 370-3, 1979.

Milner S.M., Rylah L.T.: War burns: A simplified resuscitation protocol. *Br. J. Hosp. Med.,* 50: 163-7, 1993.

Mozingo DW, Barillo DJ, Holcomb JB. The Pope Air Force Base Aircraft Crash and Burn Disaster. *J Burn Care Rehabil* 2005;26:XXX–XXX.

Murji A., Gomez M., Knighton J., Fish J.: Emotional implications of working in a burn unit. *Burn Care Research,* 27: 8-13, 2006.

Nassoura Z., Hajj H., Dajani Q., Jabbour N. *et al.*: Trauma management in a war zone: The Lebanese war experience. *J. Trauma,* 31: 1596-9, 1991.

Navy Department Library. American War and Military Operations Casualties: Lists and Statistics. Available at http://www.history.navy.mil/library/online/american %20war%20casualty.htm.

Patterson D.R., Everett J.J., Bombardier C.H., Questad K.A. *et al.*: Psychological effects of severe burn injuries. *Psychol. Bull.,* 113: 362-78, 1993.

Pearn J.: Children and war. *J. Paediatr. Child Health,* 39: 166-72, 2003.

Peleg K, Aharonson-Daniel L, Michael M, Shapira SC, and the Israel Trauma Group: Patterns of injury in hospitalized terrorist victims. *Am J Emerg Med* 2003, 21:258-262.

Peleg K, Aharonson-Daniel L, Stein M, *et al.* Gunshot and explosion injuries: characteristics, outcomes, and implications for care of terror-related injuries in Israel. *Ann Surg* 2004;239:311–8.

Peleg K, Aharonson-Daniel L, Stein M, Michaelson M, Kluger Y, Simon D, Noji EK, Israeli Trauma Group (ITG): Gunshot and explosion injuries: characteristics, outcomes and implications for care of terror-related injuries in Israel. *Ann Surg* 2004, 239: 311-318.

Phillips WJ, Reynolds PC, Lenczyk M, *et al.* Anesthesia during a mass-casualty disaster: the Army's experience at Fort Bragg, North Carolina, March 23, 1994. *Mil Med* 1997; 162:371–3.

Pizov R, Oppenheim-Eden A, Matot I, Weisss YG, Eidelman LA, Rivkind AI, Sprung CL: Blast lung injury from an explosion on a civilian bus. *Chest* 1999, 115:165-172.

Pretto E.A., Begovic M., Begovic M.: Emergency medical services during the siege of Sarajevo, Bosnia and Herzegovina: A preliminary report. *Prehosp. Dis. Med.,* 9: S39-45, 1994.

Pruitt B.A., jr: Combat casualty care and surgical progress. *Ann. Surg.,* 243: 715-29, 2006.

Purdue GF, Hunt JL. Multiple trauma and the burn patient. Am J Surg 1989;158:536–9.

Read D., Ashford B.: Surgical aspects of Operation Bali Assist: Initial wound surgery on the tarmac and in flight. *ANZ J. Surg.*, 74: 986-91, 2004.

Rew D.A., Clasper J., Kerr G.: Surgical workload from an integrated UK field hospital during the 2003 Gulf conflict. *J.R. Army Med. Corps*, 150: 99-106, 2004.

Rew D.A., Clasper J., Kerr G.: Surgical workload from an integrated UK field hospital during the 2003 Gulf conflict. *J.R. Army Med Corps*, 150: 99-106, 2004.

Rice P.: Sulphur mustard injuries of the skin. Pathophysiology and management. *Toxicol. Rev.*, 22: 111-8, 2003.

Riesgo L.G., Merino A.G.: Terrorism in Spain: Emergency medical aspects. *Prehospital Disaster Med.*, 18: 148-51, 2003.

Rignault DP, Deligny MC: The 1986 terrorist bombing experience in Paris. *Ann Surg* 1989, 209:368-373.

Rosenkranz KM, Sheridan R. Management of the burned trauma patient: balancing conflicting priorities. *Burns* 2002; 28:665–9.

Schrader E.: Wounds of war. *Los Angeles Times*, 9 Nov. 2003, A.1.

Securitydriver.com. Explosive forces of improvised explosive devices. Available at www.securitydriver.com/aic/stories/article-114.html. Accessed 2 May 2007.

Shafir R., Nili E., Kedem R.: Burn injury and prevention in the Lebanon War, 1982. *Isr. J. Med. Sci.*, 20: 311-3, 1984.

Sidel'nikov V.O., Paramonov B.A., Tatarin S.N.: Medical care for the burnt in modern local military conflicts. Voen. *Med. Zh.*, 323: 35-9, 2002.

Singer P., Cohen J., Stein M.: Conventional terrorism and critical care. *Crit. Care Med.*, 33 (suppl.): S61-5, 2005.

Sparkes B.G.: Mechanisms of immune failure in burn injury. *Vaccine*, 11: 504-10, 1993.

Sparkes B.G.: Treating mass burns in warfare, disaster or terrorist strikes. *Burns*, 23: 238-47, 1997.

Stein M and Hirshberg A Medical Consequences of Terrorism. The Conventional Weapon Threat (1999) 79(6). *Surg Clinics N Am* 1537-1552.

Stein M, Hirshberg A: Medical consequences of terrorism: the conventional weapon threat. *Surg Clin North Am* 1999, 79:1537-1552.

Taal L.A., Faber A.W.: Dissociation as a predictor of psychopathology following burns injury. *Burns*, 23: 400-3, 1997.

Teague DC: Mass casualties in the Oklahoma City bombing. *Clin Orthop* 2004, 422:77-81.

Toole M.J., Galson S., Brady W.: Are war and public health compatible? *Lancet*, 341: 1193-6, 1993.

Trunkey D.D.: History and development of trauma care in the United States. *Clin. Orthop.*, 374: 36-46, 2000.

Trunkey DD. Trauma centers and trauma systems. *JAMA* 2003;289:1566–7.

Vujovic B., Mazlagic D.: Epidemiology and surgical management of abdominal war injuries in Sarajevo: State Hospital of Sarajevo experience. *Prehosp. Dis. Med.*, 9:S 29-34, 1994.

Wachtel T. Burn disaster management. In Herndon D, editor. Total burn care. London: W.B. Saunders; 2002. p. 51–66.

Wachtel TL, Cowan ML, Reardon JD. Developing a regional and national burn disaster response. *J Burn Care Rehabil* 1989;10:561–7.

Warden GD, Heimbach D. Regionalization of burn care—a concept whose time has come. *J Burn Care Rehabil* 2003; 24:173–4.

Wightman J., Gladish S.: Explosions and blast injuries. *Ann. Emerg. Med.*, 37: 664-78, 2001.

Willebrand M., Andersson G., Ekselius L.: Prediction of psychological health after an accidental burn. *J. Trauma*, 57: 367-74, 2004.

Wong L, Grande CM, Munster AM. Burns and associated nonthermal trauma: an analysis of management, outcome, and relation to the Injury Severity Score. *J Burn Care Rehabil* 1989;10:512–6.

Yu B.H., Dimsdale J.E.: Post-traumatic stress disorder in patients with burn injuries. *J. Burn Care Rehabil.*, 20: 426-33, 1999.

Yurt B, Bessey P, Bauer G. The World Trade Center disaster: one burn center's experience [abstract]. *J Burn Care Rehabil* 2002;23:S107.

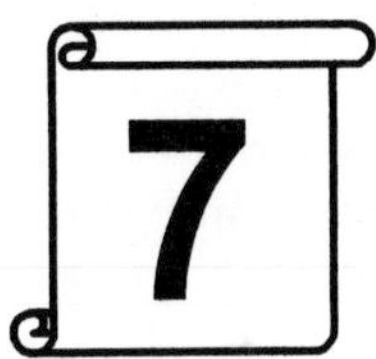

International Agencies in Relief of Natural Disasters

The international community is faced with the growing challenge of preventing, mitigating the effects of, and providing humanitarian assistance to affected populations in crises that require rapid and effective response. The 1990s saw a dramatic increase in "complex emergencies" that often involved ethnic and civil strife. In mid-1994 more than 30 million people in 29 countries were in dire need of emergency assistance. Severe drought threatening over 20 million people in sub-Saharan Africa added an additional element of suffering to that already faced by millions in Burundi, Liberia, Rwanda, Somalia, southern Sudan, and Zaire. A study released at the World Conference on Natural Disaster Reduction, convened by the General Assembly in May 1994, showed that the previous three decades had seen a steady and rapid increase in the number of significant natural disasters—and in the numbers of people affected.

NATURAL DISASTERS ARE COMMON IN ASIAN COUNTRIES

Asian natural disasters have become an opportunity for regional militaries to deploy in a disaster relief role, demonstrating their value as more than a deterrent to war or transnational threats. By employing their instruments of hard power to deliver aid to the victims of natural disasters, the United States, India, and even Japan have softened regional perceptions of their might by making humanitarian assistance a central role for their military forces in the region. The People's Liberation Army (PLA) has carefully observed the international response to recent disasters, their positive effect on public opinion and the resulting evolution of military thought. Well versed in responding to domestic disasters, such as annual floods and the recent earthquake in Sichuan Province, the PLA is carefully and cautiously assessing the future potential for international disaster relief and humanitarian assistance missions.

Cyclone Nargis struck Burma's largest city, Yangon, and the surrounding Irrawaddy Delta on May 2 and 3, 08, bringing high winds and a storm surge that resulted in an immediate estimate of 22,500 dead, tens of thousands missing and one million without food, shelter and water. Over the following days, the extent of the devastation was increasingly revealed, prompting the military government of the isolated country to issue reluctant appeals to the international community for assistance. The state, however, has been slow to allow international aid agencies and governments to send experts to assess the damage and coordinate on the ground delivery of aid, making it unlikely that regional militaries will play a significant role in delivering aid directly to affected people, and compounded the humanitarian disaster with the death poll possibly exceeding 200,000 (*Sydney Morning Herald,* May 21). While Thailand and the United States have delivered aid to Yangon by military aircraft, their militaries have not been able to deploy ships or helicopters that could deliver aid directly to affected areas. The Indian military anticipated the cyclone, pre-positioning ships in the nearby Andaman Islands, including a destroyer and a corvette that arrived with supplies in Yangon soon after the storm passed. These Indian warships, however, were not able to repeat the impressive demonstration of capabilities displayed by the amphibious assault ships, helicopters and hovercraft of several countries that deployed during the 2004 tsunami.

China appears lukewarm to disasters

The Chinese military was largely an observer to the tsunami response, choosing not to deploy abroad, delivering donated supplies by civilian charter aircraft and sending only a handful of military and civilian personnel to aid in relief efforts. China pledged $1 million worth of aid, including relief materials worth $500,000 to Burma. In contrast to the Indian Navy, the PLA did not react rapidly to this natural disaster, despite apparent aspirations to play a greater role in the region politically, economically and militarily. Sensitive to the political whims of the ruling junta, it is likely that China quickly recognized that the Burmese junta would not welcome foreign militaries operating in its territory and therefore opted instead to make modest donations. This turned out to be fortuitous, as the Sichuan earthquake struck 10 days after the Burma cyclone, creating an urgent demand for Chinese disaster recovery resources at home. Subsequently, it was expected that the PLA would prepare more robust responses to future disasters, should they strike the region. Other than donations of food and supplies, however, the Chinese military did not respond to the Bangladesh cyclone in late 2007, indicating that little progress had been made in building up or demonstrating a crisis management response mechanism or an international, military sea or airlift capacity since the tsunami.

Unlike the U.S. military, the PLA has been much more circumspect. Other than deployments on UN Peacekeeping Operations, the PLA has been reluctant to stretch its legs to perform international disaster relief or humanitarian assistance missions. There are four potential explanations for this cautious approach: the PLA is reluctant; there is existing need at home; concern an overseas deployment would expose weakness; concern about how a PLA deployment might be received internationally (China Brief, January 28, 2005; May 10, 2005; October 13, 2005). However, there are few examples of rapid reactions to domestic natural disasters. The "China International Rescue Medical Team" attached to the People's Armed Police (PAP) General Hospital responded to the Sichuan earthquake within hours and was airlifted by military aircraft to the hardest hit region. That unit is likely China's most experienced medical rescue team, having deployed abroad several times, including the tsunami and earthquakes in Iran, Pakistan and Algeria.

Humanitarian Mission in China

The Chinese government recognizes the value of humanitarian assistance, medical diplomacy and national responses to international natural disasters. Providing medical assistance to needy countries, particularly in response to natural disasters, improves international image through people-to-people diplomacy as well as effective communications campaigns. Chinese media widely broadcast the PAP General Hospital rescue unit's efforts in Indonesia following the 2004 tsunami crisis, complete with images of Chinese doctors distributing Chinese medicine and Indonesians gratefully exclaiming, "China good!" (PLA Daily, January 5, 2005). International deployments offer a real-world test of military medical response capabilities, including the opportunity to gain experience in the field, fine-tune logistics and test new equipment. Furthermore, the deployments present the opportunity to practice satellite tele-medicine consultations with doctors in the rear. In large-scale relief efforts, deployment could include exposure to other units and the opportunity to learn new techniques and technologies. These deployments can help China's military medical system become more agile and adaptable, as well as provide valuable lessons about intelligence collection, information sharing and situational awareness. It is likely that as China's military continues to modernize, its response will become more robust. The Chinese navy recently launched a new "Type 920" hospital ship, weighing 20,000 tons and purpose-built, joining a handful of existing hospital ships which are converted transports serving with each of the PLA Navy fleets. China is also improving its amphibious warfare capabilities, including commissioning new landing ships with helicopter and hovercraft capabilities. While China's "gator navy" is primarily focused on a Taiwan scenario, disaster relief operations on China's periphery are a conceivable future mission. Lastly, China's future aircraft carrier will likely also be tasked with disaster relief and humanitarian assistance missions, both for the operational experience that real-world relief missions bring, but also to reassure neighbors that China seeks to be a responsible neighbor and peaceful regional power.

United Nations Disaster Relief Coordinator (UNDRO)

Beginning in 1965, proposals were put forward in the General Assembly to increase the UN's ability to help people stricken by disasters, but it was the disasters of 1970 that brought international concern for emergency relief to a head. In 1971, the General Assembly established the Office of the United Nations Disaster Relief Coordinator (UNDRO), with headquarters in Geneva. UNDRO was not designed to assume all the responsibilities of meeting disasters from its own resources. Its principal function is that of catalyst and coordinator of donors of aid and services. Its data bank and independent telecommunications system, supplemented by the worldwide UN system, give it the capacity to define the specific needs arising from a disaster and to respond rapidly by identifying potential sources of relief. It directs and mobilizes aid emanating from the UN system and coordinates aid from other sources. UNDRO's mandate also includes assisting governments in preventing disasters or mitigating their effects by contingency planning, in association with similarly concerned voluntary organisations. It promotes the study, prevention, control, and prediction of natural disasters and gathers and disseminates information relevant to disaster relief.

The Office for the Coordination of Humanitarian Affairs (OCHA)

In December 1991, the General Assembly, by its Resolution 46/182, recognized the need to strengthen coordination for rapid response to humanitarian emergencies. Over the years ad hoc arrangements had sprung up in many of the UN departments and specialized agencies to deal with emergency relief. The General Assembly requested the Secretary-General to designate an emergency relief coordinator, supported by a secretariat, to ensure that the entire UN system was better prepared for, and more capable of rapid and coherent response to national disasters and other humanitarian emergencies. The resolution also stipulated guiding principles of humanity, neutrality and impartiality for the provision of humanitarian assistance. It also stressed respect for the sovereignty, territorial integrity and national unity of states. With UN reforms in the late 1990s, the Office for the Coordination of Humanitarian Affairs (OCHA) was established to manage complex emergencies (through the Consolidated Appeals Process), natural disasters, and other humanitarian crises.

The Consolidated Appeals Process (CAP), coordinated and monitored by OCHA, is an inter-agency exercise by which UN system organisations and other humanitarian organisations assess the full range of requirements for responding to emergencies. The CAP helps the international community to identify the most critical needs of affected people and to determine the most appropriate ways to provide assistance. This process enables donors and agencies to concentrate their efforts where they are needed most and eliminates wasteful competition among agencies for donor funds. From 1995 through 2002, appeals were launched for countries including Afghanistan, Albania, Angola, Bosnia and Herzegovina, Burundi, Colombia, Congo, Democratic Republic of the Congo, Côte d'Ivoire, Croatia, Ecuador, Eritrea, Ethiopia, Fiji, Georgia, Guinea, Guinea-Bissau, India, Indonesia, Iraq, Japan, Kenya, Democratic People's Republic of Korea, Lebanon, Liberia, the Former Yugoslav Republic of Macedonia, Occupied Palestinian territory, Pakistan, Russian Federation, Rwanda, Sierra Leone, Somalia, South Africa, Sudan, Tajikistan, Uganda, United Republic of Tanzania, and Yugoslavia. Appeals are often made by region as well—including for the Caucasus, Great Lakes Region of Africa, and Southeastern Europe (including Yugoslavia). OCHA's work takes place where the fields of international security, political affairs, and humanitarian concerns converge. OCHA's staff is involved in policy planning and early warning functions, emergency operational support and relief coordination, and disaster mitigation. The OCHA maintains close contact with the UN Departments of Political Affairs and Peacekeeping Operations in order to coordinate the security, political, and humanitarian aspects of complex emergencies. To help manage its efforts, OCHA set-up Relief Web, http://www.reliefweb.int. The Internet site provides up-to-date information on complex emergencies and natural disasters collected from over 170 sources.

International Decade for Natural Disaster Reduction

Between 1960 and 1990 deaths from natural disasters rose by a factor of 10, with 90% of casualties occurring in developing countries ill prepared to respond to natural disasters. Although the World Meteorological Organisation has shown that each dollar spent on disaster preparedness is equivalent to 100 dollars spent after a disaster, no mechanisms existed to transfer the huge body of knowledge on disaster preparedness and prevention from the industrialized countries to developing countries. For example, an earthquake of 6.6 magnitude on the Richter scale in California in January 1994 caused fewer than 100 deaths. An earthquake of6.4 magnitude in India's Maharashtra State in September 1993 caused 10,000 deaths. Most of the deaths in the Indian tragedy were caused by the collapse of homes while people slept. By contrast, California has long been a proving ground for earthquake-resistant architectural innovations.

The General Assembly declared the 1990s the International Decade for Natural Disaster Reduction to reduce loss of life and property damage resulting from natural disasters. It established a high-level council of 10 internationally renowned personalities, a scientific and technical committee of 24 scientists from around the world, and approximately 120 national committees to promote the decade and the formulation of disaster preparedness programmes. 13 October was declared "International Day for Natural Disaster Reduction," and observed by public gatherings and publicity to raise awareness of the need to implement disaster preparedness.

In May 1994, the World Conference on Natural Disaster Reduction was convened in Yokohama, Japan. Representatives from 147 countries and 37 nongovernmental organisations and observers from UN specialized agencies participated in the conference, which both reviewed implementation of the General Assembly's recommendations during the first half of the decade and adopted the "Guidelines for Natural Disaster Prevention, Preparedness and Mitigation," also called the "Yokohama Strategy." It noted that the first half of the decade had seen some improvement in the field of disaster response, but that the goals for disaster prevention and preparedness had not received wide publicity. In its "Strategy for the Year 2000 and Beyond," the conference called for a global culture of prevention and a policy of self-reliance in each vulnerable country and community. Other elements of the strategy included education and training in disaster prevention, strengthening research and development for disaster reduction and mitigation, and improving awareness in vulnerable communities through more active use of media. It also recommended an improvement in communications capabilities on natural disasters among countries for preparedness and early warning systems.

In this connection, the UN established a set of guidelines for humanitarian missions in conflict situations:

1. The need for humanitarian relief assistance to be undertaken in accordance with the principles of impartiality, neutrality, and humanity;
2. Reaffirmation of free, safe, and unimpeded access for humanitarian assistance and the role of humanitarian diplomacy in that regard;
3. The need for greater collaboration with non-governmental organisations engaged in humanitarian relief;
4. The need to ensure security and protection of all relief personnel;
5. The need to apprise the Security Council fully on relevant humanitarian issues that should be appropriately reflected in its decisions on complex emergencies;
6. The importance of shielding humanitarian assistance against the effects of sanctions, particularly in relation to vulnerable groups.

Health care costs are mounting in peace and during disaster

Almost the entire cost of health care in the developing world is borne by the developing countries themselves. Aid from international health organisations in the developed countries pays for less than 5% of the total health care costs in the developing world. This aid can be of crucial importance. Research and pilot programmes sponsored by agencies from the industrial nations have generated many of the best ideas for improving health in developing countries. Also, the international health organisations are a major source of expert technical advice and training for local health professionals. Finally, these organisations produce the major textbooks in tropical health, as well as the most important manuals for health care workers. A large number of organisations of various sizes provide international health aid. The exact roles played by these organisations can be bewildering at times, even to professionals in this field. What follows is a description of the functions of the largest international health organisations. After a look at the major organisations providing long-term health care, the focus shifts to those that specialize in giving aid to victims of war, famine and natural disasters.

Organisations Providing Long-term Health Care

International health organisations are usually divided into three groups: multilateral organisations, bilateral organisations, and non-governmental organisations (NGOs). The term multilateral means that funding comes from multiple governments and is distributed to many different countries. The major multilateral organisations are all part of the United Nations. The World Health Organisation (WHO) is the premier international health organisation. Technically it is an "inter-governmental agency related to the United Nations." The World Bank is the other major "intergovernmental agency related to the UN" heavily involved in international health. The World Bank loans money to poor countries on advantageous terms. The amount of money loaned to developing countries for human resources development,, i.e. health and education, has increased steadily over the past 10 years, from 5% of total loans in the early 1980s to 15% in the past two years, with a projected 50% increase in human resource development loans over the next three years. The total amount of loans for health, nutrition, and population activities in 1995 was approximately $1,200 million. The United Nation Children's Fund (UNICEF) spends the majority of its programme budget on health care. UNICEF makes the world's most vulnerable children its top priority, so it devotes most of its resources to the poorest countries and to children younger than 5. UNICEF runs many of the child health programmes in cooperation with WHO. The United Nations Population Fund (UNFPA) spent about $130 million of its $260 million budget for 1994 on family planning programmes, with 59 priority countries receiving 70% of this money. The United Nation Development Programmeme (UNDP) allocated $141 million, out of a total budget for field expenditures of $1 billion, to "health, education, employment." Its major health concerns are AIDS, maternal and child nutrition, and excessive maternal mortality. In conjunction with WHO and the World Bank it sponsors the Special Programmeme for Research and Training in Tropical Diseases (TDR).

Non-governmental Organisations

Non-governmental organisations (NGOs), also known as private voluntary organisations, provide approximately 20% of all external health aid to developing countries. Most of these organisations are quite small; many are church-affiliated. In the very poorest countries, hospitals and clinics run by missionary societies are especially important. The largest NGO devoted to international health in the United States is Project Hope, with an annual budget exceeding $100 million. Worldwide, the most important NGO in long-term international health is probably Oxfam, International.

Disaster Relief Organisations

In most natural disasters, e.g. earthquakes, floods, volcanic eruptions, the majority of deaths occur in the first few hours or days, and likewise most of the lives that are saved are saved early on and saved by local efforts at disaster relief. A major disaster, however, can overwhelm the resources of a poor country and, by destruction of an already somewhat tenuous economic and social infrastructure, set the stage for famine and epidemics. The aid provided by international relief organisations in the days immediately following the disaster can play a major role in averting health crises and re-establishing a functioning society. In contrast to natural disasters, famines and refugee crises tend to develop slowly, often preceded by warning signs of the impending emergency, so that international agencies can coordinate relief efforts with national agencies in a timely fashion. There are several very large NGOs active in refugee and disaster relief. Two of these, the International Committee of the Red Cross (ICRC) and Medecins Sans Frontieres, perform special functions.

United Nations Organisations

Three of the six major agencies are mentioned above in the section on long-term health care viz. UNICEF, WHO and UNDP. The World Food Programme (WFP) supplies food relief in disasters and coordinates the activities of NGOs involved in food relief, as well as assisting them with transportation and logistics. UN High Commissioner for Refugees (UNHCR) provides international protection to refugees and also attempts to find long-lasting solutions to their problems. The sixth of the UN organisations involved in relief work is the Food and Agriculture Organisation (FAO). Like the World Bank and WHO it is technically an "inter-governmental agency related to the UN."

International Red Cross and Red Crescent Movement

It is the largest and most prestigious of the world's humanitarian NGOs. It has three components: the International Committee of the Red Cross (ICRC); the International Federation of Red Cross and Red Crescent Societies; the 160 or so individual national Red Cross societies, e.g. the American Red Cross. The seven fundamental principles of the Movement are: humanity; impartiality; neutrality; independence,, i.e. autonomy *vis-à-vis* national governments; voluntary service; unity,, i.e. for each country only one national Society, open to all and serving the entire country; universality. The ICRC is a Swiss organisation, founded in 1863 and mandated by the Geneva Conventions to protect and assist prisoners of war and civilians in international armed conflicts. It may also offer its services in civil wars. Its functions include: visiting and treating prisoners of war and political detainees and providing them with a communication service with the outside world; setting up surgical hospitals or providing expatriate teams to work in existing hospitals; providing other types of medical assistance and relief, especially rehabilitation of war-disabled patients; development and dissemination of educational materials concerning health care of prisoners and victims of war. The International Federation of Red Cross and Red Crescent Societies receives its principal support from the individual national societies. Its main mission is to provide disaster relief. It works closely with the national Red Cross Societies in the affected countries.

Like the Red Cross, Medecins Sans Frontieres (MSF) provides health aid to victims of war and natural disasters. Unlike the Red Cross, MSF is willing to enter war-torn areas without the permission of authorities. Another difference between the two organisations is that MSF, although its charter includes the same principles of impartiality and neutrality followed by the Red Cross, considers one of its functions to be speaking out on human rights abuses. Usually this speaking out consists of drawing attention to cases of human rights violations that MSF considers under-reported, but on occasions MSF will take a strong stand and denounce egregious violations.

AmeriCares in disaster relief

AmeriCares is a private, non-profit international disaster relief and humanitarian aid organisation, which delivers medicines, medical supplies and aid to people in crisis around the world. Since it was established in 1982, AmeriCares has distributed more than $7.5 billion in humanitarian aid to 137 countries. It takes pride to be a part of critical relief effort, providing hope and health to the victims of devastating events. AmeriCares is continuing its efforts to provide long-term relief for people living in China's earthquake-stricken Sichuan Province and in areas most affected by Cyclone Nargis in Myanmar. This nonprofit international aid organisation announced that it has delivered a second field hospital to Sichuan Province and provided a second shipment of life-saving medicines and medical supplies to support primary health clinics serving displaced people in Myanmar's Irrawaddy Delta.

AmeriCares in China

Ameri-Cares is constructing and equipping its second field hospital in Sichuan Province. The second field hospital will be established in Wenchuan County, the epicenter of the 7.9 magnitude earthquake on the site of the Xuankou Township Hospital, which received severe structural damage. Currently, medical personnel are working out of a collection of tents on the site, seeing anywhere between 80 and 200 patients a day. The new hospital will include an operating room, a clinical laboratory, an inpatient ward and will provide comprehensive maternal health services, including ultrasounds. The hospital will also have an emergency vehicle available to provide transportation for patients from the surrounding mountainous communities. Ameri-Cares is working with local Chinese authorities to make the hospital fully operational by the middle of July. The Xuankou field hospital follows the construction of an earlier field hospital in Qingchuan, an area where 250,000 residents lost their only hospital after the initial earthquake and major aftershocks. The field hospital in Qingchuan is fully operational, seeing between 150 and 160 outpatients each day, performing operations and deliveries and treating an inpatient population. Northwest Airlines donated the transportation costs for delivering both field hospitals, which are a product of blu-med Response Systems. AmeriCares was one of the first private international relief organisations to provide aid to Chengdu, the capital of the hard-hit Sichuan Province, delivering an initial supply of medicines and providing an additional shipment of critically-needed medical supplies, including anesthetics and nutritionals for diabetics to the Sichuan Provincial People's Hospital in Chengdu, China.

Ameri-Cares in Myanmar

In the wake of Cyclone Nargis, Ameri-Cares was one of the first nonprofit organisations to fly an airlift directly into Yangon. The airlift included 15 tons of medical supplies and medicine to help operate mobile medical clinics serving victims in local communities, including the Irrawaddy Delta region. This second shipment of aid will replenish earlier supplies, allowing our partner, the International Organisation for Migration (IOM) to continue the relief effort in Myanmar and establish ten primary health clinics throughout the region. AmeriCares relief workers are in Myanmar working with locals to ensure the delivery of aid reaches those most in need. The shipment contains 7,000 pounds of medicines such as antibiotics, analgesics, IV solutions, pain relievers and other essential drugs and medical supplies to equip IOM's health clinics. In addition to this shipment, Ameri-Cares is delivering medications to treat malaria and dengue fever to The mentor Initiative and IV solutions to help combat cholera outbreaks.

ASIAN DISASTER PREPAREDNESS CENTER; US AID-Project (Programme for enhancement of emergency response (PEER))

Past experience shows that well developed Search and Rescue (SAR) capabilities of First Responders and medical assistance by them can significantly reduce the loss of life and serious disabilities after a natural disaster. While large areas and populations of many Asian countries are exposed to natural disasters, the SAR capabilities of the First Responders have not been systematically developed to undertake this critical life saving task. Recognizing this gap, and in consultation with the respective governments, the United States Office of Foreign Disaster Assistance (OFDA) has offered to assist in the process of capacity building for medical first response and urban search and rescue in selected Asian countries of India, Nepal, Indonesia and the Philippines. The Asian Disaster Preparedness Center (ADPC), with its expertise in training, capacity building and managing regional programmes in disaster management, will manage the programme. Miami-Dade Fire Rescue Department (MDFRD), will provide technical inputs to this capacity building programme.

Programme Purpose

The programme will improve the search and rescue capability and performance of first responders from government and non-government agencies. This training will enable these first responders to effectively assess, treat and transport victims of a disaster, and to plan for, undertake and manage effective search and rescue operations in the event of building collapse in earthquakes and other situations. The program will also develop the capacity in each of the four countries to organize and conduct their own training in Medical First Response (MFR) and Collapsed Structure Search and Rescue (CSSR).

Objectives

1. Train personnel of government and NGOs to respond to the immediate medical needs of victims of disasters.
2. Train personnel of agencies that have a key role to play in urban search and rescue techniques and skills to locate, stabilize, and rescue victims trapped in collapsed structures, using the most appropriate and safest procedures.
3. Equip first responders with skills and information on how to develop train and employ special task canines and handlers to locate trapped victims within collapsed structures.
4. Assist agencies to organize and conduct their own training for emergency medical response and for urban search and rescue response and management
5. Develop, adapt and translate training courses and material that are relevant to the local context
6. Strengthen coordination linkages amongst target agencies in respect to planning for and managing response efforts for urban search and rescue operations
7. Enhance the national disaster management system in its ability to effectively plan and coordinate the implementation of the government's activities in disaster preparedness and response.

Programme Components

1. Course Development and Adaptation

This will involve adaptation of OFDA's Training for Instructors (TFI) and MDFRD's Medical First Responder (MFR), Collapsed Structure Search and Rescue (CSSR). Courses will be tailored to the context and requirement of each of the four countries. During PEER implementation, new courses will be identified by partner institutions. These courses will be designed and developed for Asia. At present, two new courses have been identified: Facilitators Skills Course and a Training course on Hospital Disaster Preparedness (HosDiP), the Facilitators Skills Course is undergoing its first review and envisioned to be piloted by January 2001. The HosDiP course will be designed and developed later this year.

2. Training

Regional, Sub-Regional and National Training courses will be conducted for respective national training institutes of the four countries. Initially, training will be conducted by officials from OFDA, MDFRD and ADPC. Increasingly, trained personnel who have participated in initial courses will assist with and eventually take over conduct of training in country. The training and adaptation of courses will go through an iterative process as shown in the following diagram.

Cadre of peer trainers

One of the major outputs of PEER is the establishment of a cadre of regional and natonal trainers. Each potential trainer goes through the Training for Instructors (TFI) or MFR or CSSR. Those who would be selected to become part of the cadre of trainers will go through the Instructors Workshop. They then will be given assignments on the next training course with monitor and will be evaluated. The successful trainers will be able to act as full pledge trainer. Those who are not successful will go through more exposure and coaching from the monitor until they have successfully passed the evaluation. It is imperative that each instructor of content courses (MFR and CSSR) undergo the TFI (for training methodology) and then the MFR (or CSSR) Instrúctor's workshop.

3. Support for local level training agencies to organise and conduct their own training

Limited technical and financial assistance will be made available to organize and conduct CSSR and MFR in-house training. Support would cover training equipment, computer software, funds for material reproduction and translation costs and instructor charges.

4. institutionalization of SAR planning, preparedness and response

Technical assistance will be made available for planning interventions that will support the integration of SAR measures into national and institutional operational mechanisms. This is designed to generate a large pool of trained instructors from emergency response agencies who will in turn train others from their organisations. Emphasis will be placed on joint multi agency training. Trainers training on how to instruct and on how to teach the different SAR Courses will be conducted towards building up a cadre within the country that is capable of taking the lead on initiating and conducting SAR training. Training will be performance-based, designed around a good definition of problems to be addressed. Use of highly interactive training methods will take advantage of the knowledge and skills of participants and will minimize differences in knowledge and skill level of the target audience. Local expertise will be sought for the development, adaptation, testing and revising of all training courses and materials. Provisions to translate courses and materials will be made so training can be conducted in the national languages, and further into local dialects where needed.

USAID Mission in Partner Countries

The USAID through its staff at the country office will act as liaison agencies between the implementing institutions and the partner government agencies.

Institutions in Partner Countries

Partners in each of the participating countries have been identified for the implementation of the project. These comprise lead agencies at national level responsible for disaster management in the country; as well as emergency response services including, Police, Fire Services, Emergency Medical Services, Civil Defense, Army, Red Cross/Crescent Societies and Scouts; as well as other agencies involved in first response to a disaster.Partner Institutions include:

1. India: Ministry of Agriculture and Ministry of Homes
2. Philippines: National Disaster Coordinating Council
3. Indonesia: BAKORNAS, PMI Pusat, Ambulan 118, Jakarta Fire Service, Indonesian Scout Movement
4. Nepal: Ministry of Homes

The following are the key priority activities executed until the end of Phase 1.

BASELINE DATA COLLECTION

To have a reliable basis for evaluation of impacts, the benchmark situation in each country will have to be assessed and established. Information related to first responders and search and rescue activities, legal framework under which the first responders operate, training activities on MFR and CSSR, who provides training, the target participants, training impact evaluation and other will be collected. Data collection will also include data on hospital preparedness in disaster events with emphasis on collapsed structure due to earthquakes. A follow-up review in Nepal with those who attended the Earthquake Medicine Training Course in Kathmandu will also be done. The framework and parameters for data collection will be designed by a Senior Consultant in collaboration with OFDA and ADPC, supported by a team with training, MFR, SAR, and medical expertise. This framework will be modified for each country. OFDA will he requested to share the cost or the data collection team by providing the Senior Consultant. Several channels can be used for data collection: country visits, questionnaire, on site interviews, and review of documentation

ADPC will be involved in all stages of data collection. OFDA, will also be consulted, on the data collection and type of data to be collected. The data collection and processing, the resultant baseline situation, and the M&E design will likely take up to 3-4 months and should be undertaken as a priority activity of Phase Extension. Scope of Work for the data collection team is in the process of being finalized. Baseline data collection exercise is expected to begin in May 2000.

Design and implementation of monitoring and evaluation system

Long-term and short-term impacts of PEER can be identified based on a well designed Monitoring and Evaluation (M & E). Impacts can be measured through carefully defined performance indicators that take into account the baseline status of emergency response in each country. A monitoring plan will be designed for the entire programme based on the baseline data collection exercise. The Monitoring will be done to track Programme Progress against milestones. Monitoring will be useful as part of the management responsibility of the partner countries. Sample of illustrative monitoring activities include: training database, on-site interviews at the time of disasters to assess utility of training, tacking of a sample group over the life of the PEER, development of country priorities and programmes for each target country.

PEER management also needs to monitor the presumptions made in the initial programme design. These presumptions are the bases for identifying impact indicators. Critical assumptions represent both opportunities and constraints. Monitoring provides the information necessary for Programme managers to determine the degree to which they can influence these actions or the options that can be taken to avoid or overcome a constraint before it becomes a major obstacle to achievement

Conduct of training courses and adaptation of materials

Medical First Response (MFR) and Collapsed Structure Search and Rescue (CSSR) Courses will be piloted in the regional and sub-regional levels to be followed by course materials assessment. The Training for Instructors (TFI) course has already been conducted in various levels. Two national courses will be held to be followed by the TFI materials adaptation workshop. This workshop will start the process of materials adaptation to produce the Asia version.

New component - hospital disaster preparedness (HosDiP)

While the PEER is originally addressing the need for medical first response in the scene of the disaster, it does not address the readiness and/ or preparedness issues of hospitals. Medical doctors in hospitals and clinics are used to treating patients on individual basis. They are not used to treating patients "en masse". Thus, the questions remain. Are the hospitals or other medical facilities capable of handling mass casualty for earthquake as well as other disasters? Are the hospitals in earthquake prone areas structurally sound? Do they have operational plans in cases of earthquake disaster, and in cases of hospital collapse?

The victims of disasters can be given the pre-hospital treatment by the medical first responders but these victims will eventually be taken to hospitals for further treatment. Therefore, the complete procedure would require not only the medical first responders but also the hospital medical staff and administration. Logically, in order for the hospital to effectively respond, it has to have its capacities to respond intact after a devastating earthquake or other major disasters. In the event that the hospital is also a victim of disaster, the hospital should have a disaster response plan that allows it to still function as a hospital.

To address these, it is recommended that Hospital Disaster Preparedness (HosDiP), become another component of PEER. To introduce this component, a program design workshop is planned to take place in May 2000 while the HosDiP training course design workshop to start the course development process for a training course designed to establish HosDiP in Asia is planned to take place in October 2000 as one of the priority activities under the Phase I extension.

HosDiP will utilize some of the recommendations from the Earthquake Medicine Training Courses and other related exercise conducted in Nepal.

Hospital preparedness

The term "hospital preparedness" is a catch-all phrase, covering a multitude of inter-related areas of medical and non-medical disaster management. Although the Joint Commission on Accreditation of Health Care Organisations (JCAHO) mandates specific standards for hospital preparedness, in many institutions these standards never extend beyond the written page. Prior to September 11, 2001, hospital preparedness in US focused on man-made mass casualty events viz. accidents, earthquakes, tornadoes, commercial building collapse, airline and school bus accidents. In contrast to Israel and European countries, and despite such events as the 1993 World Trade Center bombing and the 1995 Oklahoma City bombing, the spectre of terrorism was remote from hospital disaster planning. Since September 11, 2001, the reality of U.S. vulnerability to domestic terrorism has translated into an increased sense of urgency to prepare for potential terrorist acts.

Hospital Staffing

One of the principal concerns in hospital preparedness is the determination of adequate staffing capabilities. Inter-hospital cooperation is hindered in part by fears of "poaching" of scarce nursing resources. Nursing shift "call-offs" are a routine event at many institutions, with the subsequent result of under-staffing during daily operations. Concern exists at many levels regarding staffing patterns during times of disaster hospital operations.

The Ontario Health Coalition report submitted to the SARS commission specifically noted inadequate hospital capacity and understaffed facilities. The SARS epidemic resulted in significant psychological stress for hospital staff, as noted by a survey of the hospital staff of a tertiary care facility. The four factors which most correlated with degree of concern for family and personal well-being were perception of a greater risk of death from SARS, living in a household with children, personal or family lifestyle affected by SARS outbreak, and most interestingly, being treated differently by individuals simply because of working in a hospital.

Much of the attention has been focused upon nursing issues. However, attention should also be placed upon ancillary staff and management. The former is required for the hospital to function. Without trained housekeeping and maintenance staff, there is the potential for nosocomial spread as well as potential delay in the disposition and rooming of admitted patients. Despite the critical role of these individuals in hospital functioning, these ancillary staff may be more vulnerable to absenteeism during a disaster event due to a lack of medical awareness regarding actual versus perceived personnel risks. Health care workers do not live within an insular system, and may be directly and personally affected by the disaster. Adequate staff contingency planning should take this reality into account. Health care workers may be amongst the victims, as may be their families. After a disaster that significantly affects the local infrastructure, it may be necessary to provide safe shelter and food to the families of affected staff members. Without providing this, there will be little incentive for those staff members to report to work.

The nature of the disaster may impact staffing issues. In one survey, the willingness of staff to respond to a disaster was placed in the context of whether the disaster was an airplane crash scenario, a radioactive "dirty" bomb, or a biological agent scenario. The number of staff willing to work extra hours to care for disaster victims varied depending upon the circumstances, with 98% willing to help after an airline disaster, 76.4% willing to help after a radionuclide event, and 60.9% willing to work after a infectious agent scenario. Gender, but not parental status, was an important factor in staffing.

Pharmaceutical services represent one of the most important and yet under- recognized services in mass casualty care and disaster medical services. Proper integration of pharmaceutical services can represent the difference between a successful operation and a chaotic one. Integration of pharmaceutical services is an important element in any hospital-specific, local and national disaster preparedness plan. The Agency for Health Care Quality and Research (AHQR) has developed a computer-based simulation for mass pharmaceutical distribution and mass vaccination in the disaster setting.

- Advice to Hospital and Health-system Pharmacy Directors.
- Advice to Hospital and Health-system Pharmacists.
- Advice to Hospital and Health-system Administrators.
- Advice to Emergency Preparedness Planners.
- Advice to State Societies of Health-system Pharmacists.

Whether preparing for mass antidote administration or the development of mass antibiotic prophylactic stations, hospitals in the post-9/11 in USA or 26/11 in INDIA, environment must develop hospital- and community-specific plans including the provision of adequate pharmaceutical stockpiling. This may require the formation of hospital pharmacy consortiums or vendor agreements, providing the ability to rapidly obtain and distribute needed pharmaceutical supplies during a disaster.

Outbreak of Influenza epidemic; disaster proportions

The recent outbreaks of avian influenza (H5N1) have placed a renewed emphasis on preparing for an influenza pandemic in humans. Developing plans to deal with the allocation of critical care resources, including mechanical ventilators, which will likely become scarce during a pandemic, presents a significant challenge. Models of the potential impact of a pandemic on the Ontario population predict that hospital admissions for influenza will peak at 1823 per day over a 6-week period. This translates to 72% of the total hospital capacity being used by influenza patients. Similarly, the demand for intensive care unit (ICU) resources, solely for patients with influenza, would peak at 171% of current ICU bed capacity and 118% of the ventilator capacity. When resource scarcities occur, the tenets of biomedical ethics and international law dictate that triage protocols be used to guide resource allocation. International law requires a triage plan that will equitably provide every person the "opportunity" to survive. However, such a law does not guarantee either treatment or survival. They have developed this triage protocol in an effort to ensure the equitable and efficient use of critical care resources if scarcities occur during an influenza pandemic.

Critical care triage protocol

The working group embarked on developing a critical care triage protocol. Although triage protocols were identified for trauma and chemical, biological, radiation and nuclear events, these were not felt to be generalizeable to the population or situations in critical care. However, certain features of these protocols (e.g., a colour-coded triage tool, inclusion criteria, exclusion criteria and minimum qualifications for survival were deemed useful for a triage protocol for critical care. Illness severity scoring systems used to predict critical care outcomes were also assessed for potential inclusion in the protocol. The Sequential Organ Failure Assessment (SOFA) score was felt to be the most appropriate scoring system for use in a triage protocol given its basis on physiologic parameters, ease of calculation, requirement for simple laboratory tests and its validation for use in patients with a wide variety of conditions requiring critical care.

The protocol is designed to provide guidance for making triage decisions during the initial days to weeks of an influenza pandemic if the critical care system is overwhelmed. The impetus for this triage protocol was the potential for the critical care system to be flooded by patients with influenza during a pandemic. However, it must be noted that the triage protocol would apply to all patients who are being considered for critical care, not just those with influenza, since all patients must share a single pool of resources.

The triage protocol has 4 main components: inclusion criteria, exclusion criteria, minimum qualifications for survival and a prioritization tool. The inclusion criteria identify patients who may benefit from admission to critical care and primarily focus on respiratory failure, since the provision of ventilatory support is what fundamentally differentiates the ICU from other acute care areas. It is anticipated that expanded care models will be developed as part of the surge capacity response and will permit hemodynamic support and other advanced care modalities to be provided in areas that have appropriate monitoring but do not typically provide this level of care. However, should hemodynamic support not be available elsewhere, it will qualify as an inclusion criterion for critical care admission.

The exclusion criteria can be broken down into 3 categories: patients who have a poor prognosis despite care in an ICU, patients who require resources that simply cannot be provided during a pandemic and patients with advanced medical illnesses whose underlying illness has a poor prognosis with a high likelihood of death, even without their current concomitant critical illness.

Maximizing benefits for the largest number

This triage protocol is a tool aimed at maximizing benefits for the largest number of patients presenting to an overwhelmed critical care system. The ethical values that inform this protocol were derived from the work of the Joint Centre for Bioethics, in the document Stand on Guard for Thee. They identified 10 substantive values (individual liberty, protection of the public from harm, proportionality, privacy, duty to provide care, reciprocity, equity, trust, solidarity and stewardship) and 5 procedural values (reasonable, open and transparent, inclusive, responsive and accountable). Under normal circumstances, all patients should have an equal claim to receive the health care they need. Unfortunately, during a pandemic it will not be possible for all patients to receive intensive care due to finite resources. A triage protocol will assist in distributing the available resources fairly by triaging patients who will not benefit from treatment to non-critical care management, thereby conserving critical care resources for patients who are more likely to benefit. Although it may be unfortunate that some patients do not receive all that they could possibly "use," this does not by default make it unfair. Any restrictions placed on treatment must, however, adhere to the value of proportionality, which requires that restrictions to individual liberties not exceed what is necessary to address the essential needs of the community.

The protocol was developed by experts in advance of a pandemic, to allow time for thoughtful contemplation and community input before ever employing the protocol. When the protocol is implemented, it must be used in an open and transparent manner. Its limitations must be acknowledged, with plans to revise it as information becomes available regarding prognostic factors, specifics of the influenza virus causing the pandemic and resource availability. Processes for ongoing re-evaluation and for consideration of exceptions must be developed in addition to an appeals mechanism. Aside from being an ethical imperative, a process to evaluate and refine the triage protocol prevents undertriage or overtriage, both of which increase overall deaths in disasters. This process will require a central triage committee as well as appropriate infrastructure to collect and review the information for analysis and to disseminate revisions to the protocol. This committee may serve many different and distant critical care centres. The central triage committee must assure a population-based approach with equitable resource allocation. Advanced training will be required for triage officers to effectively implement the triage protocol. This is not unique to our protocol, since most military and disaster triage guidelines also require extensive training for effective use.

References

Aiken LH, Buchan J, Sochalski J, *et al.* Trends in International Nurse Migration. *Health Aff* (Millwood) 2004; 23: 69-77.

American Society for Transplant Physicians (ASTP)/American Thoracic Society(ATS)/ European Respiratory Society(ERS)/International Society for Heart and Lung Transplantation(ISHLT). International guidelines for the selection of lung transplant candidates. *Am J Respir Crit Care Med* 1998;158:335-9.

ASHP Statement on the Role of Health-System Pharmacists in Emergency Preparedness. Retrieved from the web at: [www.ashp.org/emergency/counterte...], on January 2nd 2005.

Barthell EN, Aronsky D, Cochrane DG, Cable G, Stair T; Frontlines Work Group. The Frontlines of Medicine Project progress report: standardized communication of emergency department triage data for syndromic surveillance. *Ann Emerg Med.* 2004 Sep;44(3):247-52.

Bartram T, Joiner TA, and Stanton P. Factors Affecting the Job Stress and Job Satisfaction of Australian Nurses: Implications for Recruitment and Retention. *Contemp Nurse* 2004; 17: 293-304.

Baskett PJ. Ethics in disaster medicine. *Prehospital Disaster Med* 1994;9:4-5.[Medline]

Beigel JH, Farrar J, Han AM, *et al.* Avian influenza A (H5N1) infection in humans. *N Engl J Med* 2005;353:1374-85.[Free Full Text]

Benson M, Koenig KL, Schultz CH. Disaster triage: START, then SAVE—a new method of dynamic triage for victims of a catastrophic earthquake. *Prehospital Disaster Med* 1996;11:117-24.[Medline]

Boyd CR, Tolson MA, Copes WS. Evaluating trauma care: the TRISS method. Trauma Score and the Injury Severity Score. *J Trauma* 1987;27:370-8.[Medline]

Brindley PG, Markland DM, Mayers I, *et al.* Predictors of survival following in-hospital adult cardiopulmonary resuscitation. *CMAJ* 2002;167(4):343-8.[Abstract/ Free Full Text]

Burkle FM Jr. Mass casualty management of a large-scale bioterrorist event: an epidemiological approach that shapes triage decisions. *Emerg Med Clin North* Am 2002;20:409-36.[CrossRef][Medline]

Cabre L, Mancebo J, Solsona JF, *et al.* Multicenter study of the multiple organ dysfunction syndrome in intensive care units: the usefulness of Sequential Organ Failure Assessment scores in decision-making. *Intensive Care Med* 2005;31:927-

Canadian Association of Emergency Physicians. Guidelines for Managing Severe Acute Respiratory Syndrome (SARS) in Canadian Emergency Departments. 18 April 2003. Accessed 1/11/05. [www.caep.ca/002.policies/002-01. ...]

Cardiac Transplantation. 24th Bethesda Conference. November 5–6, 1992. *J Am Coll Cardiol* 1993;22:1-64.[Medline]

Devlin J, O'Grady J. Indications for referral and assessment in adult liver transplantation: a clinical guideline. British Society of Gastroenterology. *Gut* 1999;45 (Suppl 6):VI1-VI22.

Disaster and Hospital Functions Retrieved from the web on December 26th, 2004

Domres B, Koch M, Manger A, *et al.* Ethics and triage. *Prehospital Disaster Med* 2001;16:53-8.[Medline]

Duffield C and O'Brien-Pallas L. The Causes and Consequences of Nursing Shortages: A Helicopter View of the Research. *Aust Health Rev* 2003; 26: 186-193.

Fauci AS. Pandemic influenza threat and preparedness. *Emerg Infect Dis* 2006;12:73-7.[Medline]

Ferreira FL, Bota DP, Bross A, *et al.* Serial evaluation of the SOFA score to predict outcome in critically ill patients. *JAMA* 2001;286:1754

Fleischauer AT, Silk BJ, Schumacher M, Komatsu K, Santana S, Vaz V, Wolfe M, Hutwagner L, Cono J, Berkelman R, Treadwell T. The Validity of Chief Complaint and Discharge Diagnosis in Emergency Department-based Syndromic Surveillance. *Acad Emerg Med.* 2004 Dec;11(12):1262-7.

Foldy S, Biedrzycki PA, Barthell EN, Healy-Haney N, Baker BK, Howe DS, Gieryn D, Pemble KR. Syndromic surveillance using regional emergency medicine Internet. *Ann Emerg Med.* 2004 Sep;44(3):242-6.

Fowler RA, Lapinsky SE, Hallett D, *et al.* Critically ill patients with severe acute respiratory syndrome. *JAMA* 2003;290:367-73.[Abstract/Free Full Text]

Frykberg ER. Medical management of disasters and mass casualties from terrorist bombings: how can we cope? *J Trauma* 2002;53:201-12.[Medline]

Gardiner B. Doctors Among Victims in Tsunami-Hit Indonesia; Nordic Leaders Tour Thailand. Canadian Press Online, Accessed 1/17/05.

Garner A, Lee A, Harrison K, *et al.* Comparative analysis of multiple-casualty incident triage algorithms. *Ann Emerg Med* 2001;38:541-8.[CrossRef][Medline]

Geller RJ, Lopez GP, Cutler S, Lin D, Bachman GF, Gorman SE. Atropine availability as an antidote for nerve agent casualties: validated rapid reformulation of high-concentration atropine from bulk powder. *Ann Emerg Med.* 2003 Apr; 41(4):453-6.

Hayden F, Croisier A. Transmission of avian influenza viruses to and between humans. *J Infect Dis* 2005;192:1311-4.[CrossRef][Medline]

Hick JL, Hanfling D, Burstein JL, *et al.* Health care facility and community strategies for patient care surge capacity. *Ann Emerg Med* 2004;44:253-61.[CrossRef][Medline]

Hick JL, O'Laughlin DT. Concept of operations for triage of mechanical ventilation in an epidemic. *Acad Emerg Med* 2006;13:223-9.[CrossRef][Medline]

Irvin CB, Nouhan PP, Rice K. Syndromic analysis of computerized emergency department patients' chief complaints: an opportunity for bioterrorism and influenza surveillance. *Ann Emerg Med.* 2003 Apr;41(4):447-52.

Kilgo PD, Meredith JW, Osler TM. Incorporating recent advances to make the TRISS approach universally available. *J Trauma* 2006;60:1002-8.[Medline]

Knaus WA, Draper EA, Wagner DP, *et al.* APACHE II: a severity of disease classification system. *Crit Care Med* 1985;13:818-29.

Knaus WA, Wagner DP, Draper EA, *et al.* The APACHE III prognostic system. Risk prediction of hospital mortality for critically ill hospitalized adults. *Chest* 1991;100:1619-36.[Medline]

Knaus WA, Zimmerman JE, Wagner DP, *et al.* APACHE-acute physiology and chronic health evaluation: a physiologically based classification system. *Crit Care Med* 1981;9:591-7.

Loutfy MR, Wallington T, Rutledge T, *et al.* Hospital Preparedness and SARS. *Emerg Infect Dis* 2004; 771-776.

Marshall JC. Organ dysfunction as an outcome measure in clinical trials. *Eur J Surg Suppl* 1999;584:62-7.

Maziak DE, Lindsay TF, Marshall JC, *et al.* The impact of multiple organ dysfunction on mortality following ruptured abdominal aortic aneurysm repair. Ann Vasc Surg 1998;12:93-100.

Ministry of Health and Long-Term Care. Ontario health plan for an influenza pandemic 2006. Available: www.health.gov.on.ca/english/providers/program/emu/pan_flu/pan_flu_plan.html (accessed 2006 Sept 25).

Nagle LM and Vincent L. A SARS Postcard—Reflections of Two Health Care Leaders. *Nurs Leadership.* 2003; 16: 24-26.

Oda S, Hirasawa H, Sugai T, *et al.* Comparison of Sepsis-related Organ Failure Assessment (SOFA) score and CIS (cellular injury score) for scoring of severity for patients with multiple organ dysfunction syndrome (MODS). *Intensive Care Med.* 2000;26:1786-93.[CrossRef][Medline]

Okumura T, Suzuki K, Fukuda A, Kohama A, Takasu N, Ishimatsu S, Hinohara S.The Tokyo subway sarin attack: disaster management, Part 2: Hospital response. *Acad Emerg Med.* 1998 Jun; 5(6):618-24.

Ontario Health Coalition. Ontario Health Coalition Submission to the SARS Commission. 18 November 2003. Accessed 5 January 2005. 8. Nickell LA, Crighton EJ, Tracy CS, *et al.* Psychosocial Effects of SARS on Hospital Staff: Survey of a Large Tertiary Care Institution. *CMAJ* 2004; 170: 793-798.

Ontario Ministry of Health and Long Term Care. SARS Provincial Operations Centre: Directives to All Ontario Acute Care Hospitals Regarding Infection Control Measures. *Directive* 03-05. 20 April 2003.

Osterholm MT. Preparing for the next pandemic. *N Engl J Med* 2005;352:1839-42.[Free Full Text]

Palmer K. Librarian Sues Over SARS Duty. Toronto Star 10 July 2003. Accessed 11 January 2005. [www.thestar.com/NASApp/cs/Conten...]

Parsons L. Toronto: New SARS Outbreak Provokes Nurses' Protest. World Socialist Web Site. 10 June 2003. Accessed 5 January 2005. [www.wsws.org/articles/2003/jun20

Peres Bota D, Melot C, Lopes Ferriera F, *et al.* The Multiple Organ Dysfunction Score (MODS) versus the Sequential Organ Failure Assessment (SOFA) score in outcome prediction. *Intensive Care Med.* 2002;28:1619-24.[CrossRef][Medline]

Public Health Agency of Canada. Canadian pandemic influenza plan. 2004. Available: www.phac-aspc.gc.ca/cpip-pclcpi/(accessed 2006 Sept 25).

Risavi BL, Salen PN, Heller MB, *et al.* A two-hour intervention using START improves prehospital triage of mass casualty incidents. *Prehosp Emerg Care* 2001;5:197-9.[CrossRef][Medline]

Romig LE. Pediatric triage. A system to JumpSTART your triage of young patients at MCIs. *JEMS* 2002;27:52-8.[Medline]

Rubenfeld GD, Caldwell E, Peabody E, *et al.* Incidence and outcomes of acute lung injury. *N Engl J Med* 2005;353:1685-93.[Abstract/Free Full Text]

Rubinson L, Nuzzo JB, Talmor DS, *et al.* Augmentation of hospital critical care capacity after bioterrorist attacks or epidemics: recommendations of the Working Group on Emergency Mass Critical Care. *Crit Care Med* 2005;33:2393-403.[CrossRef][Medline]

Rubinson L, O'Toole T. Critical care during epidemics. *Critical Care* 2005;9:311-3.[CrossRef][Medline]

Ryan CM, Schoenfeld DA, Thorpe WP, *et al.* Objective estimates of the probability of death from burn injuries. *N Engl J Med* 1998;338:362-6.[Abstract/Free Full Text]

Seventeen critical benchmarks for bioterrorism preparedness planning. US Department of Health and Human Services (DHHS) June 6 2002. HSS Press Office.

Sheward L, Hunt J, Hagen S, *et al.* The Relationship Between UK Hospital Nurse Staffing and Emotional Exhaustion and Job Dissatisfaction. *J Nurs Manag* 2005; 13: 51-50. Khowaja K, Merchant RJ, and Hirani D. Registered Nurses Perception of Work Satisfaction at a Tertiary Care University Hospital. *J Nurs Manag* 2005; 13: 32-39.

Sinuff T, Kahnamoui K, Cook DJ, *et al.* Rationing critical care beds: a systematic review. *Crit Care Med.* 2004;32:1588-97.[CrossRef][Medline]

Society of Critical Care Medicine Ethics Committee. Consensus statement on the triage of critically ill patients. *JAMA* 1994;271:1200-3.[Abstract]

Steffen C, Masterson L, Christos S, *et al.* Willingness to Respond: A Survey of Emergency Department Personnel and Their Predicted Participation in Mass Casualty Terrorist events. *Ann Emerg Med* 2004; 44 (Suppl): S34.

Suyama J, Sztajnkrycer M, Lindsell C, Otten EJ, Daniels JM, Kressel Surveillance of infectious disease occurrences in the community: an analysis of symptom presentation in the emergency department.. *Acad Emerg Med.* 2003 Jul;10(7):753-63.

Tallgren M, Klepstad P, Petersson J, *et al.* Ethical issues in intensive care—a survey among Scandinavian intensivists. *Acta Anaesthesiol Scand* 2005;49:1092-100.[CrossRef][Medline]

Task Force of the American College of Critical Care Medicine, Society of Critical Care Medicine. Guidelines for intensive care unit admission, discharge, and triage. *Crit Care Med.* 1999;27:633-8.[CrossRef][Medline]

UKT Cardiothoracic Advisory Group. National protocol for the assessment of cardiothoracic transplant patients. Bristol (UK): The Group; 2002. Available: www.uktransplant.org.uk/ukt/about_transplants/organ_allocation/cardiothoracic/national_protocols_and_standards/protocols_and_standards/patient_assessment.jsp (accessed 2006 Sept 25).

United Nations Department of Peacekeeping Operations. Medical support manual for United Nations peacekeeping operations. 2nd ed. New York: Department of Peacekeeping Operations; 1999. Available: www.un.org/Depts/dpko/training/tes_publications/books/medical_support/med_support.pdf (accessed 2006 Sept 25).

University of Toronto Joint Centre for Bioethics Pandemic Influenza Working Group.

Stand on guard for thee: ethical considerations in preparedness planning for pandemic influenza. Toronto: University of Toronto Joint Centre for Bioethics; 2005. Available: www.utoronto.ca/jcb/home/documents/pandemic.pdf (accessed 2006 Sept 25).

US Centers for Disease Control and Prevention (CDC). FluSurge 2.0. Atlanta: CDC. Available: www.cdc.gov/flu/flusurge.htm (accessed 2006 Oct 16).

Verbeek PR, McClelland IW, Silverman AC, *et al.* Loss of Paramedic Availability in an Urban Emergency Medical Services System During a Severe Acute Respiratory Syndrome Outbreak. *Acad Emerg Med* 2004; 11: 973 - 978.

Vincent JL, Moreno R, Takala J, *et al.* The SOFA (Sepsis-related Organ Failure Assessment) score to describe organ dysfunction/failure. On behalf of the Working Group on Sepsis-related Problems of the European Society of Intensive Care Medicine. *Intensive Care Med.* 1996;22:707-10.[Medline]

Vollmar L.C. Military medicine in war: the Geneva Conventions today. In: Beam TE, Sparacino LR, editors. Military medical ethics. Washington, DC: Office of the Surgeon General; 2003.

Webster RG, Peiris M, Chen H, *et al.* H5N1 outbreaks and enzootic influenza. *Emerg Infect Dis* 2006;12:3-8.[Medline]

World Health Organisation Global Influenza Programme Surveillance Network. Evolution of H5N1 avian influenza viruses in Asia. *Emerg Infect Dis* 2005;11:1515-21.[Medline]

Appendix

International Organisations

European Union Humanitarian Aid Office (ECHO). Humanitarian aid office of the European Union. Site includes lists of publications and decisions.

Food and Agriculture Organisation of the United Nations, includes a section on emergency relief operations. See also the FAO Global Information and Early Warning System.

Inter-governmental Oceanographic Commission. Includes section on mitigation of marine related disasters.

International Fund for Agricultural Development. Specialized agency of the United Nations dedicated to eradicating rural poverty in developing countries.

Joint UNEP/OCHA Environment Unit. United Nations mechanism to coordinate the international response to environmental emergencies and natural disasters.

Joint United Nations Programme on HIV/AIDS (UNAIDS). The UN AIDS agency. See the section on HIV/AIDS in Emergency Settings.

United Nations Capital Development Fund. Investment fund for Least Developed Countries to help reduce poverty and achieve the Millennium Development Goals.

United Nations Children's Fund (UNICEF). United Nations children's agency. See the section for publications on children and emergencies.

United Nations Development Programme Disaster Reduction Unit. See also UNDP Publications on Disasters.

United Nations High Commissioner for Refugees (UNHCR). The United Nations Refugee Agency. Includes many online books, papers and statistics.

United Nations International Strategy for Disaster Reduction. UN agency charged with reducing human, social, economic and environmental losses due to natural hazards.

United Nations Millennium Development Goals Web Site. Outlines the background, objectives and progress to date of the eight UN Millennium Development Goals.

United Nations Office for Coordination of Humanitarian Affairs. Chief UN office for coordination of humanitarian affairs, within the UN itself and with other international agencies, especially for major emergencies and natural disasters.

United Nations Office of the High Representative for the Least Developed Countries. UN Office for Least Developed Countries, Landlocked Developing Countries, and Small Island Developing States.

United Nations Department of Peacekeeping Operations (DPKO). UN agency with responsibility for maintenance of international peace and security. Includes links to ongoing missions, e.g. in Chad and Darfur.

United Nations Social, Humanitarian and Cultural Committee. "Third Committee" of the UN General Assembly, with a mandate to address human rights, social development, refugees, advancement of women, indigenous peoples, and more.

World Food Programme (WFP). The United Nations Food Agency. The WFP is the world's largest international food aid organisation, dedicated to combating hunger in nations with severe food shortages. World Health Organisation. Activities, reports, news and events in WHO programmes and offices working on the health-related aspects of disasters.

Nongovernmental Organisations (NGOs)

There are many NonGovernmental Organisations devoted to disasters and humanitarian relief. Please see the UC Berkeley Library research guide on Non-governmental Organisations (NGOs) for additional information. The following are some of the more important NGOs in this field.

Directories

American Council for Voluntary Interaction. Links to disaster relief organisations.

Directory of Development Organisations. Over 47,000 organisations of all kinds listed by region and country. One of the most extensive compilation of NGO country directories.

Idealist.Org. Excellent online NGO directory. Includes section on "Disaster Response Resources".

OneWorld.net. Network of over 400 international agencies working in development, human rights and disaster relief.

TakingITGlobal. International non-profit organisation centered on young people interested in connecting across cultures. Good source of NGO information by country and area of focus. Go to browse organisations. USAID Directory of Private Voluntary Organisations. Pull down menu by "activity sector" includes food security, disaster relief, etc.

WANGO. World Association of Non-Governmental Organisations. Excellent NGO directory by region.

Selected Humanitarian NGOs

American National Red Cross. Mission is to save lives and ease suffering by providing relief to victims of disaster, locally and globally. Doctors Without Borders. International medical humanitarian organisation that delivers emergency aid to people affected by armed conflict, epidemics, natural or man-made disasters, or exclusion from health care in more than 70 countries.

Genocide Intervention Network. Nonprofit working to protect civilians from genocide and mass atrocities. Background and information on conflicts worldwide involving widespread civilian death and displacement.

International Crisis Group. Non-governmental organisation working to prevent and resolve deadly conflict through field analysis and advocacy. International Federation of Red Cross and Red Crescent Societies, (IFRC). Related organisation with the ICRC, the two societies share the same secretariat in Geneva. The Red Crescent is used in place of the Red Cross in many Islamic countries.

International Committee of the Red Cross (ICRC). Largest Humanitarian Organisation. See their World Disaster's Report and extensive list of online publications.

InterAction. Large alliance of U.S. based international development and humanitarian nongovernmental organisations.

International Save the Children Alliance. World's largest independent organisation for children, working in 110 countries world-wide. NetAid. Development web site dedicated to eradicating poverty worldwide Red R. Mission to select and train personnel for humanitarian programmes working in disaster situations world-wide.

Relief International. NGO providing emergency rehabilitation and development services in the areas of health, shelter, food, conflict resolution, etc.

World Vision International. Relief and development organisation working in the areas of emergency relief, education, health care, economic development and promotion of justice.

Relief Organisations for Natural Disasters

Action Against Hunger

(May 12, 2008)—Working on the ground in Myanmar since 1994, Action Against Hunger/Action Contre la Faim (ACF) teams responded immediately with rapid assessments around Yangon and in the Ayeyarwaddy delta. Based on rapid assessments, ACF launched emergency operations in Yangon and Bogalay while flying reinforcements to the region to ensure a response in the south. Current programmes: environmental clearing and clean-up; distributions of nutritional products (high protein biscuits), food (rice, oil, beans, lentils), and essential non-food items (cooking and hygiene kits); distributions of water purifying tablets, pumps, and equipment for the provision of clean water. Next phase: rehabilitation and protection of water points and hygiene education; distributions of rations, cash, and/or vouchers depending on market accessibility. Donations can be made at http://support.actionagainsthunger.org/donate.

ADRA International

Myanmar Cyclone Fund, 12501 Old Columbia Pike, Silver Spring, MD 20904, 1-800-424-ADRA (2372) (May 12, 2008)—In a continued effort to assist the survivors of Cyclone Nargis, the Adventist Development and Relief Agency (ADRA) has committed at least $235,000 in emergency funds for immediate disaster relief, and is providing food assistance and medical supplies to communities in the hard-hit Irrawaddy Delta region in southern

Myanmar. ADRA is currently accepting financial contributions to help the communities affected by this disaster. Donations can be made securely at http://www.adra.org/.

Air Serv International

(May 7, 2008)—Air Serv International is preparing to be a first responder to Myanmar disaster. With helicopters ready to deliver crucial supplies and relief workers to areas hardest hit in this devastated country, Air Serv is conducting a needs-assessment on how to deliver aid to the Myanmar people quickly and efficiently. As time is always an issue in responding to a disaster, Air Serv mobilized its Rapid Response Team the moment news broke about the events in Myanmar. Air Serv International is accepting gifts in kind of aircraft equipment, communications equipment, and fuel.

American Friends Service Committee

(May 9, 2008)—The American Friends Service Committee is responding to the flooding in Myanmar with immediate assistance to those affected. AFSC also is committed to a long-term recovery that is flexible to the needs of the Burmese people, building on our ongoing partnerships with community groups and schools.

American Jewish Joint Distribution Committee

(May 6, 2008)—JDC is collecting funds to assist the cyclone victims on a nonsectarian basis. JDC is now in contact with leaders from the local Jewish Community in Yangon and with other disaster relief partners in the region to determine an appropriate emergency response, one that reaches those who are not being served by others.

American Jewish World Service

45 West 36th Street, 11th Floor, New York, NY 10016, 1-800-889-7146.

(May 6, 2008)—AJWS has been making grants focused on Burma since 2002 and has long-standing partnerships with organisations on the eastern and northern borders of the country. These groups are providing contacts and support networks to those who are affected. AJWS is providing rapid relief funding to communities hit by the storm, particularly in the Irrawaddy River Delta. Due to their remote rural location, these communities are even less able to access aid than those in other parts of Burma.

American Red Cross

(May 12, 2008)—The American Red Cross is supporting the relief efforts of the Myanmar Red Cross, which has more than 27,000 volunteers on the ground. On May 11, the first airplane of American Red Cross supplies arrived in country. In total, the American Red Cross has made available an estimated 10,000 tarps, 20,000 mosquito nets, 3,800 kitchen sets, 30,000 jerry cans, and 15,000 hygiene kits from warehouses in Kuala Lumpur and Dubai. As of May 12, the American Red Cross has committed a total of $1.5 million in supplies and financial support, including $1 million from USAID. The American Red Cross is in close contact with the International Federation of Red Cross and Red Crescent Societies and will provide additional assistance as needed.

American Refugee Committee

(May 6, 2008)—ARC intends to respond to the emergency and is working to distribute emergency supplies. Pending approval of entry visas, a rapid assessment team will be deployed to the region. ARC will work with local partners to respond.

AmeriCares

(May 6, 2008)—AmeriCares has relief workers on the ground in Myanmar coordinating our relief efforts. Our emergency response includes over 15 tons of essential medicines and medical supplies valued at more than $1 million ready to leave our warehouse in Amsterdam. We are also looking into alternate delivery methods in order to send our aid as quickly as possible. AmeriCares aid includes emergency medicines and medical supplies essential for relief efforts after a disaster, including: antibiotics, analgesics, latex gloves, oral rehydration salts, multivitamins, anti-malarials, medications used to treat diarrheal diseases and dengue fever, as well as water purification sachets to produce potable water in the flooded region.

Giving Children Hope

(May 12, 2008)—Giving Children Hope is collecting monetary donations for the victims of the Myanmar cyclone. Monetary donations are being collected to purchase water purification tablets, antibiotics, mosquito netting, local food, and other disaster materials. Giving Children Hope is an Orange County, California, faith-based, non-profit organisation engaged in domestic and international poverty alleviation through disaster relief, medical development, vocational training, and advocacy.

Habitat for Humanity

(May 6, 2008)—Habitat for Humanity is assembling a technical team to partner with other organisations in support of long-term shelter reconstruction efforts for those affected by Cyclone Nargis in Myanmar, which left nearly one million people homeless. HFHI has played a major role in rebuilding efforts following the 2004 Indian Ocean tsunami and will bring its considerable experience in rebuilding permanent housing following disasters to the work in Myanmar.

Hands On Disater Response

(May 12, 2008)—Hands On Disaster Response has recently completed our project in Bangladesh, after cyclone Sidr, repairing and building schools and homes, and providing a broad range of volunteer based disaster assistance. We will send an assessment team to Myanmar, and are prepared for a similar response, pending visa approvals. See http://www.hodr.org/for information on the work of more than 2,000 volunteers over our past five projects and to make a secure donation.

International Medical Corps (IMC)

(May 12, 2008)—International Medical Corps (IMC) is coordinating with international and local partners to provide emergency relief for the survivors of Cyclone Nargis. IMC is working closely with the World Food Programme and other international organisations on the ground in Myanmar, as well as a local partner, to administer medicines, medical supplies, and other relief items while waiting on visas to deploy its emergency response team. Once on the ground, IMC will continue to collaborate with its partners to administer emergency medical assistance and distribute relief materials to Myanmar's most impacted populations, including Yangon and the Irrawaddy Delta region. Christian Reformed World Relief Committee (CRWRC) is responding to Cyclone Nargis with partners in Burma to provide 10,000 displaced families with emergency food, shelter, medical care, and water purification kits through July 31, 2008. CRWRC will continue to collaborate with local NGOs to assess and determine plans for additional recovery, resettlement and reconstruction phases during this time.

International Relief and Development

(May 12, 2008)—IRD is accepting donations to help victims of Cyclone Nargis. IRD is lending its regional expertise to provide humanitarian aid and support the work of local Burmese organisations responding to the disaster. IRD's response will be based on the needs on the ground and has traditionally consisted of emergency nonfood items, food, and water.

International Relief Teams

(May 6, 2008)—International Relief Teams (IRT) is collecting cash donations to help purchase relief supplies to assist the survivors of the catastrophic cyclone in Myanmar. IRT will work in collaboration with partner organisations to get aid to communities most affected.

International Rescue Committee

(May 6, 2008)—International Rescue Committee emergency experts have started arriving in Myanmar to determine the needs of cyclone survivors and launch rapid relief efforts. IRC teams initially expect to focus on supplying clean water and emergency supplies and setting up sanitation facilities for tens of thousands of vulnerable people who have been made homeless by the disaster. In addition to water, urgent needs include shelter materials, food, and special care for children.

Latter-day Saint Charities

(May 6, 2008)—Latter-day Saint Charities has been working in Myanmar since 1998 with emphasis on clean water and mother/child health. We have a field team in-country and closely cooperate with other international agencies in disaster response. Latter-day Saint Charities is accepting gifts in kind of medical supplies.

Lutheran World Relief

(May 6, 2008)—LWR is supporting the response of Action by Churches Together, a worldwide coalition of faith-based aid agencies, to the Myanmar (Burma) cyclone. The response will address emergency needs such as food, clean water, and shelter. LWR is also exploring other potential partnerships for responding to this disaster.

Medical Teams International

(May 8, 2008)—Medical Teams International is partnering with World Concern in Myanmar to purchase medicines and supplies for families devastated by Cyclone Nargis. Agency medical volunteers and staff are also on standby in various countries, waiting for visa approval to enter Myanmar. Once these approvals are received, these volunteers and staff will provide direct medical care and help local partners expand their efforts to prevent and treat disease. Medical Teams International is currently accepting donations and gifts in kind of antibiotics, analgesics, antifungals, and malaria and cholera drugs.

MAP International

(May 12, 2008)—MAP International is currently working with partner organisations on the ground in Myanmar to provide emergency medicines and relief supplies. MAP has shipped medicines to Bangkok, which will be hand-carried into Myanmar. In addition to delivering medicines to medical teams, MAP is also purchasing medicines from local sources. MAP is planning to remain involved in Myanmar for at least the next 12 to 15 months.

Mercy Corps

(May 12, 2008)—Mercy Corps is sending its top European official to Myanmar and hopes to have several other members of an emergency-response team in country in the coming week. Mervyn Lee, executive director of Mercy Corps Europe, is expected to arrive early next week in Myanmar. Once on the ground, Mercy Corps staff will work with partner agencies to help assess needs and explore opportunities to ease suffering in the aftermath of Cyclone Nargis. Mercy Corps will explore ways to provide clean water and reduce disease risks through improved sanitation. The agency will also consider Cash-for-Work programmes that pay residents to clear debris, repair infrastructure, and fill other immediate needs.

Operation USA

(May 12, 2008)—Operation USA has a team on the Thailand-Myanmar border awaiting entry visas and is partnering with IOs and NGOs active inside Myanmar. OpUSA has worked for 15 years with Burmese refugees in the border areas and is purchasing relief supplies locally as well as preparing medical shipments from its U.S. warehouse.

Pact (May 8, 2008)—Pact has more than 1,300 local staff working in Myanmar. Four hundred of them are in the Delta region working from 34 branch offices (mostly intact due to sturdier construction) in more than 1,500 villages. Pact is the only NGO with such reach and, in two of the hardest hit townships, the only operating NGO. Because of the local, on-the-ground network, Pact is being asked to take on a role as distributors of immediate assistance—most importantly food, water, and shelter. Pact anticipates initially to be able to mobilize efforts to reach 75,000 households with food aid, 50,000 with oral rehydration solution, and 20,000 with plastic water containers. Down the road, Pact hopes to be able also to help survivors of the cyclone to rebuild their lives.

Project HOPE

(May 6, 2008)—Project HOPE will respond with appropriate medical assistance when the needs have been assessed and requirements identified. We will work with donor companies to secure donations of medical product, with individuals to secure cash donations to support our response, and with partner organisations to ensure that the medicines are properly stored and utilized. If a longer-term response is warranted, HOPE will make a determination as to what role it can play.

Relief International

(May 6, 2008)—Relief International (RI) is assessing the extent of damage and evaluating appropriate emergency response strategies to provide aid, following a massive Category 3 cyclone in southeast Myanmar. RI is reaching out to local partners to provide emergency assistance to relief operations. RI programme response will be expanded as emergency and long-term needs are detailed. The RI Rapid Emergency Deployment (RED) team is currently on standby at our Los Angeles headquarters to provide additional assistance. To help, please donate now to RI's Emergency Response Fund (ERF). The ERF is RI's revolving emergency fund, drawn upon only for emergencies throughout the world, including the current crisis in Myanmar.

Salvation Army World Services Army

(May 12, 2008)—The Salvation Army has been in Burma (Myanmar) since 1915. Personnel there are providing cooked meals from their own store of food for those in desperate need. They are also dispensing rice and other available relief materials. Two Salvation Army children's homes in Yangon have artesian wells and personnel are running the generators to pump water from the wells almost non-stop. The public is coming to these compounds to receive water. An assessment team from the region is currently determining the most immediate needs to be met and will plan accordingly. SAWSO is committed to supporting the Salvation Army in meeting urgent and other needs as they emerge over the long haul.

Save the Children USA

(May 12, 2008)—During the first week of relief operations, Save the Children's 500-person staff based in Myanmar has reached 100,000 survivors of the cyclone in 12 Yangon townships and the Irrawaddy Delta region. Supplies have included rice, water, oral solution, water purification devices, blankets, materials for cooking, and shelter. The first plane load of relief supplies arrived in Myanmar this weekend. Government officials approved the shipment and the materials are now on their way to the delta region. During the past week Save the Children has been purchasing relief materials within the country to supplement its massive relief operation.

Unitarian Universalist Service Committee

(May 6, 2008)—The Unitarian Universalist Service Committee, an international human rights organisation based in Cambridge, MA, responds strategically to natural or man-made humanitarian crises, especially when rights are threatened or when those in need are overlooked or neglected by traditional relief strategies.

United Methodist Committee on Relief

(May 12, 2008)—UMCOR is responding to the Myanmar cyclone by working through Action by Churches Together, a worldwide coalition of faith-based aid agencies. The response addresses needs such as water, food, and shelter. UMCOR continues to explore other partnerships to respond to this disaster.

International disaster relief organisations and agencies

Organisation or Agency Name	Services
Adventist Development and Relief Agency International (ADRA)	Provides immediate disaster relief; supports development programmes in community development, construction, and agriculture
Church World Service (CWS)	Provides material aid to refugees and disaster victims; supports development programmes in agriculture, energy, soil

	conservation, reforestation, preventive medicine, sanitation, and potable water supply
Cooperative for Assistance Relief Everywhere (CARE)	Provides refugee and disaster relief; and supports development programmes in reforestation, conservation, and agriculture
Direct Relief International (DRI)	Specializes in emergency health care, providing pharmaceuticals, medical supplies, and equipment in famine, refugee, and disaster-affected areas
Disaster Preparedness and Emergency Response Association (DERA)	Assists international communities in disaster preparedness, response, and recovery; serves as a professional association linking disaster relief personnel
Food for the Hungry (FH)	Provides food aid and disaster relief supplies; provides technological support to eliminate hunger
League of Red Cross and Red Crescent Societies (LICROSS)	Coordinates relief activities for disaster victims; provides assistance to refugees; helps countries increase their capacity to respond to humanitarian needs of victims
Lutheran World Federation (LWF)	Provides emergency relief for disaster victims; supports refugee settlement programmes and a variety of development assistance activities
OXFAM International (formerly Oxford Committee for Famine Relief)	Provides assistance to people affected by emergencies, disease, famine, earthquakes, war, and civil conflict; supports long-term development programmes in impoverished nations
Salvation Army World Service Office (SAWSO)	Supports a variety of programmes in disaster relief, community development, food production, public health, and social welfare
United Nations Children's Fund (UNICEF)	Provides disaster and refugee assistance, particularly to children; supports programmes in sanitation and water supply; promotes training and education to improve child health care

United Nations Office for the Coordination of Humanitarian Affairs (OCHA)	Responsible for the coordination of UN assistance in humanitarian crises; provides support for international policy development; advocates humanitarian issues
United States Agency for International Development (USAID)	Provides humanitarian, economic, and development assistance to the international community; houses the Office of U.S. Foreign Disaster Assistance

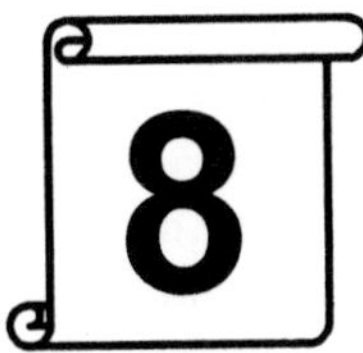

Lapses in Health Care of Disaster Victims

When we talk of disaster and the management of its victims in hospitals, many lapses are bound to occur. In fact the lapses are inherently built in the term 'disaster'. There would be lapses at every stage. The delay in extricating the injured and the dead, the delay in transport, delay or denial in the resuscitation on way to hospital, delay or under-triage before treatment, delay in getting the attention of the skilled medical men, paucity of materials, lack of coordination, breakdown of the communication systems, paucity of hospital space and beds, paucity of food and so on. Certain disasters destroy the hospitals of the area and the result is another disaster for the victims.

Disasters such as the earthquakes in Turkey (1999), Gujarat, India (2001) and Bam, Iran (2003) or the cyclones in Grenada, Haiti and the Philippines (2004) call to mind images of a large number of injured victims awaiting medical treatment and make-shift facilities operating under war-like conditions on the grounds of a severely damaged hospital. However, the medical impact of a damaged health facility runs far deeper. Health services facing the challenge of resuming treatment of normal medical emergencies and providing routine care must, at the same time, offer follow-up care to the disaster victims. As the issue of mass casualties fades from the international conscience (sometimes in a matter of days) and the initial groundswell of support ebbs, an even greater segment of the population will be affected, just when the country needs all its strength to recover. In Gujurat, India, a massive 7.9 magnitude earthquake killed 20,000 and injured 30,000 in 2001. In the most affected district, Kutch, all health facilities collapsed.

In Bam, Iran, the 2003 earthquake left a death toll of 26,271, tens of thousands injured. Public memory faded fast and we started waiting for another disaster.

LIFE PROTECTION IS EXPECTED IN ANY HOSPITAL

Life protection is the minimum level of protection that every hospital structure must comply with. It ensures that a building will not collapse and harm its occupants. Many hospitals in developing countries do not comply with this requirement. However, years ago this was also the case in developed countries. In the 1971 San Fernando, California earthquake, more than 90% of the deaths occurred in hospitals. Investment protection involves safeguarding infrastructure and equipment. From a health point of view, protecting the investment means that repairs can be made more rapidly, leading to much faster rehabilitation. Post-disaster reconstruction can be a very long process. Operational protection is meant to ensure that health facilities can function in the aftermath of a disaster. This is the optimal level of protection for the most essential hospitals. Making hospitals safe from natural disasters requires the multidisciplinary expertise of a variety of experts, from engineers to architects to administrators and others. Specialized engineering skills are required to design or evaluate the structural elements, which include the load-bearing components that make a building stand—columns, beams, roofs and the walls.

New action plan has been launched

The global disaster community has come together for a second World Conference in Kobe, Japan to increase the profile of disaster risk reduction and craft a Plan of Action for 2005-15. This also entails safe hospitals and disaster friendly hospitals, where the lapses would be minimal. Why should the global multi-sectoral Plan of Action include a strong focus on mitigating disaster damage in hospitals and health facilities? Hospitals are much more than just another "critical" facility. Their importance extends far beyond the role they play in saving lives and safeguarding public health in the aftermath of disasters. Health facilities are powerful symbols of social progress and a prerequisite for economic development. There are compelling reasons for all sectors to pay special attention to reducing the physical vulnerability of all health facilities. We have to assess and obviate the lapses to the maximum possible, at all stages in the care of mass casualties.

Let us study some aspects of the lapses that can occur in the pre-disaster stage, during the disaster and the post-disaster phase in relation to an air disaster, which occurred in Nigeria. Indian airports are better than Nigerian airports, but still a few lessons to be learnt.

Lapses in the Pre-Disaster Phase

Starting from the airports, a number of problems were already existent which might have prevented or at least reduced the effects of these disasters if only they had been corrected earlier. The airport infrastructure was in a very poor state. The runways were poorly maintained to the extent that some of them are riddled with potholes. The runway lights, which are especially necessary in the night and in poor weather, are mostly not functional. The radar is epileptic and does not work on weekends. There's also poor security with little or no perimeter fencing in most Nigerian airports. This lack of perimeter fencing was responsible for the July 7, 2005 Air France Airbus taxiing into a herd of cows on the runway of the Port Harcourt International Airport, killing 7 of the cows.

Water supply and electricity at the airports is at best epileptic. Based on anecdotal reports it is said that the airport at Bauchi spent 15 million naira on water in 2005. In fact, one of the major delays in extinguishing the fire from the Sosoliso Airline crash was the unavailability of water at the Port-Harcourt International Airport where the crash occurred. Also, there was no electricity supply in this airport for 6 hours prior to the air-crash. The beacons currently in use at our airports are mostly out-dated and are in fact known to transmit false signals or no signals at all. About 3 hrs after the crash, NEMA got an initial alert on the 121.5 Beacon. However, this particular beacon habitually transmits false signals and instead of getting it changed or at the worst repaired, the practice over time has been to wait until the satellite resolves the alert before swinging into action. (*The Daily Sun*, Wed. 26/10/05). It took a disaster to showcase the hazards of such a laissez-faire attitude. The tower consoles are also reported to be bad.

International Airport at the nation's capital, Abuja, had been operating for the past 23 years without formal registration with the IATA. Their facilities were found not to be up to par with international standards and their staffs were described as incompetent. The Port Harcourt international Airport was also noted by the same Task force to be below standard. (The Punch, 24/12/05) This can only be explained by gross mismanagement and oversight on the part of Airport authority and any other person in charge of the day-to-day running of these airports. Most Nigerian airports are understaffed.

Most aircraft in Nigeria are old. No fewer than 29 aircraft out of 53 operating commercial flights in the country have exceed the 22 year age limit stipulated by the Ministry of aviation. However, owners of overage aircraft that were already registered were given 5 years to get rid of them. There's a poor maintenance culture in the aviation industry. Maintenance logs are not kept for the planes and there's a tendency to 'manage' planes instead of repairing them. This unwillingness to spend money in maintenance, regular check-up and repair of aircraft signifies indiscipline and a lack of value fore human lives.

Since the industry is generally understaffed, flight and ground crew (including technical staff) are overworked. The International civil aviation organisation standards on flying hours state that if a pilot is on duty for 12 hours, he must also rest for 12 hours before the next flight. Staffs are poorly trained and there's hardly any retraining, recertification or upgrading of technical staff including pilots. Operating protocol are arbitrarily breached thus unduly placing human lives at risk. The conditions of service are poor and it is no wonder that the staffs are poorly motivated as well.

With all the above time bombs ticking away, it is unfortunate that the emergency services currently on ground are practically useless. There's apparently no coordination between the staff and between all agencies in some way involved with handling such disasters. To top it off, emergency equipment are bad or absent, and communication within the airport and with planes in transit is also poor.

Lapses in the Disaster Phase

In the Nigerian situation, a lot of the previously mentioned lapses still come into play and that a disaster necessarily results in massive property destruction and death. First of all, there isn't adequate communication at the time of a disaster both within and outside the airport. In most airports there are no emergency radios to speak of. In fact there are anecdotal reports that something might be happening at one section of the airport with another section being in total oblivion. This inadequacy in communication results in delay of arrival of the fire service, police and emergency medical service at the time of a disaster. Emergency services at the airport are so poor as to be declared absent. This is in marked contrast to the Chang-Kai Chek airport crash on 31st Oct. 2000. Here, the airport alert was almost immediate, and the 32 men at the airport's fire brigade, who 4 months earlier had trained on a similar scenario, were prepared. They responded instantly by being at the scene of the accident in 1 minute, 38 seconds. The disaster alert also was sent to the dispatch centre in the county of Tao-Yuan, which further alerted the 17 emergency hospitals in the area. Emergency medical teams from each hospital were gathered rapidly and sent to the airport. The Sosoliso aircraft that crashed may not have had any lightning deflectors as eyewitnesses present at the airport reported that it sustained a direct lightning strike. Radio beacons/ transponders also play a role in the disaster phase as they could help locate a missing plane immediately. Unfortunately, as previously explained the beacons currently available in the country are obsolete, faulty or simply not working. It was the Shell Petroleum Fire Brigade that provided fire support to the airport, as the airport's fire service was ill-equipped to handle the inferno especially as it had no water. The Airport Medical Center, major hospitals and trauma centers in Port Harcourt were ill-equipped to deal with the mass casualty situation and the dead victims were not treated with dignity and professional care (*Saturday Punch*, Dec. 24, 2005).

Lapses in the Post-disaster Phase

Some of the lapses mentioned in the pre-disaster and disaster phases continue to play a role in the post-disaster phase. Transportation, both for medical evacuation and for search and rescue was also a major lapse in this phase. There were no helicopters for medical evacuation. It appears that NEMA has one helicopter, which they use for search and rescue. However, it is said that this helicopter is not even meant for search and rescue, being of the type used in transporting relief materials like blankets, rice and other foodstuffs.

The public relations information management left much to be desired. It was the African Independent Television that eventually gave the first accurate reports on the Bellview air crash but were immediately shut down for their effort by the National Broadcasting Commission who accused them of 'professional misconduct' in showing offensive photographs to the public and reporting that all aboard had died when foreign media and our own top government officials were reporting that there were survivors. In fact the handling of information about the Bellview air crash was disorganised, uncoordinated and downright embarrassing. Of course, this mishandling of information further compounded the psychological trauma experienced by relatives of victims.

Since the crash occurred at night, and there was no electricity, it was too dark to go out and investigate what the loud explosion they had heard signified. When the villagers discovered the crashed plane the next morning (Sunday, 23/10/05), the absence of telephone services delayed the transmission of this information to the police station in nearby Sango. Also, poverty, lack of enlightenment and respect for human lives resulted in the massive looting that characterized this crash. It is hoped that these recent spate of crashes and the increased awareness will finally effect the speedy rectification of the abnormalities in the aviation sector.

Lapses in Disaster Preparedness in Rural Hospitals; a US study

Disaster preparedness has always been an area of major concern for the medical community, but recent world events have prompted an increased interest. This study examines the experiences of rural hospital emergency departments with threat preparedness. Analysis of preparedness activities will help identify common themes to better prioritize preparedness activities and maximize a hospital's response capabilities, a Research Study by William G. *et al.* says. It is clear that barriers and challenges to hospital disaster preparedness are significantly different for rural and urban hospitals. Barriers for rural hospitals include smaller or non-existent local public health departments, less capacity, fewer resources, inferior communication technology, reliance on volunteers, poorly equipped ambulances and life-support devices, fewer health care professionals (particularly experts in mental health, infectious diseases, and burn treatment), minimal surge capacity, downsizing and hospital closures, and greater distances from other needed resources. The situation in Indian rural hospitals is worse than most of the rural hospitals of US.

Even if hospitals are well prepared, it appears reasonable to assume that there will still be chaos, inadequate resources, deaths and injuries, and confusion and contention over who is in command, often exacerbated by lapses in security and breakdowns in communication. Preparedness standards to which hospitals are to be held accountable also are not clear and provide no guarantees or assurances that the response will be adequate. In fact, no outcome measures exist to determine whether, during a disaster, the hospital's written plan will be followed or is effective.

Far more hospitals are conducting terrorism training than there are hospitals that have had to deal with an actual terrorist event. This finding is not unexpected, given the amount of money that has been made available for terrorism training. Certainly some skills and actions are common to any disaster, but terrorism training requires a great deal of specialized knowledge. Information that is specific to a weaponized agent, including symptoms, prognosis, triage protocols, remedies, treatments, and personal protective strategies, likely are not applicable to motor vehicle crashes, school bus wrecks, and extreme weather conditions. Given the rarity of terrorism events, it is unlikely that specialized skills and knowledge will be retained until there is an opportunity to use them. This problem is only exacerbated in rural hospitals that are struggling with high staff turnover and personnel shortages. It may not be advisable to provide hospital staff with advanced terrorism training if skills are lagging in basic and advanced life support and trauma care, which would enhance their ability to respond to disasters that occur more often.

An incident that has just 10 critically ill or injured victims would quickly overwhelm the resources of many small rural hospitals. A relatively routine emergency situation in an urban setting easily could be considered a full-scale disaster in a rural setting. A majority of the respondents felt unprepared for events that involve a large number of victims. A mass casualty incident involving 50 to 100 patients, injured in any way, would be a burden that most rural hospitals could not deal with. The fact that 95% of the responding hospitals reported that their emergency departments would be overwhelmed by 10 or fewer critically ill or injured patients arriving simultaneously indicates that these hospitals do not have the ability to take on a very large, sudden surge of patients. Rural hospitals need to find a way to realistically assess their actual surge capacity and make decisions as to how they can best improve this capacity. Surge capacity, by definition, involves committing financial resources to capabilities that may sit unused the majority of the time. In Indian conditions the rural hospitals are almost non-existent and even the hospitals at the district level are unable to handle the load of disaster victims. It has become a practice to refer all seriously injured cases to regional hospitals like AIIMS in New Delhi or PGI at Chandigarh. No doubt these hospitals remain always over-burdened and in case of a disaster they can hardly take more loads. Where do the victims go?

Because resources are limited and staff turnover and burnout are high, hospitals need to make sure that personnel are trained in the basic life-support skills common to all disasters. It seems most prudent that preparedness training in rural environments needs to concentrate on the common elements that can improve a system's response to any disaster. These elements include communications, command and control, and interagency cooperation.

Disaster Management in Indian Railways

In India, the railways are the most preferred mode of transport both for the movement of people and goods consignments in bulk. Unlike in other countries where the role of Railways, in the event of a disaster, is restricted to clearing and restoring the traffic, in our country Indian Railways handles the rescue and relief operations. Increasing traffic density, longer length of trains with a large number of passengers on board, higher operational speeds of trains, emerging technologies, etc., called for a paradigm shift from the existing level of preparedness and readiness to combat any disastrous situation to a much higher level of an effective 'Disaster Management System'. The Disaster Management Act, 2005 stipulates that Ministries of Government of India shall be responsible for taking measures necessary for prevention, mitigation, capacity building and to respond effectively to any threatening disaster situation or a disaster. Disasters on the railway network are a consequence of human and equipment failures, natural calamities and acts of sabotage and comprise collisions and derailments of trains, accidents at level crossings, fires on trains; floods, cyclones, earthquakes, bomb blasts, terror attacks and other destructive/disruptive activities.

Various studies revealed the following points for discussion and improvements.

Poor coordination in arrangements

Lack of proper co-ordination was evident in the post incidence response to various disasters as Railways could not harness the infrastructure and support of the civic/private agencies in 46 out of the 94 incidents that required external support.

- In the absence of an MoU, the private hospitals refused medical help in the bomb blasts that took place on 11 July 2006 in the Mumbai suburban section and consequently WR was left to face court cases, claims and criticism.
- In a major accident where Rajdhani express derailed and fell on river bank on 9 September 2002 in ER, the injured were taken to Howrah by train. Enquiring into the incident the CRS observed that the Railways could have hired helicopters/planes to move them to hospitals.
- In SCR, when the Delta Fast Passenger derailed on 29 October 2005 and fell into a water body flowing underneath the bridge, the assistance of an Air Force helicopter, naval divers, army battalion, boats and trained personnel were sought for. While the Air Force helicopter reached the site six hours after it was requisitioned, the boats and trained personnel reached after five hours by which time all the victims were extricated and those surviving were sent to nearby hospitals. The naval divers from Visakhapatnam arrived at 14:30 hours the next day (34 hours after the disaster).

- Even when Deccan Queen express and two other suburban trains were wrecked by a violent mob on 30 November 2006 at 10:22 hours in CR, fire extinguishers were called at 11:30 hours and two fire tenders reached only by 13:00 hours, by which time most of the coaches were gutted by the fire.
- Poor communication system and faulty communication equipment hampered rescue work and effective transmission of information. The information about an accident was communicated by the Guard of the train to the nearest station master using the mobile phone of a passenger. Similarly, the Guard of train No. 5273 Satyagraha express could not use the portable communication phone provided to him, when the train collided with a loader of a JCV machine on 10 April 2006 at Jahanighera station on NR.

.Safety aids play a crucial role in prevention of disasters such as collisions and accidents at level crossings. Corporate Safety Plan envisaged installation of modern devices and warning systems to prevent collisions, modernisation of signalling system and maintenance of signalling equipment. Audit observed that safety aids were yet to be comprehensively provided.

- The Corporate Safety Plan envisaged provision of Anti Collision Device (ACD) for comprehensive safety coverage to eliminate collisions and consequent fatalities. This device provided in the trains, stations and level crossing gates assists in detecting train partings and provides audible and visual warnings at level crossing gates when trains approach them. Even after four years of finalization of the Corporate Safety Plan, IR was yet to implement the ACD.
- Track circuiting is one of the most important safety aids to be provided at all stations to reduce collisions in station area. Track circuiting eliminates the chance of reception of trains on the occupied lines at stations. Full track circuiting was not implemented in as many as 1,784 out of 6,211 signaling stations in 67 divisions across IR.
- Axle counters are electronic devices employed for detecting the presence of a vehicle on a block section, i.e., the section of a track between two adjacent stations. This is a critical device that detects presence of parted load (bogies and wagons) that get disconnected from the running trains and remain dangerously on the track. Tracks used even for 'A' class routes, on which super fast trains are operated, did not have the facility of block proving (process of proving that there are no vehicles in the entire block section) by axle counters.
- Train Actuated Warning Devices (TAWDs) are provided at

unmanned level crossings to warn about an approaching train and to prevent accidents at unmanned level crossings. There were as many as 18,976 unmanned level crossings in all the 67 divisions; and even though accidents at level crossings were identified as a serious concern, only 43 unmanned level crossings in seven divisions were provided with TAWDs.

- Modernization of points and signals through Panel Interlocking (PI), Route Relay Interlocking (RRI), and Solid State Interlocking (SSI) were not completed. Out of 6,211 signaling stations only 2,959, 288 and 164 stations respectively were provided with PI, RRI and SSI.
- Numerous instances of signal gear failures were noticed across all zonal railways. For the year 2006-07 alone 2,08,966 failures in signal gears were reported across IR, with Bilaspur Division of SECR, Howrah Division of ER, Lucknow, Delhi and Moradabad Divisions of NR accounting for the maximum failures.
- Auxiliary Warning System (AWS) eliminates human error in passing signals. Even though AWS was working satisfactorily in the Mumbai suburban sections of CR and WR, the system was not implemented in any route across IR.

Thus, IR was neither able to rapidly access the disaster sites nor could they provide organised rescue and relief through effective coordinated arrangements with civil/other agencies. Providing rescue and relief during the 'Golden hour' was the exception rather than the rule. Delayed arrival of relief equipments at the disaster sites also led to delayed restoration of rail traffic, causing diversions and cancellation of trains. The response time of Indian Railways warranted significant improvement. The provision of safety aids and maintenance of infrastructure to enhance safety of the traveling passengers was inadequate and the measures adopted to enhance security at stations for prevention and mitigation of disasters were not commensurate with the number of passengers.

Recommendations

1. IR should augment its infrastructure of relief equipments-SPARTs, ARTs, ARMVs, break down cranes and rescue ambulances, etc. facilities in hospitals and in trains to the envisaged scale.
2. IR should initiate effective measures in maintaining the relief equipments, in a state of operational readiness at all times.
3. IR should quickly provide communication system in trains and in relief trains for transmission of real time information from the disaster site, which is essential in assessing the gravity of the disaster and in organizing rescue and relief. The facilities in the control rooms need to be enhanced.

4. IR should on priority, address the issues of operational constraints imposing speed restrictions, positioning the relief trains/medical vans, cranes, etc. in a manner that optimizes the response time, which is the essence of any response mechanism.
5. IR should enter into formal coordination arrangements with the State Governments/District authorities, civil/private hospitals and other agencies so as to effectively leverage their infrastructure while responding to disasters.
6. Most of the trauma patients could be saved (i) if bleeding was effectively stopped and blood pressure restored within one hour, i.e. golden hour, (ii) victims remaining in a state of shock for long duration would die and therefore surgical intervention in the first hour was crucial for increasing the patients' chances of survival.
7. IR needs to improve their response time in order to provide effective post incidence response to disasters. Co-ordination with private agencies/NGOs and harnessing the infrastructure of the district authorities are vital in promptly responding to disasters. IR also needs to effectively monitor the movement of relief equipments so as to ensure their timely availability at the disaster sites.
8. IR needs to enhance their state of preparedness in handling disasters involving water bodies.
9. Facilities in terms of collapsible coffins, air conditioned mortuaries and embalming gums and chemicals for preservation of the dead bodies for a reasonable time need to be provided in all the railway divisional hospitals.
10. Ideally every victim who is alive should be labeled by color coding system, i.e. white strips for non-critical cases, yellow with blue strips for more serious cases and yellow with the red strips for emergency cases. These are helpful in identifying and isolating case according to seriousness of injuries to provide first-aid merit-wise.
11. To take care of the dead bodies the disaster plan must include setting up of temporary emergency mortuary. The use of the hospital mortuary is not recommended. Air conditioned tents, which may be erected conveniently at any place may be considered at every 500 and above bedded hospital. The medical man has an important role in the management of dead bodies. He may be involved in the following ways:
    * Proper scientific numbering and tagging of the dead bodies for future identification purpose by the relatives.
    * Identification of body as far as possible by noting down the identification features.
    * Issuing of death certificates.
    * Conduction of medico-legal autopsy.

12. Need for Pathological autopsy. Here the doctor seeks to learn the extent of the disease or cause of death for which they were treating the deceased patient. Any body kept for autopsy should not be kept in a frozen cabin. It hinders the microscopic examination of tissue by destroying cells. Here it is important to mention that any sort of disrespect or unnecessary mutilation of dead body may amount to an offence under section 297 I.P.C.
13. The legal authority may waive of the postmortems to minimize the inconvenience to the relatives of the victims. For example, in "Uphar tragedy", where about 58 peoples died the post-mortems was waived off by the Lieutenant Governor of Delhi.

Bhopal Gas Tragedy: A tale of lapses from the word go

Bhopal Gas Tragedy, the worst 'Mega Industrial Disaster' of the world happened in the night of 2nd and 3rd December 1984 when a pesticide plant of Union Carbide spewed about forty five tons of highly lethal MIC gas. One Thousand and five hundred persons were killed instantaneously and lakhs were taken seriously sick but not a single person of Union Carbide died. The gas had started trickling slowly long before midnight, may be around ten, but its effect was not felt by the people at large. Union Carbide people were struggling unsuccessfully to plug the leakage. Ultimately around one, the entire gas of one tank, about forty-five tons, escaped into the air and created havoc. The pungent gas was suffocating, irritating in the eyes and was like flames on the skin, face in particular. Thus gas went on slowly moving and changing its southward courses as per variation in wind directions, went on settling down in densely inhabited areas and went on inflicting people. Nobody could bear the gas and had to flee away as fast as one could. Those who had their own vehicles, fled quickly; others ran on foot. Those running on foot mobbed and forcibly occupied available space in buses, trucks, cars, scooters, etc. All cooperated in crisis though stampede had its own casualties. Institutions running round the clock, i.e. even in the night like Hospitals, Police Stations, etc. were deserted. Under trials in police station lock-ups were let out to save their lives. Police control room's wireless conversation became silent. People who inhaled the gas excessively, died instantaneously—either in homes or while fleeing or elsewhere; others went on dying gradually as per the severity of exposure to this gas. Nothing happened to those who remained indoors sleeping with doors and windows tightly closed as gas could not enter. JP District Hospital in south Bhopal about 12 KM away from Union Carbide factory was the first to be flooded with gas victims and first to report casualties—first two casualties, then three more and so on. Realization that the gas was toxic and lethal dawned only after getting information about the casualties from JP hospital. Ambulance from JP hospital was the first to be sent to Union Carbide area and then other resources were mobilized to transport gas victims to hospitals. True macabre/dreadful scenario unfolded only after daybreak. The biggest hospital in old Bhopal, i.e. Gandhi Medical College and Hospital, deserted in the night, became operational by daybreak and gave symptomatic treatment to gas victims on a massive scale. All philanthropic people and NGOs turned up with enough eatables, milk, tea, fruits etc at major centers. District administration guided them to needy people and places. NGOs opened community kitchens at several central places and ran them round the clock.

After decades of Bhopal gas leak disaster; an apology of care

The situation speaks volumes about the present government's "concern" for the survivors, around two lakhs of them suffering from long-term effects of the MIC gas leak and one lakh afflicted with permanent or temporary disability. Action Plan-I for the medical and economic rehabilitation of the survivors envisaged completion of all referral hospitals by 1995. It has not been done. As Action Plan-I has not been completed, the Central government has not released funds for Action Plan-II (1996-2000). The Supreme Court had, in its order of January 25, 2000, directed the state government to make all the hospitals and dispensaries fully operational by May 25, 2000, but the government has failed in this respect also. The gas-affected people suffering from cancer were getting free medical aid at the cancer hospital. The state government last year amended the rules to permit free medical aid to only those gas victims who were found to be living below the poverty line.

On November 27, 2001, a state government announcement said the Chief Minister had directed the Bhopal Gas Disaster Relief Department to issue identity cards to the December, 1984, gas leak victims for their speedy treatment in the department-run hospitals. Mr Digvijay Singh's concern for providing proper treatment to the gas victims was splashed in the newspapers across the state and beyond. (Opinion, N.D. Sharma, *The Tribune*, Dec. 3, 2001). In fact, it was the Supreme Court that had directed the state government—on July 25 this year—to issue identity cards to the gas victims in need of medical aid. The Supreme Court had left it to the state government to work out the modalities in this regard. The three-month period expired on October 25 without the government moving an inch towards complying with the apex court directive. Now for all publicity purposes it becomes Mr Digvijay Singh's concern.

As Madhya Pradesh Congress Committee chief in the early nineties, Mr Digvijay Singh appeared to have made the welfare of the gas victims his major objective, if not the only one, of his life. He was so moved by the plight that he did everything except committing suicide. In its 1993 Assembly election manifesto prepared under Mr Digvijay Singh's guidance, the Congress said: "the Bhopal gas victims are today feeling utterly harassed and frustrated because of the cumbersome procedure of distribution of interim relief and compensation. The grievances of the victims will be redressed by speeding up the payment of compensation. Besides, schemes for providing jobs to the gas-affected women will be implemented". It will not be inappropriate to say that Mr Digvijay Singh forgot the gas victims after becoming the Chief Minister. Eight years of his rule have been full of scandals involving the money meant for medicines and rehabilitation of the gas victims. The hospitals were constructed but these were not equipped. Costly equipment was purchased but the staff to operate them were not recruited. Medicines purchased in bulk for the gas victims were sold in the black market. Rampant corruption was reported in the payment of compensation. Mr Digvijay Singh had started distancing himself from the gas victims soon after becoming Chief Minister in December, 1993. There was no word about them in his party's 1998 manifesto.

At least five cases of corruption involving crores of rupees meant for the welfare of the survivors have been pending with the Madhya Pradesh Lokayukta since 1995. Major conduits for the misappropriation of gas relief money have been civil works and purchase of medicines. Tragically, the victims going to the hospitals and dispensaries for the gas-affected people do not get the medicines they need and are asked to purchase these from the market.

The government claimed to have spent Rs. 70 crore till 1994 on economic rehabilitation. Not even 70 persons have been provided with jobs, according to Abdul Jabbar. Mr Motilal Vora had initiated a scheme for setting up a special industrial area where 10,000 gas-affected persons were to be provided employment suitable to their physical condition. After spending Rs. 8 crore on its development, the whole project stands practically abandoned. Those who survived the December, 1984, MIC leak from the pesticides plant of the Union Carbide are facing another hazard in the form of huge quantities of toxic wastes left behind by the US multinational. A report prepared by a group of Bhopal citizens after visiting the site and submitted to the Chief Minister says that 21 tonnes of residue has been stored at the south-western end of the factory adjacent to Arif Nagar. More than 50 tonnes of Naphthol and other chemicals are stored in other areas. About three acres of land at the eastern end of the factory are covered with tonnes of solid toxic wastes which only means that the management of the erstwhile pesticides factory had been constantly dumping hazardous material there. The total quantity of the deadly chemicals dumped by the Union Carbide is estimated at 4000 tonnes. The people living around the erstwhile pesticide plant have been drinking water contaminated with these toxic chemicals.

The state government had washed its hands off the task removing the waste. The recent verdict of the Appellate Court of the USA gives some hope to the people living around the erstwhile pesticide factory. As a consequence of the decision of the Appellate Court, Union Carbide and its then Chairman Warren Anderson are now answerable to the charges of contaminating the ground water and soil in and around the Bhopal factory premises and causing health damage to thousands of people.

Steps towards disaster management of animals

Land being limited the number of marginal farmers and Landless people are increasing every year. This section by and large depends on animals for their livelihood. "Gujjar, Bakharwal or Raikas" of India are a large number of nomads who by and large depend on animals for their livelihood.

22 out of 32 states and Union Territories of India are vulnerable to some disaster or other. The cyclone in the state of Andhra Pradesh, of November 14 to 20, 1977, caused an estimated loss of 2,30,146 cattle and 3,44,056 other livestock, as against 8,515 human deaths. Similarly in Orissa cyclone during the 4th of June, 1982 there had been 11,468 cattle lost against 243 human deaths. Earthquake has comparatively less impact on animals; but in Uttarkashi earthquake, 3100 cattle heads were lost as against 770 human lives. Between 1953-1990 we lost 1,02,905 cattle against 1532 human lives because of earthquakes. It is apparent that even though animals are the main source of livelihood to the poorest of the poor and to the landless, concrete steps towards disaster management of livestock and other animals are yet to be taken.

In India as high as 70% of livestock is owned by 67% of small and marginal farmers and by the landless people. Living on edge, the small holders generate milk, meat, wool, etc. for the community with virtually no capital resource or training; but they contribute significantly to the GDP. In India these people contribute 62% of the total milk procured. 60% of livestock farming labor is provided by women and more than 90% of work related to care of animals is rendered by womenfolk of the family. Though poultry rearing has assumed the role of an industry in some pockets, 70% of the poultry of India are still reared in the backyards, where these birds produce eggs and meat by scavenging around their habitation.

Animals' role in disaster (mitigation, search, rescue, relief or rehabilitation)

It is assumed that animal can fore-warn an incumbent disaster. Animals like the dogs are used for search and rescue operations. During flash floods people escape holding on to animals; all animals are natural swimmers. Animals and animal driven carts are the available means of transport of injured and invalid people when no other transport is possible. Animals are also used for clearance of debris. During disaster the people loose their property and livelihood. Loss of crops, infrastructure or machinery takes time to recoup. Animals if salvaged can provide the community with food, energy, transport and the other utilities immediately (as long as they are healthy and cared for). Unlike standing crops or infrastructure, the animals can be salvaged and brought to safer places, where a disaster can be predicted. In transit camps or in rehabilitated dwellings too the animals can be utilised for milk, manure, transport, fuel (dung cakes). Animals are used for fetching water or for lifting water from the water sources, where machine or manpower are not available or can not be used. Even in their death animals serve the community; they provide some material gain through, their hide, bonelard and carcass. Partially damaged crops and grains unfit for human consumption can be gainfully used as animal feed. Since there is major participation of women and children in the care of animals, this activity can be a major diversion to tide over the gloom and depression that fall over the victims during a disaster. Flooded areas where drainage is slow can be used for duck rearing and fish farming. These help in clearing pests that usually breeds during floods. Free living animals like the pigs play an important role in clearing garbage, waste materials, etc.; they provide livelihood to economically weaker section and can be a cheap source of protein to these communities especially when other sources of food become scarce. Dogs (pets and community animals) keep the creeping reptiles and straying wild animals at bay or at least forewarn the community of their intrusion. People marooned during floods or earth quakes during winter have survived chilly nights taking refuge among herds of sheep and goats. During war animals play a key role. Horses and mules are used for transport in difficult terrain around the border. Dogs are used in the army for reconnaissance, tracking, guarding and combat. Animal rearing is the only dependable vocation for the border villagers who are under constant threat of disturbances and dislodgment. Animal rearing can generate protein food for army and a source of income for the poor border dweller, thus building a positive rapport and mutual dependence between the two. Stray dogs consume discarded food, crows clear a spoilt material that is thrown around vultures devour the dead animals, snakes control rodents; cats do the same.

A disaster management plan for animals shall essentially include:

1. Retrospective epidemiological study of the disasters in the area and this shall include,

(a) *Data Collected* interpreted and analysed (i.e. information), on the basis of which some prediction can be made.

(b) *Disaster Vignetting* is a means by which mapping is done on the basis of incidence frequency magnitude, epicentre, vulnerable areas.

(c) *Herd profile*:, the total animal population (herd number), vulnerable animal population as per their species, breed, age, sex, etc.

(d) *Community Profile,* the total population, animal owning population their age, sex, socio-economic status, education, cultural distribution, etc.

(e) *Animals at risk*; the nature of hazard, the intensity of impact and mortality rate (immediate or delayed).

(f) *Risk factor analyses* is the analysis of type of risk (identification and analyses).

2. Action Plan

Since following disaster animals are to be rescued and collected in relief camps, the immediate priority would be controlling and combating disease. The animal health component of disaster mitigation will include

(a) Promotional herd health care such as nutrition, pregnant animal care, care of new-born and young animal, etc.
(b) Prevention of risk is through vaccination, pest/vector, control, sanitation, etc.
(c) Specific therapy by way of early diagnosis and treatment.
(d) *Rehabilitation* help animals to recover from any trauma or fear.
(e) *Disposal of dead animals*: Carcass utilisation is one method. Many animals in which treatment is unlikely to be beneficial may have to be put to sleep, i.e. Euthanasia ("mercy killing")

3. Resources Planning

(a) Assessment of available man power, i.e. Veterinary doctors, Paraveterinary staff, ancillary staff.
(b) Store and equipment include the medicine, surgical and medical appliances, diagnostics, life saving equipment, etc.
(c) Logistical needs: that is the need for fuels, lighting equipment, tents, sheds, Grass bedding, trolleys, material for sanitation, storage of feed and fodder and water.
(d) Ambulance and out reach facility, transporting animals is more cumbersome when they are sick, injured and non-ambulatory.
(e) Veterinary medical facilities as veterinary hospital, mobile veterinary units, etc.
Grazing and watering facility.

4. Training Plan

(a) Training veterinary personnel, paravets, attendants, etc.
(b) Training administrators like B.D.O., telephones and Fire Service personel, Civil defence personel, Sarpanch/Village headmen, administrators.
(c) Animal Health awareness for trainees such as social workers, volunteers.

5. Allied Planning (Organisation)

(a) Augmenting political and administrative support.
(b) Involving N.G.O.'s, C.B.O's, media, Goshalas, animal welfare organisations and other volunteer groups.
(c) Eliciting commitment and allocation of funds.
(d) Formation of veterinary service groups at State and Central Government level.

(e) Organisation of district/area level bodies, assigning specific tasks and responsibilities.
(f) Establishing communication channels, alternate channels like ham radios.
(g) Establishing alternate source of power, energy, etc.
(h) Plan for monitoring and supervision.
(i) Publicity and public relation activities (Vet-PR)
(j) Plan for mitigation and rehabilitation of animal owners along with animals

6. Execution of short and long-term plan

Plan implimentation include estimation of animals involved, damage assessment. One may make use of media to help locating remote areas where often organisers' attention may not easily reach. Monitoring is part of implementation.

7. Impact assessment of the past disasters, preparedness and mitigation measures

Disaster need not repeat every-time

Experience gained from similar hazards of nearby areas are positively helpful. This is especially useful in animal disaster management which is still in its infancy.

8. Post-execution evaluation of plan

Follow-up of disaster management especially that of animal management is valuable experience, that need be shared among disaster prone areas. Unfortunately this is not forthcoming. Linking with allied agencies for uniformity in all regions is part of disaster management programmeme as unbiased and uniform measures help transparency and hence would instill confidence of the community in the system. Temporary Vety. hospitals.

The equipment and other infrastructure are provided along with stock pile of emergency, equipment and drugs. All veterinary personnel may not be used at a time. It would be important to plan shifts to avoid mental and physical fatigue. Early phases would need more work force and in all departments of activity viz. Specialists like surgeons, anesthesiologists (pain mangers), diagnosticians as well as task force like para-veterinary personnel and physical workers. Supervision and monitoring would be important and demands all qualities of leadership (like confidence, competence, experience, patience, communication skill, etc.). As search and rescue would be over, relief and rehabilitation would acquire importance.

Recovery and Rehabilitation

The impact of disaster being calamitous one may come across a number of cases which are beyond mere physical injuries or contagious disease. The mental trauma due to the loss of a sibling or a partner where bullocks are used in pair, can be encountered and will have to be handled at appropriate stage. Many of the cases of extensive trauma that cannot be handled may have to be put to sleep (mercy killing). Doing so under full public view where the public is already surcharged with losses of life and property may set in depression or even public outcry. Overenthusiastic and ill trained animal activists often can blow things out of proportion, specially because in many parts of India religious sentiments are attached with some animals. There is a role for Veterinary extension specialists to placate such situations.

Control Rooms

For the information exchange and co-ordination of veterinary support, control rooms are used. These handle co-ordination information among directorate of Animal Husbandry, district Vet. hospitals, rural hospitals of the affected area, etc. Control rooms keep link with and co-ordinate supplies from agencies. The control room would be working on feed back from affected area on the extent and nature of emergency, the need for special equipment, emergency equipment (pain killer, sedatives, antibiotics, fracture equipments, etc.) The role of a veterinary public relation man (Vet PR) assume significance.

Control of diseases

Immediate task after the first emergency, treatments are completed would be taking care of diseases that may spread. Since animal fares are part of village life in many areas of India "health care precautions" and "disease control" programmes are already available in many state departments of Animal Husbandry. Melas like the "Pushkar mela" of Rajasthan and the state and regional cattle shows are already held regularly in many states. Armed with retrospective epidemiology, authorities would identify emergency diseases and sanitation measures. This would include digging manure pits, drainage facilities (more important in floods, cyclone, etc.), drinking water and water troughs. This will have to be simultaneously established in hospitals, temporary shelter camps as well as in the affected areas from time to time and as per priority.

For health care operations there is a need for discipline; public co-operation is also essential. Animal welfare agencies working in the areas can help arranging stockpiles. Media can help by providing feed-backs from field.

Animal waste disposal

The methods of animal waste disposal/recycling vary with animals. Cow and buffalo dung is used as manure or can be caked and dried for use as fuel. Horse, goat and poultry waste is also used as manure. Where possible small manure gas (or gobar gas) units can be organised. Improper disposal can enhance pest or vector problems. Preparation of compost or digging the manure pit be considered. Manure pits should be layered with dry waste and lime regularly. During prolonged stagnation of flood water, duck rearing and fish farming can be considered as the means of pest control.

Disposal of dead animals

An important problem that has to be faced during disaster management of animals is the disposal of dead animals. This poses acute problems during floods and cyclone, as the number of animals dying would be enormous. Most states have fallen animal management programmes and carcass utilization programme. Admittedly, one administrative group does not uniformly handle these.

Disaster management of animals

Earthquake: Since in India animals are tied outside or in thatched sheds, chances of physical injuries are low. But when tied or caged their chances of escape are minimized.

Flood: Animals are natural swimmers; therefore can escape drowning if they are not tied or caged.

Cyclone: Though cyclone can be predicted with some accuracy, salvaging animals has never been a priority. Cyclone shelters are not designed to house animals.

Drought and famine: Meteorological or Agricultural drought, need not necessarily affect animals as they can survive without agriculture. Animal stand the stress of the famine better than humans. They can use most sources of the water which may be unclean by human standards. Dry fodder reserves, urea molasses licks, bricks made of fodder urea and molasses, etc. can be part of the stock pile. Scarcity fodder can be grown as part of the preventive action.

Cold famine: An incidence famine has occurred in the alpine pastures of J&K due to unusual snow that covered grass. The sheep easily withstood the snow but starved for want of pastures. Stores were subsequently established by storing the dry fodder in pits; the low ambient temperature prevents spoilage. Cold famines are known in the snow deserts or part of Ladakh; but Yaks do survive these.

Landslides and snow avalanches: Tied or caged animals stand a higher risk during these disasters. Care of animals is often a low priority in disaster management. Though animals stand better chance of survival during disasters, much less efforts have been made in this direction.

Fire, Forest fire: Animals are more prone to fire as they are usually housed in thatched sheds. The practice of smoking the sheds to repel pests is a common practice. Proximity of the chaff or the paddy straw makes conditions vulnerable to fire accidents. Forest fire affect wild animals and birds though many of them are more lucky than their domestic counterparts, being more athletic and free to escape from fire.

Industrial and technological: Animals are not frequent direct victims, though indirectly they can be trapped/affected any time. During Bhopal gas tragedy many animals including livestock , were affected; but poultry is known to have escaped from the impact of the hazard.

Epidemics: By and large ethnic animals can withstand the stress and disease, though endemic diseases and chronic conditions like worm infestations or ticks are not uncommon. Preventive health care therefore assumes special significance. Some states have a high percentage of crossbred animals, specially cattle whose health perspective will have to be considered independent of ethnic animals.

Psychosocial counseling; essential in the management of disaster victims

While some care is provided/planned for the physical ills of the disaster victims, the aspect of mental care is generally ignored. The Bangalore-based National Institute of Mental Health and Neurological Sciences (NIMHANS) is helped the tsunami-affected people in the country by offering them psychosocial counseling. Over 70 psychiatrists, doctors and social workers, including those from the Institute's Disaster Management Group, were drafted for the task. Just back from Cuddalore, worse affected spot in Tamil Nadu, Director Dr. D. Nagaraja spoke to Ravi Sharma on the Institute's initiatives.

Q. Is intervention and counseling the key ingredient in treating people affected by disasters ?

Yes. Once the affected people realize the gravity of the situation they go into depression and develop panic anxiety. You see a number of those affected complaining that nothing is being done for them. In reality it may not be completely accurate. But since their emotions are so heightened, even a minor lapse becomes a major issue. Even a small disturbance, makes them anxious, panicky and they get palpitations. It disturbs their routine and interferes with their ability to go back to their normal work. They can have problems in establishing a pattern of life, getting proper sleep, concentrating on anything and even develop a guilt complex that they survived while others died. If it is very severe, some can also become suicidal.

Q. How do you tackle this?

It must be remembered that what we are tackling is not a mental illness. It is a natural emotional reaction to an abnormal situation. It is not psychiatric but a psychological problem. That is why medicines are not the major items with only a few persons requiring medication. What is required is a healing touch. We have to make the affected people cope with the abnormal situation. The major fear for entire communities is that the disaster [tsunami] will occur again and that they will be wiped out. So they are always in a state of tension. They have to be convinced that it won't occur all the time.

Q. How do you convince them?

By talking to them. The moment they start accepting their emotions, half their tensions will abate. But though their emotions are heightened, they can't express this to anybody. Probably there is nobody at home and neighbours may not be prepared to listen since they also are in a similar predicament. So it is important to get them to talk about their experiences. Another important thing in the management of these patients is to normalise, as soon as it is possible, their day to day activities. Even if housed in a relief camp, children should be made to attend school, adults encouraged to do the work they normally do at home such as cooking and washing. The tendency should not be to house them in camps, feeding them morning to night. Activities should be started at the earliest. A normalisation of their activities at the earliest will help them recover quickly. If not, they will keep brooding.

Q. Is there a difference in the way children and adults react to disasters?

Adults may have experienced bereavements, but in the case of children it will be for the first time that they are seeing so much of destruction and death, family members dying in front of them. All of a sudden they are on the streets, their homes and schools destroyed. They are in a worse state of anxiety. It is essential that they are not left in the same emotional state. They should be made to play, sent to school, so that normal emotions come into the picture.

Q. How difficult is the situation on the ground?

Some people are severely disturbed, they stop talking, eating and working. They are not able to tolerate the situation and become depressed. But the number is small, say 10 or 15 people in a camp of a 1,000. They need immediate intervention. So our psychiatrists, doctors and social workers start handling them straight away. But since the tsunamis have affected people on a massive scale it cannot be tackled by one or two psychiatrists, or even just by psychiatrists. So we need a team and it has to work in tandem with the existing personnel. What NIMHANS has developed is a Disaster Management Group that trains volunteers/officials/social workers to provide this psychosocial help even as they are distributing other relief materials.

But volunteers cannot help people ventilate their feelings unless they themselves are trained. Everybody can't listen. Our training helps volunteers to learn how to get the affected people to ventilate their feelings and emotions. Normally when somebody relates something the other person also starts reacting to it, putting his own emotions into the conversation. What is required here is a patient listener, someone who can encourage the affected person to speak, ventilate without inhibition, while at the same time ensuring that none of the listener's negative feelings is introduced into the conversation. This has to be taught to the volunteers.

Q. So the volunteers themselves need counseling?

Yes. Initially, most of the volunteers are in a heroic phase, being prepared to work without proper shelter and even food. But after a week or so, fatigue sets in. By then they would have seen so many dead bodies, got a first-hand experience of the disaster and seen things which most of them would never have seen in their lives. This will not only shatter their morale to work and provide relief, but worse, make them go into depression.

Q. The training, which is chiefly imparted by the Institute's Psychiatric Social Work Department, seeks to augment resources on the ground... ?

Yes. The department has started conducting programmes for non-governmental organisations (NGOs), volunteers and employees of hospitals and the government. This sort of training is not required for too long but it is needed to prepare the volunteers and others to handle a situation that will last not a week but at least a year to get back to near normal. The three-tier training entails training master trainers who are professionals, doctors, psychologists, psychiatrists and social workers. They in turn train the trainers. Each trainer will then train about 25 people at a time. This way we hope to train around 26,000 people by the end of January.

Q. Where are the programmes being conducted?

We plan to conduct one in Chennai. Thereafter the trained people will conduct programmes in every district that has been affected in Tamil Nadu (13), Kerala (two) and Andhra Pradesh (two). The six-day programmes are open to local psychiatrists, government officials and volunteer organisations.

Q. Are there any programmes for the Andaman and Nicobar islands?

There is only one psychiatrist for the whole island. So we had to develop the whole machinery. Six of our people are presently there working in tandem with 10 staff members from the All India Institute of Medical Sciences.

Q. How different is the present disaster from other calamities such as the Latur earthquake (1993) or the Gujarat earthquake (2001)?

In the other two disasters there were a lot of injured people and a massive effort in medical attention was required. In this disaster, there are mostly only two categories of victims—those who are dead and those who have survived. There are not so many injured victims.

Q. NIMHANS has also provided its expertise in dealing with disasters such as Latur, Gujarat and the Orissa cyclone. What lessons have been learnt?

The government, after any such calamity, plans to build shelters, provides food, create jobs, and so on. But that alone in not enough. You've got to talk to the people about their emotions, support them, draw out their negative emotions and strengthen the positive aspects. This will go a long way in their recovery and normalisation.

Q. What are the long-term effects of such disasters?

We have clearly established from our experience in Gujarat and Latur and from other studies that these disasters result in a significant degree of psychosocial morbidity, which interferes with the recovery, production and quality of life. And unless it is tackled and normalization restored recovery will take much longer. We are learning after all the concept of psychosocial rehabilitation is only around 15 years old. Earlier it was known as acute care but not seen as a medical concept. The recent terror attack on CST Mumbai on 26/11/08 exposed the security lapse and the total carelessness on part of the authorities to tackle such emergencies.

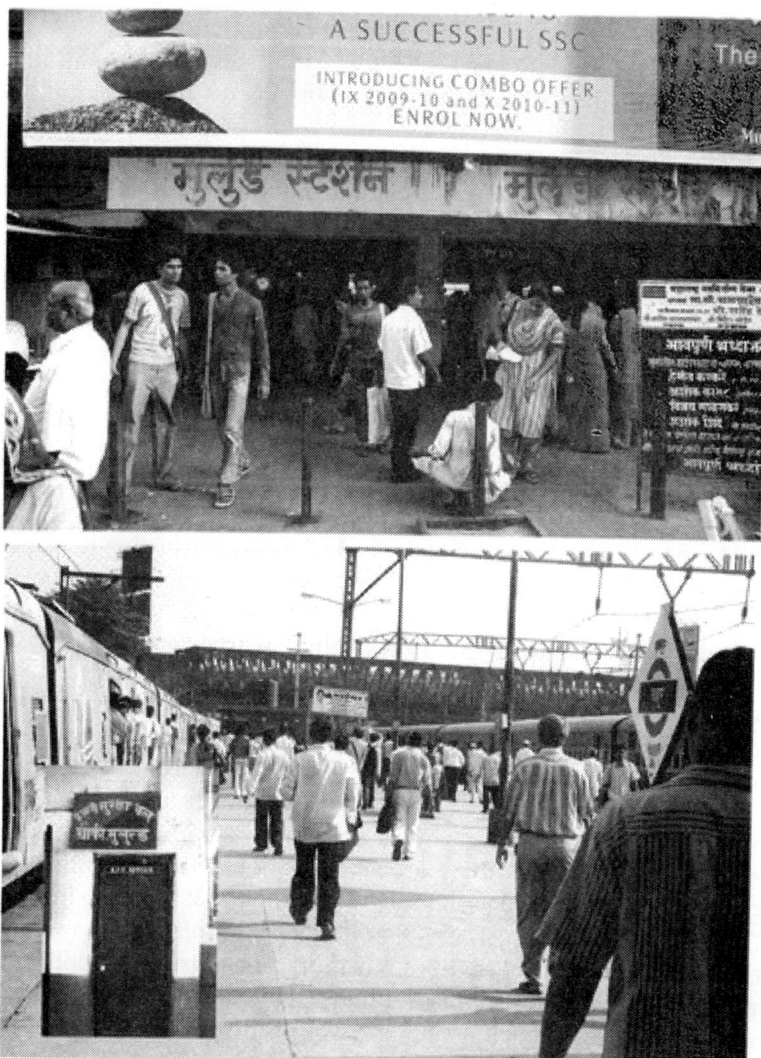

At Mulund station, they found the RPF room locked and this is where the CCTV cameras are monitored. S.N. More, the station master in charge of Mulund was on leave and his deputy Sawant was in a meeting at the CST. Moreover, Mulund station has already witnessed a bomb blast. P.A. Rajaram, a commuter says, "There is no attempt made by the police officials to step up the security measures. I do not find even routine checking during the peak hours." Like him several other commuters also echo the same sentiment. Madhu Kotian, a Mulund resident who is nominated for the third year as Divisional Railway Users Consultative Committee (DRUCC) informs, "We have almost half a dozen close circuit cameras installed at prominent places like the ticket counters and platforms. The monitoring is done by Railway Protection Force (RPF). Sometimes when they are taking rounds or accompanying the staff while they are depositing cash then the camera/control room is locked." This startling bit of information simply means the public are travelling at their own risk, as the security measures are not adequate in this station.

In the wake of the recent terror attacks, members of the Mulund Pravasi Sangh, a commuter's association has dashed a letter to J.N. Lal, divisional railway manager at CST demanding the removal of all hawkers from the railway premises. He states, "Hawking inside railway premises is unauthorized. Secondly, it attracts a large crowd which in turn means huge loss of lives during emergencies. One more demand is to shift the railway stalls and canteens from the platforms to one side of the station so that public movement is not restricted. These stalls are not frequented by the railway commuters and also it can be misused by the militants to study the movements in a particular station. Even the garbage bins pose a security risk, as garbage remains unattended for many days and can easily be used for placing explosives and bombs."

At Bhandup station, the station master A. Singh openly admits that the station is ill-equipped to deal with major calamity. "Forget terror attacks, even accident victims cannot be transported to hospitals because we do not have licensed porters to shift the victims. Last week a passenger met with an accident, a private nursing home located close to the station refused to admit the patient. We had to take him to Byculla railway hospital. In the process, precious time was lost and the patient died," he bemoans.

Interestingly, Mulund, Bhandup and Vikhroli are termed as major stations in railway parlance, while Kanjurmarg and Nahur are known as halt stations which means these are small stations without station masters. The chief booking clerk done the role of a station master here. In the words of U. Saxena from Nahur, "There are only two RPF officials to man the area stretching from Kanjurmarg up to Nahur. The city local police do not generally enter railway premises unless they are specifically instructed during emergencies. In such a situation, we need more RPF staff to man the stations." Apart from the RPF, the railways have GRP and home guards posted in every station.

Though the city is in red alert, none of these stations have metal detectors which are usually seen at prominent public places like malls and airports. Inadequate security measures arising on account of shortage of police personnel, lack of proper arms to tackle the terror attack and absence of mock drills as part of disaster management programme has put the commuters at a great risk.

Lapses in Dead Body Recovery and Storage

Body recovery is the first phase of the management of dead bodies. In all countries it was characterised as being initially chaotic and uncoordinated, involving a large number of different actors. In Thailand, body recovery was done by foreign tourists, local volunteers, Thai non-governmental organisations that specialise in body recovery following disasters (Po-Tek-Tung Foundation and Ruam-Ka-Tan-Yu Foundation), the military, and the police. In Indonesia, the body recovery phase lasted several months (Figure 1), and, under the coordination of the military, 42 different organisations were involved. In Sri Lanka, body recovery was done almost exclusively by the affected communities themselves. In all cases, bodies were taken to multiple locations, and relatives did not know where their family members had been taken.

None of the countries had sufficient refrigerated storage immediately available. In Thailand, the only country able to mobilize large numbers of refrigerated containers, it took about 2 wk to provide about 100 containers needed to store around 3,600 bodies. Temporary burial in shallow trench graves (about 1 m deep) was used effectively to store about 600 bodies. Effective use of dry ice proved difficult: when placed on top of the bodies it damaged them because of its low temperature, while not providing sufficient overall cooling to stop decomposition. Handling large quantities of dry ice also caused many skin burns among individuals handling it. However, it was found that an effective method was to build a small wall of dry ice surrounding a group of bodies, and then to cover the group with a tent or tarpaulin.

Identification

Victim identification differed considerably between the three countries. In Indonesia, simple visual identification was attempted in the first few days. However, the sheer number of bodies meant that it was impossible to arrange viewing for all bodies or store the bodies for later identification. Nevertheless, the body recovery teams successfully identified over 500 victims using personal effects such as identity cards and jewellery, and even mobile telephone SIM cards.

In Sri Lanka, the Centre for National Operations (an *ad hoc* governmental disaster management committee) mandated that local authorities take photographs and collect fingerprints of all the victims. However, because of damaged communications infrastructure, these instructions only arrived after 2 or 3 days, by which time decomposition had distorted facial features. In all, many hundreds of photographs were taken by police photographers, medical staff, journalists, and freelance photographers. In some cases, the films were not developed as there were insufficient funds to pay either the developer or freelance photographers. There were, however, outstanding examples, such as the hospital at Matara, where digital photographs were taken and basic information recorded (sex, height, and personal effects) for each body as it was brought into the hospital. Over 87% of the 547 victims handled by the hospital were identified. Foreign victims, largely found in the eastern part of the country, were sent directly to the capital city Colombo, where an Identification Centre was established with support from the British government. During 2005, the Identification Centre also supervised six major exhumations to search for missing foreigners who were buried along with Sri Lankan nationals. A total of 155 bodies were examined by the disaster victim identification team. Analysis of DNA and dental records was used to successfully identify these individuals, who came from 18 different countries.

On 27 December, the first Thai forensic teams, many traveling independently under their institutes, started arriving in the affected areas of southern Thailand. They rapidly set-up basic identification facilities in local temples. During the first 7-10 days of operations, Thai forensic teams examined around 3,600 bodies. The examination included external examination, photography, and recording of all personal effects. Fingerprints were taken from about 600 cadavers. DNA samples were collected from almost all bodies during the first few days, and included hair and soft tissues and, later, ribs and teeth. During this initial phase, Thai forensic teams identified about 1,100 human remains and released them to the families. In addition, about 500 bodies were identified and released to relatives by local physicians and police without the support of forensic specialists.

After the first week, forensic teams from other countries started to arrive in Thailand. They formed an international disaster victim identification committee to work in collaboration with the Royal Thai Police. In Phuket, the committee's information centre was established with the financial support of the Australian government. The Thai government decided to combine the efforts of the Thai forensic experts, the Thai Royal Police, and international disaster victim identification committee teams, and on 13 January the Thai Tsunami Victim Identification (TTVI) centre was established in Phuket. In collaboration with Interpol, the TTVI established a central mortuary in Phuket, sponsored by the Norwegian government. It was decided to examine or re-examine all 3,777 remaining victims using Interpol's standard protocol. This included external examination, personal effects, photographs, fingerprints, forensic pathological examination, dental examination, and DNA sampling from bone and teeth. As of 27 July 2005, 7 months after the disaster, TTVI had identified 2,010 victims, with over 1,800 cadavers remaining unidentified. Sixty-one percent of victims were identified by TTVI using dental examinations (n = 1,235), 19% using fingerprint records (n = 378), 1.3% using DNA analysis (n = 26), and 0.3% using physical evidence (n = 6). In a further 18% of cases (n = 365), more than one type of evidence was used.

Disposal of Human Remains

In Thailand, unidentified victims were stored in refrigerated containers during identification activities. Bodies that were identified were disposed of by cremation or burial according to local custom. Bodies of foreign victims were repatriated by their respective embassies. Around Banda Aceh, Indonesia, there were 14 mass graves, the largest, at Lambarro, reportedly containing 60,000-70,000 victims. Finding suitable government land for these large graves was difficult, and in some instances graves were sited very close to communities. In the areas surrounding Banda Aceh, smaller village-level graves were often used. Many were constructed rapidly, sometimes within the village itself. This has caused difficulty for returning survivors wanting to exhume and re-locate the graves to outside the village. In many rural areas, there was no formal body recovery and disposal of remains. In Sri Lanka, most human remains were buried after 3 or 4 days. Common graves, in which bodies were buried haphazardly in several layers, were sited largely within existing cemeteries. However, within some Muslim communities the deceased were buried within the first 24 hours according to custom, making it difficult for the local authorities to identify and count the dead. Additionally, there were concerns that some of the deceased, who were buried as Muslims, may have been from other religious groups.

Health Impact from Dead Bodies

Shortly after the tsunami, WHO and national governments established early warning disease surveillance. No epidemics among the surviving populations were identified in the weeks after the tsunami. In Banda Aceh, Indonesia, it took some 2 months to bury the thousands of bodies. In spite of the prolonged presence of dead bodies, no epidemics occurred. Among individuals handling human remains (recovery, identification, and disposal), we did not identify any reports of "occupational" infections. A health and safety assessment of temporary morgues in Thailand by the United States Centers for Disease Control and Prevention and the Thai Ministry of Public Health reported sharp-implement injuries and mucosal splashes with body fluids as well as heat stress and dehydration due to overuse of personal protective equipment such as respirators. A questionnaire survey conducted by the Thai Ministry of Public Health of around 200 individuals involved in body recovery did not identify any reports of infectious disease. Back injuries, caused by lifting bodies into trucks, were reported by Indonesian military. Body recovery teams faced potential injury risk from working among debris, especially from earthquake-damaged buildings. In Sri Lanka, most dead bodies were taken to local hospitals, which had an indirect health impact by disrupting the provision of medical assistance to survivors and threatening to close hospitals because of the smell of decomposition.

Coordination and Preparedness

In each country, a large number of individuals and organisations were involved in managing the dead. Body recovery involved the affected community, voluntary organisations, the police, and the military. Doctors, medical staff, and forensic specialists were involved in death certification and collecting post-mortem data. National police forces and consulates or embassies were involved in collecting ante-mortem data (information about the deceased collected before death, such as dental or fingerprint records). Disposal of the bodies was done by the military or police, who also had legal responsibility for victim identification. No single person or organisation had a clear mandate to coordinate the process of collecting, identifying, and disposing of the dead, either nationally or locally. None of the countries had mass fatality plans.

Internal organs were secretly removed from some of the bodies of victims of the Marchioness disaster without the consent of relatives, the Independent on Sunday can reveal. For more than 10 years since the sinking of the pleasure craft, relatives have nursed fears that their sons' and daughters' bodies were not complete when they were released for burial. Now, a report to ministers by Lord Justice Clarke has confirmed that body parts were removed for storage at a London hospital. The gruesome discovery has echoes of the scandal at Alder Hey, the children's hospital in Liverpool where a pathologist, Professor Dick Van Velzen, stored 3,000 organs from dead babies. The discovery that organ parts were also removed in the Marchioness tragedy will add to the pain of the relatives' loss. Some are still coming to terms with the violent deaths that their children suffered. "We are all upset. We have been traumatized for years, but I have always thought that this could happen," she said. "But I personally couldn't be hurt any more than I have already been hurt."

Margaret Lockwood Croft, the mother of one victim and administrator of the Marchioness Action Group (MAG), said she was "shocked and angry" at the report's findings. She said medical authorities were banned under the 1961 Human Tissues Act and coroner's rules from removing tissue without relatives' consent. But she had suspected that organs from her son, Shaun, 26, had been secretly removed during post-mortems. "I'm upset about it," she said last night. "People who know the law should uphold the law. These organs were stolen."

Many protested that their feelings had been trampled on by the authorities after the disaster, but their agony has gone on. It was the outcry by distraught relatives at the discovery that the pathologist, Dr Paul Knapman, had ordered 25 of the 51 victims' hands to be cut-off—apparently for identification purposes—that led to a public inquiry under Lord Justice Clarke. Now they face a fresh trauma, over his report which is due to be published. It is understood that Lord Justice Clarke's very thorough investigation uncovered a code word in a medical computer file which led him to Guy's hospital mortuary where organs from the Marchioness victims were stored. They had been removed without permission from relatives and without the knowledge of ministers, until the damning report was delivered. The families have been told that they can choose whether they want a second burial with the organs. Families have been told the organs included lungs, brains, livers, kidneys, hearts, spleens and tonsils, said Mrs Lockwood Croft, adding: "None of these needed to be removed to verify the cause of death. Drowning can be confirmed by an external post-mortem."

On Monday, ministers will announce that a new legal limit for drinking while in charge of a vessel is to be introduced. The same limit imposed on car drivers is to be applied to all skippers from small yachts to liners in British waters.

References

Ajmani, M.L. Embalming—Principles and legal aspects. Jaypee Publishers, 1998:81-91.

Alexander GC, Wynia MK. Ready and willing? Physicians' sense of preparedness for bioterrorism. *Health Aff* 2003;22:189-97.

American College of Emergency Physicians. Positioning America's emergency health care system to respond to acts of terrorism: a report of the Terrorism Response Task Force. Dallas, TX: The College; 2002. Greenberg MI, Jurgens SM, Gracely EJ. Emergency department preparedness for the evaluation and treatment of victims of biological or chemical terrorist attack. *J Emerg Med* 2002;22:273-8.

Arnold JL. Risk and Risk Assessment in Health Emergency Management. *Prehosp Disast Med* 2005; 20: 143-154.

Arnold JL. The 2005 London Bombings and the Haddon Matrix. *Prehosp Disast Med* 2005; 20: 279-281.

Bernard Knight. Forensic Pathology. Arnold Publisher, London. 2nd edn, 1996:10.

Boer J, Brismar B, Eldar R, Rutherford WH. The medical severity index of disasters. *J Emerg Med* 1989;7: 269-73.

Booz-Allen and Hamilton. Bioterrorism Emergency Planning and Preparedness Questionnaire for Health Care Facilities. Questionnaire developed under contract No. 290-00-0019 from AHRQ, March 10, 2002.

"Brewing cataclysm" in emergency response? *Hosp Peer Rev* 2003;28:85.

British Broadcasting Corporation. Fact of the Day. Available at [www.bbc.co.uk/]. Accessed 9 December 2005.

Case GG, West BM, McHugh CJ. Hospital preparedness for biological and chemical terrorism in central New Jersey. *N J Med* 2001;98:23-33.

Celentano J, Fruhwirth K, Gunter C. Hospital bioterrorism preparedness. Discussion of the National Bioterrorism Hospital Preparedness Programme, presented to the County of Los Angeles Emergency Medical Services Agency. September 2003. Available at http://www. ladhs.org/ems/disaster/2Year2OrientationtoHRSAGrant-Nonparticipating.pdf. Accessed April 12, 2004.

Centers for Disease Control and Prevention. Influenza fact sheet. Available from http://www.cdc.gov/flu/keyfacts.htm. Accessed July 28, 2005.

Ciraulo DL, Frykberg ER, Feliciano DV, Knuth TE, Richart CM, Westmoreland CD, *et al.* A survey assessment of the level of preparedness for domestic terrorism and mass casualty incidents among Eastern Association for the Surgery of Trauma members. *J Trauma* 2004;56:1033-9.

Cohen A. The Big Easy on the brink. *Time* 2000;156:91.

Daub EM. Hospital emergency preparedness assessment: a framework for integrated bioterrorism planning and response. Tucson (AZ): Science Technologies Corporation; January 7, 2002.

Economic Research Service, USDA. Measuring rurality: new definitions in 2003. .Available from http://www. ers.usda.gov/Briefing/Rurality/New Definitions. Accessed October 12, 2004.

Edi J: Bellview put us in the dark-NEMA. In: Daily Sun (Nigeria), 26 October 2005, Vol.2, No.572, p. 3. Also available at [www.sunnewsonline.com/].

Flowers LK, Mothershead JL, Blackwell TH. Bioterrorism preparedness II: the community and emergency medical services systems. *Emerg Med Clin North Am* 2002;20: 457-76.

Franz DR, Zajtchuk R. Biological terrorism: understanding the threat, preparation, and medical response. *DisMon* 2002;48:493-564.

Gerberding JL, Hughes JM, Koplan JP. Bioterrorism preparedness and response: clinicians and public health agencies as essential partners. *JAMA* 2002;287:898-900.

Greenberg MI, Hendrickson RG. Report of the CIMERC/Drexel University Emergency Department Terrorism Preparedness Consensus Panel. Acad Emerg Med 2003; 10:783-8.

Gresham, G.A., Postmortem procedures. World Medical Publications Ltd. London. 1979: 16-28.

Grow RW, Rubinson L. The challenge of hospital infection control during a response to bioterrorist attacks. *Biosecurity Bioterrorism Biodefense Strategy Practice Sci* 2003;1:1-6.

Gursky EA. Hometown hospitals: the weakest link? Bioterrorism readiness in America's rural hospitals. Washington, DC: Center for Technology and National Security Policy; 2004.

Heinrich J. Infectious disease outbreaks: bioterrorism preparedness efforts have improved public health response capacity, but gaps remain. Government Reform, House of Representatives, United States General Accounting Office. April 9, 2003.

Heller O, Aldar Y, Vosk M, Shemer J. An argument for equipping civilian hospitals with a multiple respirator DMR 86 Disaster Management and Response/Manley et al Volume 4, Number 3 system for a chemical warfare mass casualty situation. J Med Sci 1991;27:652-5.

Hick J.L., Leitheiser A. Integrated planning for disaster: a model for Minnesota hospitals. *Minn Med* 2002;85:44-7.

Hirsch GB. Modeling the consequences of major incidents for health care systems. Available from http://www.systemdynamics.org/publications.htm. Accessed July 22, 2005.

Hoard M, Homer J, Manley W, Furbee P, Haque A, Helm-kamp J. Systems modeling in support of evidence-based disaster planning for rural areas. *Int J Hyg Environ Health* 2005;208:117-25.

Insider Weekly, Nov. 7, 2005.

Kienstra AJ, Endom EE. Disaster medicine: bioterrorism and its impact on the emergency department. *Clin Pe-diatr Emerg Med* 2002;3:231-8.

Koenig KL, Dinerman N, Kuehl AE. Disaster nomenclatureda functional impact approach: the PICE system. *Acad Emerg Med* 1996;3:723-7.

Koshy, K. Punjab Police rules, Vol. III. The Bright Law House. 1992: 1078-83.

L. Riddez Air line Accident at the Chang-Kai Chek Airport, 31 October, 2000. *Prehosp Disast Med* 2001; 16(2): s60.

Louisiana Water Resources Research Institute, Louisiana Water Resources Research Institute: NSEL Products 1998-2002. Available from http://www.lawater.lsu.edu/. Accessed October 4, 2005.

Lovern E. Whatever the number, it's big. AHA spreads confusion with differing costs for hospitals' terrorism preparedness. Mod Health Care 2001;31:6-13. Tommet P. Hospital assessment survey for biological emergencies in Minnesota (Minnesota Department of Health Survey). St Paul, MN: Minnesota Department of Health; 2003.

Manley W, Homer J, Hoard M, Roy S, Furbee P, Summers D, *et al.* A dynamic model to support surge capacity planning in a rural hospital. Available from http://www.systemsdynamics.org/publications.htm. Accessed July 25, 2005.

Manual for control of hospital associated infections. NACO, Ministry of Health and Family Welfare, Govt. of India.

Mobilizing America's health care reservoir. Joint Commission on Accreditation of Health Care Organisations. *Joint Commission Perspect* 2001;21:1-23.

Odebode N et al: Bellview: Lisa village head arested. In: *The Punch* (Nigeria), 4 November 2005, Vol. 17, No. 19469, p. 6.

Olatuyi O: 29 planes are overage. In: The Punch (Nigeria), 4 November 2005, Vol.17, No. 19469, pp. 1-2. Also available at [www.punchng.com/].

Parikh, C.K. Medicolegal Postmortems in India. Medical Publications, Bombay. 1985: 157-160.

Polson, C.J. The essentials of Forensic medicine. Pergamon press, Oxford. 4th edn., 1985: 677-94.

Public Safety Wireless Network Programme. Answering the call: communications lessons learned from the Pentagon attack. January 2002. Available at http://www. safecomprogram.gov/SAFECOM/library/interoperability casestudies/1063_AnsweringCall.htm. Accessed June 22,2005.

Richards CF, Burstein JL, Waeckerle JF, Hutson HR. Emergency physicians and biological terrorism. *Ann Emerg Med* 1999;34:183-90.

Rinnert KJ. An approach to terrorism preparedness: Parkland Health and Hospital System. *Baylor Univ Med Center Proc* 2001;14:231-5.

Rubin J.N. Recurring pitfalls in hospital preparedness and response. Available from http://www.homelandsecurity. org/journal/Articles/rubin.html. Accessed October 12, 2004.

Sarkar, P.C. Criminal major acts. Orient Law House, New Delhi. 6th edn., 1999.

Schultz CH, Mothershead JL, Field M. Bioterrorism pre-paredness I: the emergency department and hospital. *Emerg Med Clin North Am* 2002;20:437-55.

Schur C.L. Understanding the role of the rural hospital emergency department in responding to bioterrorist attacks and other emergencies: a review of the literature and guide to the issues (No. 5U1CRH0002604). Bethesda, MD: National Opinion Research Center of the University of Chicago, Walsh Center for Rural Health Analysis; 2004.

Schur CL, Berk ML, Mueller CD. Perspectives of rural hospitals on bioterrorism preparedness planning. Political analysis brief (W Series, No. 4). Bethesda, MD: National Opinion Research Center of the University of Chicago, Walsh Center for Rural Health Analysis; April 2004.

Siegelson HJ. Preparing for a terrorist attack: mass casualty management focus on soft targets. Indianapolis, IN: Disaster Planning International; 2002.

Stein M, Hirshberg A. Medical consequences of terrorism. The conventional weapon threat. *Surg Clin North Am* 1999;79:1537-52.

Subrahmanyam, B.V. Modi's medical jurisprudence and toxicology. Butterworths. 22nd edn, 724-27.

TFQCDM, Sundnes KO, Birnbaum ML(eds): Health Disaster Management: Guidelines for Evaluation and Research in the Utstein Style. 1st ed. Madison, Wisconsin: *Prehosp Disast Med*, 1003, pp. 1-177.

The Guardian, Oct. 24, 2005.

The Guardian, Wed. 14th Dec. 2005.

The National Commission on Terrorist Attacks Upon the United States. The 9-11 Commission report. 2004; 1:383-98. Available from http://www.9-11 commission. gov/report/index.htm. Accessed October 12, 2004.

The News, Vol. 25, No. 18, Nov. 7, 2005.

The Punch, 24/12/05.

The Punch, Friday Dec. 30, 2005.

The Punch, Thursday, 27/10/05.

Thorne CD, Curbow B, Oliver M, al Ibrahim M, McDiarmid M. Terrorism preparedness training for non-clinical hospital workers: empowering them to take action. *J Occup Environ Med* 2003;45:333-7.

Tur-Kaspa I, Lev EI, Hendler I, Siebner R, Shapira Y, Shemer J. Preparing hospitals for toxicological mass casualties events. *Crit Care Med* 1999;27:1004-

Washington State Department of Health and Bioterrorism. Washington State Department of Health and Bioterrorism Hospital Preparedness Programme. Washington, State Implementation Plan. Needs assessment. Available From http://www.doh.wa.gov/phepr/FedApps2003/

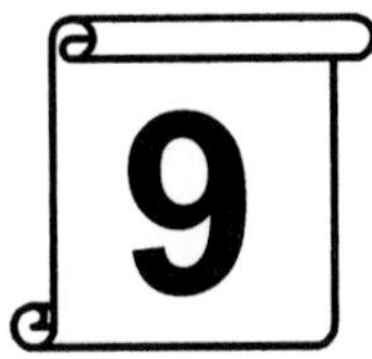

Weapons of Mass Destruction and Hospital Preparedness

Weapons of Mass Destruction (WMD) include chemical, biological, and radiological (CBR) agents. Our knowledge of weapons of mass destruction (WMD) is based upon our experience with Hiroshima, Nagasaki, and Chernobyl, where large number of people had died suddenly due to radiation exposure. Radiation injuries can be caused by four possibilities: localized exposure, resulting in a burn; whole body exposure, resulting in acute radiation syndrome; internal contamination via inhalation, ingestion, skin, and/or wounds, resulting in radio iodine accumulation in the thyroid; and external contamination, whereby removal of the clothing alone results in 90% elimination of the contamination (Mettler and Voelz, 2002). It is estimated that a one-megaton nuclear warhead would kill almost two million people in the Washington, DC area (Richards et al, 1999). The 1995 sarin nerve gas attack in Tokyo, Japan demonstrated the lethal consequences of an organophosphate nerve agent. This attack utilized plastic bags containing diluted sarin that were placed on subway trains, and subsequently activated when terrorists pierced them with the tips of umbrellas (Lee, 2003). Twelve passengers died as a result of this attack and thousands were injured. A biological agent is "any organism or toxin found in nature that can be used to incapacitate, kill, or impede an adversary". The Greeks practiced biological warfare as early as 300 BC, when they polluted wells by filling them with dead animals (Slater and Trunkey, 1997). Biological agents may be disseminated by aerosol, sprays, explosives, food, or water contamination (Richards *et al.*). The United States experienced the adverse effects of a biological agent in 2001, when 22 individuals contracted anthrax in the Washington, DC area, resulting in five deaths (Gerberding, Hughes, and Koplan, 2002). It is now estimated that 100 kg of anthrax released in Washington, DC could kill over one million people (Richards et al). Chemical agents consist of nerve, blister, blood, choking, and incapacitating agents. Generally the WMDs are used by terrorists to destroy large areas or kill many people to create scare. Sometimes these are used in war and occasionally it could be accidental. See appendix attached to this chapter for some facts about WMDs.

WHAT IS TERRORISM?

There are many definitions of terrorism, but the one developed by Cunningham (2003) is one of the most useful: 'Terrorism is defined as the illegitimate use or threat of violence to further political objectives. It is illegitimate in that it targets civilians and/or non-combatants and it is perpetrated by clandestine agents of state and non-state actors in contravention of the laws of war and criminal statutes. It is symbolic and premeditated violence whose purpose is to communicate a message to a wider population than the immediate victims of violence. It is designed to affect this audience by creating psychological states of fear in order to influence decision-makers to change policies, practices or systems that are related to the perpetrators' political objectives. These objectives can be either systemic or sub-systemic and may be motivated by complex social forces including, but not limited to, ideology, ethno-nationalism or religious extremism'. They use weapons of all kinds to kill/injure the innocent civilians, including weapons of mass destruction. Terrorism threatens the public with widespread death and disease, fear, panic, and disruption to society—both psychologically and economically (Richards, Burstein, Waeckerle, and Hutson, 1999).

Suicide bombs detonate in close proximity to victims, with two-thirds exploding in confined/closed spaces (Hiss and Kahana, 2000). To increase injuries, some bombs contain numerous metal fragments (e.g., nails), or even pellets of rodent poison, to introduce bleeding coagulopathies in injured victims (Wolf and Rivkind, 2002). A study of suicide bombings involving 892 victims in Israel from 1994-1997 revealed a mortality rate of 17%, with 30% of the fatalities having no obvious external cause of death (Wolf and Rivkind); this suggests that immediate death was probably related to massive pulmonary bleeding or a pulmonary embolism (Stein and Hirshberg, 1999).

Common injuries after a bomb attack

A typical scenario of a blast injury related to the bombing of a building would begin with direct exposure to air gas, followed by the displacement of mass movement of air; a penetrating and non-penetrating impact of blast-energized debris; burns from flash and hot gases; inhalation of noxious gases; and finally the possible collapse of the building (Cooper, Maynard, Cross, and Hill, 1983). A pulmonary blast injury is the most common form of thoracic trauma found in immediate blast fatalities, but it is rare to find among injured survivors (Stein and Hirshberg, 1999). A study of thoracic blast injuries in rats may explain this lethality, in which a reflex of apnea, bradycardia, and hypotension occurred in the rats after the injury (which did not occur when abdominal blast injuries were tested) (Guy, Kirkman, Watkins, and Cooper, 1998). Incidentally, the presence of blood in a victim's airway is a dependable sign that a blast lung injury has been sustained (Alfici, *et al.*, 2006). Patients suffering from primary blast injury to the lungs are challenging to manage. Based on the Israelis' experience, respiratory support has included volume-controlled, pressure-controlled, individual lung, or high frequency ventilation (Stein and Hirshberg). Extracorporeal membrane oxygenator was unsuccessful the only time it was used, and nitric oxide improved the respiratory status of a just few patients. Alfici *et al.* recommend securing the airway by means of a rapid sequence induction and intubation, followed by positive pressure ventilation (PPV); however, the authors caution that PPV may actually cause further barotrauma to the lungs, so it might not be an option for all patients. Head injuries are the most common contributor to both immediate and late fatality for victims of terrorist bombings, and abdominal and chest injuries contribute to late fatality in immediate survivors (Frykberg and Tepas, 1988). Patients with closed head injuries require the expertise of neurosurgery and patients with ocular injuries need to have an ophthalmologist as a part of the health care team. Abdominal trauma patients may require nasogastric tubes, intravenous fluids, and colostomies, and all patients require superb post-op care management, including antibiotics (Stein and Hirshberg, 1999).

There is an overwhelming prevalence of minor, non-life-threatening trauma. Flash burns, fractures, and eardrum injuries are seen in those closest to the bomb. Eighty-four percent of all surgeries performed on survivors of bombings are to repair soft tissue and bone injuries, which do not contribute to mortality unless a traumatic amputation is involved. These patients need labor-intensive wound cleansing and debridement, and may benefit from the use of vacuum-assisted closure to promote wound healing. Crush injuries can result from massive soft tissue injury in victims trapped in buildings. With a crush injury, myoglobin is released from muscle tissue, which induces rhabdo-myolosis; thus, to optimize renal hemo-dynamics and prevent accompanying acute renal failure, survivors of crush injuries need to be aggressively hydrated and diuresed, along with alkalizing their urine (Criddle, 2003).

Essentials in the management of mass casualties from terrorist bombings

- *Protection of medical assets*: Medical assets (e.g., first responders, including ambulance personnel) need to be protected, based on the "second hit" principle whereby snipers may fire on first responders. This was the case in the evacuation of victims after the bombing of the Marine Barracks in Beirut, Lebanon in 1983.
- *Record keeping*: Record keeping has to be exceptional because it

is the major means of leaving an audit trail that contributes to continuity of patient care and tracking the location of victims. Accurate records also contribute to retrospective review to explore "lessons learned."

- *Triage*: During a mass casualty incident, advanced triage systems are activated since a large number of victims will overwhelm existing resources of personnel, equipment, and supplies. The challenge of this form of triage is to differentiate the minority of casualties who are critically injured and need immediate care from the majority of victims who do not have life-threatening injuries. Nurses may struggle morally with triaging patients to the "expectant" category as they have to shift their mindset from the normal management of day-to-day trauma to mass casualty management (which targets care of the population). This decision-making process may result in some immediate survivors in extremis (e.g., with respiratory failure and profound shock) not being treated and then dying—an event for which many nurses find themselves unprepared.

Disaster response

While there are many aspects to disaster response, such as security, transportation, and reconstruction, the medical response directly affects the people most impacted by the disaster. Providing nursing care during a disaster presents numerous challenges, such as an uncertain physical environment, scarce human and material resources, personal risk, and most certainly, patients who are at their most vulnerable. Registered nurses are often the single largest group of responders in any major disaster. Now is the time for nursing-power response to be harnessed, cultivated, and deliberately managed so that it can be deployed in a manner that will be of greatest benefit to this nation during a major disaster (Cheryl A. Peterson).

The success of any response is dependent on all individuals or teams understanding their roles, responsibilities, and the chain of command within the disaster response. Disaster respondents who deploy within a system that is part of the overall disaster planning usually come with the essential equipment that is needed to complete their mission and to keep the responder safe from hazards that might result from the disaster. A spontaneous volunteer who shows up on the disaster scene may not have the necessary equipment and may also easily become a distraction to those leading the response effort. Any volunteer/nurse who believes that he/she will want to respond at the time of a disaster should pre-register with one of the many disaster registries and response organisations that already exist.

With WMD the dead outnumber the injured

Tragically, in major terrorist events, many people die at the time of the incident, as was the case after the September 11 attacks in the United

States—but 48 hours after the tragedy only 18 patients remained in hospital. Hospitals must have contingency plans to corral less-injured patients in advance of the arrival of ambulances bringing the more severely injured. No plan is effective unless tested periodically by practice drills. There have been extensive exercises at a jurisdictional and national level for a number of disaster scenarios that test hospital systems. Hospitals' ability to manage a sudden surge in casualties and ensure that the most critically injured patients receive timely resuscitation and life-saving surgery.

Chemical or Biological Terrorism; An American study

Hospital emergency departments generally are not prepared in an organised fashion to treat victims of WMD due to chemical or biological terrorism. (*Am J Public Health*, 2001;91:710–716) There is growing concern about possible terrorist use of chemical or biological weapons against civilian populations. In the 1984 incident in Oregon, members of a religious commune deliberately contaminated restaurant salad bars with Salmonella typhi bacteria, causing 751 cases of gastroenteritis. One theoretical model predicted that a terrorist attack releasing Bacillus anthracis spores in prevailing winds toward the suburb of a major city could cause up to 50,000 cases of anthrax, with more than 32000 deaths, in an exposed population of 1,00,000 people. True preparedness to reduce loss of life from an incident involving a biological or chemical weapon is critically dependent on the availability of resources at the local level. The Domestic Preparedness Programme, however, has included no systematic efforts to integrate hospitals into response plans, and it has provided only limited funds to acquire resources for state and local responders and none for hospitals.

A large proportion of hospitals probably are poorly prepared to handle victims of chemical or biological terrorism. Commonly, hospitals are not fully prepared to respond to massive casualty disasters of any kind, either in their capacity to care for large numbers of victims or in their ability to provide care in coordination with a regional or federal incident command structure. Surveys of hospital emergency departments (EDs) have found broadly prevalent deficiencies in knowledge, plans, or resources for responding to hazardous materials or radiation incidents. Levels of preparedness were relatively low in all areas examined—awareness, plans and training, physical resources, and medication inventories. In general, urban hospitals were better prepared than rural hospitals, and urban hospitals with busier EDs tended to be better prepared than hospitals with EDs serving smaller populations. Very few hospitals, however, fully met the conservative criteria used in this study to assess preparedness for hypothetical incidents involving 50 individuals exposed to sarin or anthrax. Most surveyed hospitals did have plans and training for response to a community or hospital hazardous materials incident, and it is conceivable that those plans could provide a foundation for the eventual development of plans for response to incidents involving chemical or biological weapons. Respondents may have underreported preparedness, but the findings are comparable to those in other surveys of preparedness for hazardous materials incidents in Philadelphia and Washington State.

It is foreseeable that even the better-prepared hospitals could be overwhelmed by the potentially large number of victims in a chemical weapons incident.

A well-fitting respirator with an organic vapor or high-efficiency particulate air cartridge could provide a meaningful level of protection against some chemical agents, and it might be better than using no respiratory protection in a crisis situation.

The surveyed hospitals were universally unprepared to provide pralidoxime to a group of 50 victims in a hypothetical sarin incident, (May 2001, Vol. 91, No. 5, *American Journal of Public Health*) and only 29% had sufficient atropine. These findings mirror those of another study of antidote supplies in Colorado, Montana, and Nevada: 62% of 137 hospital pharmacies did not have adequate pralidoxime to provide the necessary 2-g dose for even 170 kg. individual poisoned by an organophosphate insecticide, which causes the same symptoms and pathophysiology as sarin or VX nerve agent.

Not surprisingly, hospitals close to the Umatilla chemical weapons depot were more likely than other hospitals to have plans for responding to incidents involving chemical weapons. These survey responses may not have included military antidote kits or protective equipment stockpiled near the hospitals, and they may under-represent the true level of preparedness. However, the availability of isolation areas, decontamination facilities, and identified personal protective resources was comparable to that of other hospitals.

The quality of effort-dependent responses could have been adversely affected by the frequently expressed opinion of respondents that biological and chemical weapons do not present a real threat to their community. Some respondents may have portrayed their institution in an overly positive manner, especially given that many administrative actions and physical resources covered by the survey are required under existing regulations pertaining to chemical hazards (D.C. Wetter, W.E. Daniell, C.D. Treser).

What does preparedness mean?

Consider tourists visiting San Jose, California. Even warm locales may on some rare occasion experience a snow flurry. From this, one can imagine hypothetical snowstorm. Conduct a poll of such travelers to determine if any have packed snowshoes and you might determine a woefully low level of preparedness for a blizzard. A more reasonable conclusion might be that owing to the low risk of snow and even much lower risk of a blizzard, the travelers were best prepared by leaving the snowshoes at home.

Mass Casualty Event in Netherlands: Lessons Learnt

The overall worldwide incidence of MCEs or disasters is increasing. the three most deadly misconceptions in dealing with MCEs are: (1) "it will not happen here," (2) "it will not happen to me," and (3) "someone else will take care of the problem". Upon evaluating MCEs in the Netherlands over the last 60 years, it is worth noting that 39 major events occurred, with an average of 59 (0–947) wounded and 67 (2–1,836) fatal casualties. Statistically speaking, there is a chance of being confronted with an MCE every two years in Netherlands (Michael Bemelman, Luke Leenen).

In general, the sudden surge of casualties in an MCE presents two challenges. The first is the logistic challenge: a large number of casualties need to be processed through the system. The second challenge is the medical challenge: how can we provide the greatest level of care for the greatest number of patients? Preparation is essential to cope with these challenges. The only way to prepare for these events is to learn from our past and try to train for the future.

Our response also corresponds to the four recognized phases viz. First, there was chaos: the mechanism contributing to the event was not clear and the amount of casualties was initially unknown. During this phase, the first reports of casualties were greatly overestimated—"more than one hundred." This is a well-known phenomenon, especially in man-made disasters, showing that the initial estimation is higher than the true number of victims. After 20 min. the paramedics at the scene had eventually obtained an adequate estimate of the number of victims. The second phase, response, is defined by the response of the emergency services: the deployment of the ambulances, MMT, police and fire brigade at the scene, and the installation of the trauma teams at the hospital. The third phase, recovery, is defined by the actions taken by the emergency services and trauma teams. However, this phase does embrace more than only taking care of the patients; it also means cleaning up at the scene, restoring infrastructure, and providing post-traumatic psychological support. The fourth and final phase, mitigation, is characterized by evaluating the event and taking precautions for the future; for instance, in the present case all staircases in the city were checked and were replaced as necessary. The initial field triage during this event had a considerable over-triage; this is a well-described problem. Over-triage rates of 8–80% have been reported in the literature. The danger of over-triage is that the limited resources will be exhausted for the wrong patients. The opposite problem, under-triage, leads to unnecessary deaths because critically ill patients are not recognized and are assigned to a less urgent scale.

Priority-1 are patients with life-threatening injuries needing immediate treatment; Priority-2 are patients with serious injuries, but who can tolerate some delay (6 hrs.) in treatment; Priority-3 are ambulant patients with minor injuries who, in general, can be treated by physician assistants; Priority-4 are patients who have died or who are not expected to survive. Based on other disasters, it is accepted that approximately 10–

15% of the total casualty count will have serious injuries requiring immediate treatment.

References

Rosenfeld JV, Fitzgerald M, Kossmann T, *et al.* Is the Australian hospital system adequately prepared for terrorism? *Med J Aust 2005*; 183: 567-570.

Emergency Management Australia. Emergency management. Assistance to the states and territories (COMDISPLAN). (accessed Nov 2005).

NSW Health. Disaster mental health response handbook. Sydney: NSW Health, 2000. Available at: (accessed Nov 2005).

Council of Australian Governments (COAG). Council of Australian Governments' meeting. 3 June 2005. (accessed Nov 2005).

Cooper D. AusBurnPLAN strategy paper. Australian Mass Casualty Burn Disaster Plan. Final draft. 2004. (accessed Nov 2005).

Arnold JL, Tsai MC, Halpern P, *et al.* Mass-casualty terrorist bombings: epidemiological outcomes, resource utilization and time course of emergency needs. *Prehospital Disaster Med* 2004; 18: 220-234.

Frykberg ER. Medical management of disasters and mass casualties from terrorist bombings: how can we cope? *J Trauma* 2002; 53: 201-212.

Edwards NA. Exercise: Supreme Truth—the report. Adelaide: Mediflight, 2003.

AAP. Car bomb explodes in simulated terror attack. The Sydney Morning Herald 2004; 31 May. (accessed Nov 2005).

Landstinget i Östergötland. Senior instructor course—simulation exercising in disaster medicine. (accessed Nov 2005).

Alfici, R., Ashkenazi, I., and Kessel, B. (2006). Management of victims in a mass casualty incident caused by a terrorist bombing: treatment algorithms for stable, unstable, and in extremis victims. *Military Medicine*, 171, 1155-1162.

Atran, S. (2003). Genesis of suicide terrorism. *Science*, 299(5612), 1534-1539.

Auf der Heide, E. (2006). The importance of evidence-based disaster planning. *Annals of Emergency Medicine*. 47(1), 34-49.

Centers for Disease Control and Prevention (CDC). (2002a). Injuries and illnesses among New York City fire department rescue workers after responding to the World Trade Center Attacks. *MMWR*, 51, 1-5.

Centers for Disease Control and Prevention (CDC). (2002b). New classification for deaths and injuries involving terrorism. *MMWR*, 51, 18-19.

Centers for Disease Control and Prevention (CDC). (n.d.a). Bioterrorism.Retrieved July 10, 2007, from www.bt.cdc.gov/bioterrorism/.

Centers for Disease Control and Prevention (CDC). (n.d.b). Chemical emergencies.Retrieved July 10, 2007, from www.bt.cdc.gov/chemical/.

Centers for Disease Control and Prevention (CDC). (n.d.c). Radiation emergencies.Retrieved July 10, 2007, from http://www.bt.cdc.gov/radiation/.

Cooper, G.J.,Maynard, R.L., Cross, N.L., and Hill, J.F. (1983). Casualties from terrorist bombings. *Journal of Trauma-Injury Infection and Critical Care*, 23(11), 955-967.

Criddle, L.M. (2003). Rhabdomyolysis. Pathophysiology, recognition, and management. *Critical Care Nurse*, 23(6), 14-22, 24-26, 28, 31-32.

Cunningham, W. G. (2003). Terrorism: Definitions and typologies. Terrorism: Concepts, Causes, and Conflict Resolution. Fort Belvoir, VA: Defense Threat Reduction Agency and George Mason University's Institute for Conflict Analysis and Resolution.

Department of Homeland Security (DHS). (2007). Ready.gov.Retrieved May 21, 2007, from www.ready.gov/america/index.html.

Eiseman, B. (2001). Combat casualty management for tomorrow's battlefield: Urban terrorism. *Journal of Trauma-Injury Infection and Critical Care,* 51(5), 821-823.

Friedman, A. (2003). Terrorism in context. Terrorism: Concepts, Causes, and Conflict Resolution. Fort Belvoir, VA: Defense Threat Reduction Agency and George Mason University's Institute for Conflict Analysis and Resolution.

Frykberg, E.R. (2002). Medical management of disasters and mass casualties from terrorist bombings: How can we cope? *Journal of Trauma-Injury Infection and Critical Care,* 53(2), 201-12.

Gebbie, K., and Qureshi, K. (2006). A historical challenge: Nurses and emergencies. OJIN: *The Online Journal of Issues in Nursing,* 11(3).

Gerberding, J.L., Hughes, J.M., and Koplan, J.P. (2002). Bioterrorism preparedness and response: clinicians and public health agencies as essential partners. *JAMA,* 287(7), 898-900.

Guy, R.J., Kirkman, E., Watkins, P.E., and Cooper, G.J. (1998). Physiologic responses to primary blast. *Journal of Trauma-Injury Infection and Critical Care,* 45(6), 983-987.

Hiss, J., andKahana, T. (2000). Trauma and identification of victims of suicidal terrorism in Israel. Military Medicine, 165(11), 889-893.

Hoffman, B. (2006). Inside terrorism. NY: Columbia University Press.

Lee, E.C. (2003). Clinical manifestations of sarin nerve gas exposure. *JAMA,* 290(5), 659-662.

Leibovici, D., Gofrit, O.N., Stein, M., Shapira, S.C., Noga, Y., Heruti, R.J., *et al.* (1996). Blast injuries: Bus versus open-air bombings—a comparative study of injuries in survivors of open-air versus confined-space explosions. *Journal of Trauma-Injury Infection and Critical Care,* 41(6), 1030-1035.

Markon, J., and Dwyer, T. (2006). Moussaoui says he was to fly fifth plane on 9/11. Washington Post, March 28, A1, A16.

Mettler, F.A., Jr., andVoelz, G.L. (2002). Major radiation exposure—what to expect and how to respond. *New England Journal of Medicine,* 346(20), 1554-1561.

Mintz, J. (2004). The world after 911: The biological threat. Washington Post, A1, A6.

Moore, J. (2001). The evolution of Islamic terrorism: an overview. Frontline: Target America. Retrieved May 24, 2007.

Moore, S.R. (2003). Characteristics of terrorism. Terrorism: Concepts, Causes, and Conflict Resolution. Fort Belvoir, VA: Defense Threat Reduction Agency and George Mason University's Institute for Conflict Analysis and Resolution.

National Institutes of Health (NIH). (2007). NIH Funding Opportunities and Notices in the NIH guide for Grants and Contracts: Behavioral and Social Research on Disasters and Health (R21) PA-06-452. Retrieved June 4, 2007

Parry, W. (2007). Store clerk key to Fort Dix plot arrests. ABCNEWS.com. Retrieved May 9, 2007 from http://abcnews.go.com/US/wireStory?id=3154608.

Pavlin, J.A., Eitzen, E.M., and Caudle, L.C. (1997). Chapter 28: Biological warfare defense. In Sidell, F.R., Takafuji, E.T., Franz, DR (Eds.), Medical Aspects of Chemical and Biological Warfare (pp. 627-654). Washington, DC: Office of the Surgeon General at TMM Publications Borden Institute.

Peterson, C. (2006). Be safe, be prepared: Emergency system for advance registration of volunteer health professionals in disaster response. OJIN: The Online Journal of Issues in Nursing, 11(3).

Richards, C.F., Burstein, J.L.,Waeckerle, J.F., and Hutson, H.R. (1999). Emergency physicians and biological terrorism. Annals of Emergency Medicine, 34(2), 183-190.

Romano, C.A. (2007). Nursing leadership and outreach. A Message from the Chief Nurse. Retrieved June 2, 2007 from http://phs-nurse.org/chiefnurse/april_28_2007.html.

Silver, R.C., Holman, E.A., McIntosh, D.N.,Poulin, M., and Gil-Rivas, V. (2002).

Nationwide longitudinal study of psychological responses to September 11. *JAMA*, 288(10), 1235-1244.

Slater, M.S., and Trunkey D.D. (1997). Terrorism in America. An evolving threat. Archives of Surgery, 132(10), 1059-1066.

Stein, M. andHirshberg, A. (1999). Medical consequences of terrorism. The conventional weapon threat. Surgical Clinics of North America, 79(6), 1537-1552.

Thomas, E. (2006). The new age of terror: Soldiers in the war on terror have learned much since 9/11. So, too, has the enemy. How the London plot was foiled—and where we are in the five-year struggle. Newsweek, August 21, 43 – 53.

American Hospital Association. (2005). Emergency system for advanced registration of volunteer health care personnel—Hospital implementation issues and solutions focus group meeting report. Retrieved August 22, 2006,

American Nurses Association. (2002a). Registered nurses' rights and responsibilities related to work release during a disaster. Retrieved May 15, 2006,

American Nurses Association. (2002b). Work release during a disaster—guidelines for employers. Retrieved May 15, 2006,

Health Resources and Services Administration. (2006). Bioterrorism hospital preparedness—Emergency system for advance registration of volunteer health professionals (ESAR-VHP). Retrieved on February 6, 2006

Hoard, M. L. and Tosatto, R. J. (2005). Medical reserve corps: Strengthening public health and improving preparedness. Disaster Management and Response, 3(2), 48-52.

National Disaster Medical System. (2006). Welcome to NDMS: Our mission. Retrieved July 29, 2006 from www.oep-ndms.dhhs.gov.

Weiner, E. (2006). Preparing nurses internationally for emergency planning and response. OJIN: The Online Journal of Issues in Nursing, 11(3).

Wikipedia. (2006b). Plot of the Rue Saint-Nicaise. Retrieved March 30, 2006 from http://en.wikipedia.org/wiki/Infernal_machine.

Wolf, Y.G., andRivkind, A. (2002). Vascular trauma in high-velocity gunshot wounds and shrapnel-blast injuries in Israel. *Surgical Clinics of North America*, 82(1), 237-244.

Wynd, C. (2006). A proposed model for military disaster nursing. OJIN: The Online Journal of Issues in Nursing, 11(3). May 2001, Vol. 91, No. 5 710 *American Journal of Public Health.*

LCDR Donald Clark Wetter, PA-C, MPH, USPHS, William Edward Daniell, MD, MPH, and Charles David Treser, MPH.

Okumura T, Suzuki K, Fukuda A, *et al.* The Tokyo subway sarin attack: disaster management, part 1: community emergency response. *Acad Emerg Med.* 1998;5:613

Okumura T, Suzuki K, Fukuda A, *et al.* The Tokyo subway sarin attack: disaster management, part 2: hospital response. *Acad Emerg Med.* 1998;5:618–624.

Torok TJ, Tauxe RV, Wise RP, *et al.* A large community outbreak of salmonellosis caused by intentional contamination of restaurant salad bars. *JAMA.* 1997;278:389–395.

Kaufmann AF, Meltzer MI, Schmid GP. The economic impact of a bioterrorist attack: are prevention and postattack intervention programmes justifiable? *Emerg Infect Dis.* 1997;3:83–94.

Tucker JB. National health and medical services response to incidents of chemical and biological terrorism. *JAMA.* 1997;278:362–368.

US Congress. National Defense Authorization Act for Fiscal Year 1997. Pub L No. 104-201, Title XIV, Defense Against Weapons of Mass Destruction, Subtitle A, Domestic Preparedness (September 1996).

Hearings Before the Strategic Forces Subcommittee of the Senate Armed Services Committee, 105th Congr, 2nd Sess (1998) (testimony of H.A. Holmes, assistant secretary for defense).

Simon JT. Biological terrorism: preparing to meet the threat. *JAMA.* 1997;278:428–430.

Henderson DA. The looming threat of bioterrorism. *Science.* 1999;283:1279–1282.

Hauf der Heide E. Disaster planning, II: disaster problems, issues, and challenges identified in the research literature. *Disaster Med.* 1996;14: 453–479.

Landesman LY, Leonard RB. SARA three years later: emergency physicians'knowledge, beliefs, and actions. *Prehospital Disaster Med.* 1993;8: 39–44.

Edgell M, James MR. Contaminated casualties: are we prepared to receive them? *J Accid Emerg Med.* 1994;11:172–174.

Burgess JL, Blackmon GM, Brodkin CA, Robertson WO. Hospital preparedness for hazardous materials incidents and treatment of contaminated patients. *West J Med.* 1997;167: 387–391.

Cone DC, Davidson SJ. Hazardous materials preparedness in the emergency department. *Prehosp Emerg Care.* 1997;1:85–90.

Merritt NL, Anderson MJ. Case review: malathion overdose: when one patient creates a departmental hazard. *J Emerg Nurs.* 1989;15: 463–465.

Thanabalasingham T, Beckett MW, Murray V. Hospital response to a chemical incident: report on casualties of an ethyldichlorosilane spill. *BMJ.* 1991;302:101–102.

Burgess JL. Hospital evacuations due to hazardous materials incidents. *Am J Emerg Med.* 1999;17:50–52.

Waeckerle JF. Domestic preparedness for events involving weapons of mass destruction [editorial]. *JAMA.* 2000;283:252–254.

Centers for Disease Control and Prevention. CDC recommendations for civilian communities near chemical weapons depots: guidelines for medical preparedness. 60 Federal Register 33307–33312 (1995).

Brennan R, Waeckerle J, Sharp T, Lillibridge S. Chemical warfare agents: emergency medical and emergency public health issues. *Ann Emerg Med.* 1999;34:191–204. May 2001, Vol. 91, No. 5, 716. *American Journal of Public Health.*

Keim M, Kaufmann A. Principles for emergency response to bioterrorism. *Ann Emerg Med.* 1999; 34:177–182.

Sharp TW, Brennan RJ, Keim M,Williams RJ, Eitzen E, Lillibridge S. Medical preparedness for a terrorist incident involving chemical or biological agents during the 1996 Atlanta Olympic games. *Ann Emerg Med.* 1998;32:214–223.

Richards CF, Burstein JL, Waeckerle JF, Hutson HR. Emergency physicians and biological terrorism. *Ann Emerg Med.* 1999;34:183–190.

McIntyre AG, Christopher GW, Gum R, *et al.* Weapons of mass destruction events with contaminated casualties: effective planning for health care facilities. *JAMA.* 2000;283:242–249.

Cohen HW, Gould RM, Sidel VW. Bioterrorism initiatives: public health in reverse? *Am J Public Health.* 1999;89:1629–1631.

American Hospital Association. Guide to Health Care Field 1997–98. Chicago, Ill: Health Care InfoSource; 1997.

1990 Census: Detailed Housing Demographics. Washington, DC: Bureau of the Census, US Dept of Commerce; January 1993.

Larson KL. Public health and medical planning for chemical weapons agent releases. Paper presented at: Third Annual Disaster Health and Medical Conference; September 18, 1997; Richland, Wash. 29. Epidemiology Programme Office, Centers for Disease.

Okumura T, Takasu N, Ishimatsu S, *et al.* Report of 640 victims of the Tokyo subway sarin attack. *Ann Emerg Med.* 1996;28:129–135.

Management of Chemical Casualties Handbook. 2nd ed. Aberdeen Proving Grounds, Md: Chemical Casualty Care Office, US Army Medical Research Institute of Chemical Defense; September 1995.

Medical Management of Biological Casualties. 3rd ed. Fort Detrick, Md: US Army Medical Research Institute of Infectious Diseases; June 1998.

Centers for Disease Control and Prevention. Bioterrorism alleging use of anthrax and interim guidelines for management—United States, 1998. *MMWR Morb Mortal Wkly Rep*. 1999;48: 69–74.

Inglesby TV, Henderson DA, Bartlett JG, *et al*. Anthrax as a biological weapon: medical and public health management. *JAMA*. 1999;281: 1735–1745.

Meselson M, Guillemin J, Hugh-Jones M, *et al*. The Sverdlovsk anthrax outbreak of 1979. *Science*. 1994;266:1202–1208.

Pile JC, Malone JD, Eitzen EM, Friedlander A. Anthrax as a potential biological warfare agent. *Arch Intern Med*. 1998;158:429–434.

Levitin HW, Siegelson HL. Hazardous materials: disaster medical planning and response. *Emerg Med Clin North Am*. 1996;14:327–348.

Hospital Emergency Departments: A Planning Guide for the Management of Contaminated Patients. Atlanta, Ga: Agency for Toxic Substances and Disease Registry; 1992. *Managing Hazardous Materials Incidents*; Vol 2.

Nozaki H, Hori S, Shinozawa Y, *et al*. Secondary exposure of medical staff to sarin vapor in the emergency room. *Intensive Care Med*. 1995;21: 1032–1035.

Gough AR, Markus K. Hazardous materials protections in ED practice: laws and logistics. *J Emerg Nurs*. 1989;15:447–480.

Dart RC, Stark Y, Fulton B, Koziol-McLain J, Lowenstein SR. Insufficient stocking of poisoning antidotes in hospital pharmacies. *JAMA*. 1996; 276:1508–1510.

FEMA Report to GAO for CSEPP. Washington,DC: Federal Emergency Management Agency, Region X; September 28, 1998.

Hearings Before the Subcommittee on National Security, Veterans Affairs, and International Relations, US House of Representatives Committee on Government Reform, 106th Congr, 2nd Sess (2000) (testimony of S.M. Ostroff, associate director for epidemiologic science, National Center for Infectious Diseases, Centers for Disease Control and Prevention).

Wikipedia. (2006c). September 11, 2001 attacks. Retrieved March 30, 2006 from http://en.wikipedia.org/wiki/9/11.

Wikipedia. (2007). 2004 Madrid train bombings. Retrieved May 9, 2007 from http://en.wikipedia.org/wiki/2004_Madrid_train_bombings.

Raddatz, M. (October 29, 2002). Stronger than heroin. US believes form of fentanyl killed hostages in Russian theater. ABCNEWS.com. Retrieved November 8, 2003 from www.abcnews.com.

CNN Wolf Blitzer Reports (February 13, 2004). CNN.com—Transcripts. Retrieved March 30, 2006, from http://edition.cnn.com/TRANSCRIPTS/0402/13/wbr.00.html.

Health Resources and Services Administration. (June 2005). Emergency system for advance registration of volunteer health professionals (ESAR-VHP) programme—Interim technical and policy guidelines, standards, and definitions. Retrieved February 6, 2006

Health Resources and Services Administration. (September 2005). Emergency System for Advance Registration of Volunteer Health Professionals (ESAR-VHP)—Legal and Regulatory Issues. Retrieved on February 6, 2006 www.hrsa.gov/bioterrorism/esarvhp.

Wikipedia. (2006a). Megaton. Retrieved March 30, 2006 from http://en.wikipedia.org/wiki/Megaton.

Peterson, C. (September 30, 2006). "Be Safe, Be Prepared: Emergency System for Advance Registration of Volunteer Health Professionals in Disaster Response" *OJIN: The Online Journal of Issues in Nursing*. Vol. 11, No. 3, Manuscript 2.

Cox, C.W., (Jan. 31, 2008) "Manmade Disasters: A Historical Review of Terrorism and Implications for the Future" *OJIN: The Online Journal of Issues in Nursing*. Vol. 13, No. 1.

Control and Prevention. Epi Info, Version 6.04b. Atlanta, Ga: Centers for Disease Control and Prevention; 1997.

Appendix

Defense Measures Against Biological Warfare

(Based on the military defense model) as adapted from Richards *et al.* (1999) and Pavlin, Eitzen, and Caudle (1997).

Note that examples noted with an asterisk (*) denote measures that may specifically involve nurses.

Measure	*Examples*
Active Defenses—with the exception of Good Intelligence, these measures are outside the scope of practice for most health care professionals	* Good Intelligence—early knowledge of specific threats allows for timely countermeasures; surveillance is the key here • Rapid maneuver of forces—this measure is exercised against the enemy before it has time to become positioned or well-organised • Counterattack against those with bio-weapons—entails eliminating the biological threat
Passive Defenses—these are physical countermeasures that are implemented to reduce exposure and to minimize the effects of biological agents	• Environmental detection—this is the first step in identifying if an event has even occurred. Additionally, the rate of illness should be compared to previous years to determine any abnormalities. Early recognition will lead to the prompt mobilization of prophylactic antibiotics or vaccines • *Individual protective gear—consists of clothing and masks that are donned for protection from chemical, biological, or radiological agents. The military version of this protective wear is known as "MOPP gear." MOPP = Mission-Oriented Protective Posture

Medical Defenses—these are the foundation of a proper response to biological agents in the civilian sector	• Contamination avoidance—includes the development of multi-agent sensors to detect, identify, and warn individuals of an agent, in order to avoid exposure to the agent • *Rapid decontamination—depends on the suspected agent, but in most cases is not necessary since most biological agents do not affect the skin and do not form secondary aerosols • *Laboratory diagnosis—includes obtaining specimens and institutional support for bacteriology, including a back-up plan for agents that cannot be diagnosed in a routine lab • *Vaccines—includes the administration of vaccines as well as the development of new ones based on the impending threat of bioterrorism • *Medications and Medical Supplies—involves administering medications and may include accessing CDC's Strategic National Stockpile (SNS) for a catastrophic event. The SNS is a national repository for antibiotics, chemical antidotes, antitoxins, and life-saving medications as well as medical-surgical items. For more information on the SNS, explore www.bt.cdc.gov/stockpile (CDC, 2007). • *Isolation or quarantine—involves enforcing infection control practices, keeping in mind that most agents are not transmitted from person to person (except for smallpox and pneumonic plague) so that nearly all patients can be managed with standard universal precautions

Immediate Actions in a Suicide Bombing Event, Based on the Experience of the Israelis

(adapted from ; Stein and Hirshberg, 1999).

- Secure the scene
- Have a bomb squad sweep the area prior to treating the casualties (so that rescue personnel do not become victims themselves if terrorists have booby-trapped the site with more explosive devices)
- Prohibit responders from entering the scene if sniper fire exists
- Direct the wounded to pre-identified trauma centers
- Photograph and videotape the scene
- Rapidly remove victims from the scene
- Number the human remains sequentially and place in body bags, then transport to the medical examiner's office
- Provide rapid cadaver identification, so that the victims may be identified, released to their families, and buried according to religious customs
- Establish a command information center, so that relatives have one source to contact, rather than calling individual hospitals in search of their loved ones

Management Phases at a Disaster Scene (adapted from Stein and Hirshberg, 1999)

Chaotic Phase	Lasts approximately 15–20 minutes after a terrorist event
Reorganisation Phase	Lasts about 60 minutes and begins once a leader is clearly identified and takes charge
Site-clearing Phase	Lasts 100-180 minutes and involves the evacuation of victims
Late Phase	Can persist up to 48 hours after the event and is the period utilized for evidence collection, reconstruction of the event, and clearing of all debris

Disaster Management Triage Categories (adapted from Frykberg, 2002)

Category	Color Code	Description
Immediate/Urgent	Red	Injuries that unless urgently treated will result in death (e.g., tension pneumothorax, exsanguinating hemorrhage, airway compromise)

Delayed Yellow	Involves patients who are expected to survive, but have life-threatening wounds, but in whom delay is acceptable (e.g., open fractures, mild flash burns)
Minor, Minimal, or Ambulatory Green	"Walking wounded"—injuries are minimal and require little or no treatment
Expectant/Unsalvageable/Dead Black	Injuries are so severe that they are anticipated to die, even if multiple resources are available (e.g., penetrating head wounds, large burns, cardiac arrest)

Suggestions for In-hospital Care of Victims of Mass Casualties Caused by Terrorist Bombings (adapted from Alfici *et al.*, 2006)

Stable Victims	• The main concern with a large numbers of victims is that some will have a life-threatening injury that will be missed with initial triage; however, this rarely happens • These patients constitute 90% of casualties, with half of them having an acute psychological reaction • Primary and secondary surveys are critical in the evaluation of these patients • Ancillary services (e.g., laboratory and radiology) should be utilized for unstable victims first • Hemodynamically stable patients with fragment penetration from bombs should be hospitalized for observation, because it is not possible to explore all wounds at this time when assessing penetration
Unstable Victims	• A patient's respiratory rate and oxygen saturation are more reliable that a chest x-ray when evaluating lung blast injuries • The presence of blood in a victim's airway is a dependable

sign that a blast lung injury has been sustained

- Avoid an emergency room thoracotomy in patients with a primary blast lung injury, since visualization of where to safely place the aortic clamp is hindered
- After stabilizing lung blast injuries, a secondary survey needs to be done to rule out other injuries
- Patients with head, neck, or trunk fragment penetration should have a chest X-ray and a computerized tomography (CT) scan; the CT scan is useful in identifying foreign bodies as well as sometimes projecting the tract that the foreign body has taken
- Those with a solitary entry wound to the neck, abdomen, or extremity should be taken immediately to the operating room to explore and control bleeding
- Protocol for unstable victims includes:
  1. Obtaining immediate airway control via rapid sequence induction and intubation , all the while supporting the c-spine.
  2. Using positive pressure ventilation (PPV) with intubated patients, keeping in mind that PPV may further induce barotrauma to the lungs
  3. Controlling external hemorrhages, including those on the back of the trunk; considering temporarily packing skin wounds to tamponade hemorrhages

4. Inserting two intravenous (IV) lines and drawing baseline labs
5. Infusing blood products and crystalloids per Advanced Trauma Life Support (ATLS) protocols
6. Reevaluating the patient with consideration of inserting chest tubes to rule out hemothoraxes
7. In most cases, disregarding diagnostic peritoneal lavage (DPL) and focused abdominal sonography (FAST) since these patients need to have a laparotomy to rule out significant abdominal injury

In Extremis Victims

- These are not common in-hospital patients, since most die at the disaster site
- If these patients do make it to the hospital, the results of any immediate treatment are usually unfavorable
- Isolated reports of survival for in extremis patients do exist, so resuscitation may be considered if resources are available

APPENDIX I

INCIDENT COMMAND SYSTEM (ICS)

The existing framework to deal with the disaster management whether natural or made-made has failed to respond quickly and efficiently to save the human lives, property, infrastructure causing a great loss to development of the country. Shivaraj Patil, Minister of Home Affairs has rightly said that the increasing incidents of disasters have been hampering poverty reduction, environmental protection and sustainable development. Disasters wipe out years of development and consumer resources that could have been used for development and social welfare of the people. Disasters and poverty compound each other in vicious cycle.

In spite of this understanding our organisational framework in India has not been effective to deal promptly with disasters. Hari Jai Singh states in his article, "Faulty System and Poor Response: Technology as a Tool For Disaster Management" in the *Daily Tribune* (Feb. 9, 2001) said that despite numerous natural calamities in the past, a viable disaster management system is missing. There is no point in boasting about our information technology revolution. We have hardly used UT power for the service of the people. It needs to be realized that information technology has made today's statecraft and politico-economic management virtually outdated. It is, therefore, necessary to shed the old mindset. It is not the people but the system, the persons at the helm and the poor standard of governance which have invariably failed the nation. This has once again been proved by the way of the people, here and abroad have responded to one of the biggest disasters ever to hit the country in the wake of the devastating earthquake in Gujarat.

Amit Sengupta in his article "Dumbstruck by *Hindustan Times* (February 8, 2001) painfully remarks that: While the bureaucracy in Bhuj and Gandhinagar had let us not forget New Delhi—twiddles its thumbs, making false claims and utterly hollow promise, reality tells a dark tale of a democracy where the political class has proved its cold insensitivity and professional inefficiency even in the face of such a disaster. There is a lesson for the people of India after this catastrophe: the hallucinatory patriotic euphoria of India being a nuclear power and a potential superpower in the new millennium is a lot of hogwash. When it comes to the mighty Indian State, it is nothing but a clueless paper tiger, a dumb, monolith. It is nowhere in sight when it comes to coping with mass tragedy as we now see in the dead cities and villages of Kutch.

There will always be damage, deaths, grief and terror. That no one can prevent. But it can be minimized, to the extent that an effective government can, with a system that responds quickly, has access to what is needed, gets it there, mobilizes personnel and—very importantly—makes as much information available as possible.

Ajit Seth in his article, "Trauma in Gujarat" (*Economics Times,* January 30, 2001) rightly suggests the need of co-ordination among NGOs to tackle the problems of earthquake. In this context, the role of NGOs deserves mention. No doubt these organisations often perform a yeoman service. But past experience in the wake of other earthquake calamities show that NGOs and individual volunteers in their anxiety and even zeal often bountifully give away relief material at sites nearest to the road. This leads to inequitable distribution. The moral: coordinate and guide the efforts of different voluntary agencies and individuals.

Co-ordination within and among various agencies/departments of the state/central governments is, of course, paramount. No doubt, this is being done. But let us remember that in the confusion and chaos which follows such devastation, it is not unknown for such coordination to collapse, particularly at the district level. This sometimes can even lead to an erosion of the hierarchal structure which is most effective for decision-making under such disaster conditions.

Based upon past experiences in dealing with disasters, we mention a number of problems and weaknesses that are visible—

(a) Professional teams with training are not provided to authorities at all levels.
(b) Specific teams with specialized tasks are not ready, rather teams carry out all types of activities causing confusion.
(c) Inadequate Resource Inventory.
(d) Action takes place only after the disaster as no exercises of professional teams is done like military operations.
(e) Lack of effective communication in Net work.
(f) Absence of unity of command and wide span of control.
(g) Lack of designated facilities.
(h) No financial discipline.

INCIDIENT COMMAND SYSETM (ICS)

Evaluation

Incident Command System (ICS) was developed in early 1970s in the United States in response to a series of major wild land fires in southern California. As a response, several agencies collaborated to form the (FIRESCOPE) Firefighting Resources of California Organised for Potential Emergencies to address these difficulties and this interagency effort resulted in the development of ICS model of management.

Command System (ICS) is an on-scene, all-risk flexible moundar system adaptable to any scale of natural as well as mandate emergency/ incidents. The ICS seeks to strengthen the existing disaster response management system by ensuring that the designated controlling/

responsible authorities at different levels are backed by trained Incident Command Teams (ICTs), whose members have been, trained in the different facets of emergency/disaster response management. The ICS will not put in place any new hierarchy or supplant the existing system, but will only reinforce it. The Members of the ICT will not jointly trained for development as a team. When an ICT is deployed for an incident, all concerned agencies of the Government will respond as per the assessment of the Team. This system therefore enables proper co-ordination amongst the different agencies of the Government.

(i) Incident Command

Has overall responsibility as the incident determines objectives and establishes priorities based on the nature of the incident, available resources and agency policy. Under this, the commander has the main responsibility to define objectives, prioritise them and take overall responsibility. The Incident commander must posses emotional intelligence. Emotional intelligence is concerned with achieving one's goals through the ability to manage one's own feelings and emotions, to be sensitive to, and influence other key people, and to balance one's motives and drives with conscientious and ethical behaviours. The following area its characteristics:

(i) Inter-personal sensitivity covering competencies like listening and sensitivity.
(ii) Motivating, including impact and energy.
(iii) Emotional Resilence.
(iv) Influence and Adaptability covering both influencing and negotiating ability and being adaptable in various types of situations and cultures.
(v) Decisiveness and assertiveness.
(vi) Integrity.
(vii) Leadership including motivating other people.

Peter Drucker defined it as the lifting of man's visions to higher sihts, the raising of man's performance to higher standard, the building of man's personality beyond its normal limitations. According to Chester I. Bernard "It refers to the quality of the behaviour of the individuals whereby they guide people on their activities in organised efforts."

(ii) Operations

Develops tactical organisation and directs all resources to carry out the Incident Action Plan. Likert has beautifully brought forth this point. To quote him:

The performance and output of any enterprise depend entirely upon the quality of the human organisation and its capacity to function as a tightly knot, highly motivated, technically competent entity,, i.e. as a highly effective interaction-influence system. High productivity, high quality products, high earnings, and successful use of research and development are not accomplished by impersonal equipment or computers. These goals are achieved by human beings. Successful organisations are those making the best use of competent personnel to perform efficiently all the tasks required by the enterprises.[1]

(iii) Planning:

Develops the Incident Action Plan to accomplish the objectives Collects and evaluates information, and maintain status of assigned resources. Cyril, L. Hudson has given a comprehensive definition of planning in the following terms:

To plan is to produce a scheme for future action, to bring about specified results, at specified cost, in a specified period of time. It is a deliberate attempt to—influences, exploit, bring about, and control the nature, direction, extent, speed and effects of change. It may even attempt deliberately to create change. It is a carefully controlled and co-ordinated activity. Plan implementation is an integral part of planning process. It requires responsibility for translating the objectives of plan into action. However, looking from the broader point of view, the plan implementation requires cooperation, coordination and commitment at all levels of the implementing machinery, starting with the ministries at the Union and State Levels, through to various non-secretariat organisations in the field at district, block or village level. It is at the implementation level that the difficulties creep in, resulting into the lower output Implementation must be watched properly and timely action should be taken to improve administrative, technical, financial or personnel inadequacies. Planning and implementation are intimately connected. To Mr. Goetz: "Plans alone cannot make an enterprise successful. Action is required; the enterprise must operate. Plans can, however, focus action on purposes. They can forecast which actions will tend towards the ultimate objective ... which tend away, which will likely offset one another, and which are merely irrelevant. Managerial Planning seeks to achieve a consistent and coordinated structure of operations focussed on desired ends. Without plans, action must become merely random activity producing nothing but chaos."

A common tautology that permeates the field of Planning is that implementation is one of the most crucial aspects of any planning exercise. Within the development context, where resources of all types are generally scarce successful implementation can represent the most critical of all issues in the process of planning, growth and development.

Experience with the Five Year Plans has demonstrated that form the very start of the planning process, implementation is generally slow even half-hearted, and there is a wide gap between the results achieved and the

1. GOI, Ministry of Home Affairs, LBSNAA, Source Book on "District Management", p. 85.

planned targets. Many of the schemes have consequently to be carried over to the next plan. It is a happy sign that the Government of India is keen to lay greater stress on implementation and that the highest priority is being given in the Plans to "Operationalize the Plan."

(iv) Logistics

Logistic provides resources and all other services needed to support the organisation. Resources are an essential requirement to take immediate action for disaster management. Without Logistics, commander and his staff cannot function. The exercise of the availability and need of resources are an essential exercise. In emergency situation, we must know before hand where the resources are stored or from where these can be purchased. A tentative performed containing the list of articles is given in Appendices 3.1, 3.2 and 3.3.

We must ensure that all the logistics are available and are, functional form. We have failed in logistics in previous disasters causing great loss to people and property.

(v) Finance/Administration

Monitors costs related to the incident, provides accounting procurement, time recording, cost analysis and overall fiscal guidance. Administration is at the core of all human affairs. Its principal aspects are the formulation of policy and then its implementation for the attainment of the stated objectives in an optimum manner. It is the systematic ordering of affairs and the calculated use of resources aimed at making the desired things happen and forestalling everything to the contrary. According to a World Bank Report, Robert McNamara, former President of the World Bank, " Management is in the end, the most creative of all the arts-for its medium is human talent itself[2]

Financial Administration is a branch of Public Administration which can help an organisation in the 'management' of financial resources through the application of well thought out principles, practices and rationalized techniques of raising, allocating and utilizing financial resources for the fulfilment of organisational objectives, systematically and scientifically. It may be defined as the art and science of policy-making, planning, decision-making, coordination, control of the processes of securing adequate resources, ensuring their safe custody, genuine allocations among different areas of socio-economic development, effective utilization and avoiding the pilferage of resources and duplication of efforts to attain the objectives of the disaster management Government in Government. In short, we may define financial administration as the technique of maximizing financial output and the optimization of financial resources.

---

2. Speech of Millsap's College, Jackson, Mississippi, February 24, 1960.

According to Prof. M.J.K. Thavraj: "Finance is the lifeblood of all magnetized socio-economic formations ranging from nuclear families complex, national and international organisations. Financial administration relates to the system, which generates, regulates and distributes the monetary resources needed for the sustenance and growth of an organisation. In this respect, financial administration is similar to to the circulatory system in complex living organisms.[3]

Financial administration is a systematized and specialized branch of knowledge of the techniques, which can help in administering financial resources for optimum performance. It is becoming more and more complex day-by-day. Until and unless we understand all the implications of such an administrations, we may not be able to reap the potential benefits of the financial resources employed in an organisation like ICA. A large number of training institutes have sprung up in all the countries at all levels to impart training in financial administration. Thus, financial administration is a definite art, which can be learnt and practiced to produce pre-designed output. It is an art as it can help to direct and guide the administrators in the formulation and implementation of financial policies of an organisation efficiently and systematically.

In his preface, Shri Rajiv Raj Mishra, IAS to. Introductory Workshop and Brainstorming Consultation at Colombo, Sri Lanka observed that Incident Command System is essentially a management system that seeks to organize various emergency functions in a single framework. The significance of this framework lies in its provision for smooth coordination between different management components. The approach in ICS is to appreciate that emergency functions such as rescue, relief, logistics, information and communication, etc. are specialized task which differ substantially in content from routine administrative jobs and therefore require adequate training beforehand. Further all such functions need to be integrated in a management framework so that such response does not suffer from disjointed efforts and affect overall performance.[4]

Sh S.S.L. Hettiarachchi in an Introductory Workshop and Brainstorming consultation at Colombo, observes that the Incident Command System (ICS) by definition as a Standardized Emergency Management System designed to allow users to adopt an integrated organisational structure equal to the complexity and demands of any emergency, irrespective of its type and magnitude. We recognize the fact that all emergencies are highly chaotic, very dynamic in character and on many occasions associated with an unparalleled degree of surprise. The ICS by its very functional mechanism provides accurate information, high

---

3. M.J.K. Thavraj, Financial Management of Government, New Delhi, Sultan Chand, 1978, p. 1.
4. Centre for Disaster Management, LBSNAA, Mussoire, Introductory Workshop and Brainstorming at Colombo, Sri Lanka, 11-12 January, 2006, Preface.

degree of accountability, and a platform for planning cost effective operations and logistical support for any emergencies.[5]

David Summer from US Department of Agricultural, Forest Services underlines the important features of ICS in the above mentioned workshop.

- Clear Objectives and priorities
- Incident Action Plan.
- Common Terminology.
- Common communications.
- Uniform Position Descriptions.
    - o Roles and responsibilities defined.
    - o Clear lines of authority, chain of command and reporting requirements.
- Standardized personnel qualifications and training—national coordinating group.[6]

ICS in India

The Government of India has collaborated with the United States Agency for International Development (USAID) for institutionalizing ICS in India after making required adaptation to make it suitable for our system of administration. This is one of the important components of GOI-USAID 'Disaster Management Support Programme'.[7]

It must be clearly understood that ICS is not to be set-up as an independent agency, rather its main principles can be incorporated in the existing set-up which can make our existing disaster management machinery competent, efficient and responsive. This work has been entrusted to Lal Bahadur National Academy of Administration Mussorie (LBSNAA) as a nodal agency. Let us discuss the components of ICS.

I. Training

Training in new technology is the most important function under ICS. For this purpose, training of Master trainers has been done in stipulated modules in the first instance, while training of trainers in the second phase for which six regional training hubs have been set-up and training of district officials in the third phase. To implement this programme a core group of 20 master trainers were identified for training in India and abroad. In addition, all the officers holding important positions like District Magistrates, relief commissioners, trainers at Union and State level civil services institutes are included. In addition, basic elements of ICS are included in the training of civil services.

---

5. Introductory Workshop and Brainstorming Consultation at Colombo, Sri Lanka, 12 Jan. 2006.
6. David Sumer, *Ibid.*, p. 19.
7. Centre for Disaster Management, LBSNAA, .Introduction to Incident Command System, First Edition, 2006, p. 6.

2. Selecting Incident Commander and Command Staff

The success and failure of ICS would depend mainly upon the right selection of Incident commander and his staff as he is to discharge all the functions and take decisions to face any incident or disaster. A commander is a person who plans, organizes, makes decisions and influences people and has a positive attitude towards people and towards their work. A number of factors are involved in the ability to lead, including the following:

(a) Insight into human behaviour.
(b) Ability to plan, organize and direct effort of others.
(c) Decision-making ability on a practical and realistic basis.
(d) Ability to co-ordinate the efforts of others.
(e) Keep the environment of work place stimulating.

Stoggill gives the following traits for commander:

Intelligence, Dependability, Responsibility, Scholarship, Social Participation and Socio-Economic status.[8]

Gheselli identifies the following traits:

Intelligence, supervisory ability, initiative, self-assurance, and self-perceived occupational level.[9]

Understanding and Directing Change

New millennium is going to be different and the new millennium needs leaders who can understand and redirect this change into fruitful changes. Leadship and change are closely linked. An awareness of the changing atmosphere at the workplace calls for leaders who can understand and deal with the changing paradigms of corporate culture. No longer is it enough for a manager to limit his job to doing thin things on time, within budget and the way they were done yesterday, only five percent better Leaders are today treading on completely unfamiliar territory where yesterday's rules no longer apply. Uncertainty is now an inescapable fact and things no longer happen in a predictable in Innovation is the new mantra for the leaders of today. They make new rules almost as fast as the old ones become redundant. Under circumstances, it is imperative for a leader to have a clear vision where his organisation is headed. In the absence of such vision, it is all too easy for orgnization, both old and new, to flounder and fail.

Norman Vincent Peale has advised the leaders to be highly charged. To quote him: Think Excitement, talk excitement, act excitement, act out excitement and you are bound to become an excited person. Life will take on a new zest, deeper interest, and greater meaning.

8. R.M. Stogill, Personal Factors Associated with Leadership: A Survey of Literature, *Journal of Psychology,* Vol. 25, 1948, pp. 35-71.
9. Ghesill, The Validity of Management Traits, related to *Occupational Self-Personnel Psychology,* Vol. 16, No. 2, 1963, pp. 109-14.

Incident commander as per the scheme of ICS has the following duties to perform:

- Determine incident objectives and strategy.
- Establish the immediate priorities.
- Establish an Incident Command Post.
- Establish an appropriate organisation.
- Ensure planning meetings are scheduled as required.
- Approve and authorize the implementation of incident action plan.
- Ensure the adequate safety measures are in place.
- Coordinate activity for all Command and General Staff.
- Coordinate with key people and officials.
- Approve requests for additional resources or for the release of resources.
- Keep agency administrator informed of incident status.
- Approve the use of students, volunteers, and auxiliary personnel.
- Authorize release of information to the news media.
- Order the demobilization of the incident when appropriate.[10]

3. Incident and Team Work—Management by Objectives

The emphasis in team building is on improving the effectiveness and efficiency of the group and not of the individuals alone or group. It of is a set of techniques by which personnel in an organisational group diagnose as to how they work together and plan the needed changes that will improve their performance and ultimately organisational efficiency.

Organisations produce very little solely from individual effort. According to Margulies and Raia.[11] "Most effective team action is not easy to achieve in which Tom, Dick and Harry are trained independently or separately .... "

The research in the utility of this technique has clearly indicated that properly planned Team Building Approach has positive impact and influence. Michael Beer concluded optimistically: "Team building or group development is perhaps the most powerful and pervasive OD technology available to the change agent. Its design provides data for diagnosis and unfreezing, incorporates experimental learning, and provides the means for refreezing new behaviour. Furthermore, the process of team development is likely to change organisational inputs (needs, values and skills) and a wide variety of group (cohesiveness, communication, planning). Through

10. Centre for Disaster Management, LBSNAA, Introduction to Incident Command System, 2005, pp. 23-24.
11. N. Margulies and Raja, A.P., "Organisation Development: Values, Process Technology", New York: McGraw Hill, 1972, p. 263.

problems identification, it can also immediate change in organisational output.[12]

According to Mike Lohre, "Advantages of Pre-established teams for ICS are:

- Local 'teams' and first responders often become 'victims' of large disasters.
- Standing teams have the advantage of experience based upon effectiveness and efficiencies.
- Standing teams maintain a 'core knowledge' by ensuring that no more than a 20% turnover of team member per year.
- Rapid mobilization through 'one call'.
- Pre-established teams ensures availability when the need exists.
- Background of diversity and experiences in incident management leads to knowledge-knowledge leads to wisdom—wisdom leads to the ability to anticipate and meets the needs of the Responsible Officials, those affected, and the public.
- Ability to meet Commander's Intent.
- Development of teamwork through years of experiences in working together on complex, challenging assignments."[13]

4. Unity and Chain of Command

In ICS commander issues command through line of authority to ensure compliance of order and effective communication.

5. Incident and Organisational Competence: A Flexibility

Even the best machine gets rusty without timely maintenance. Many aspects of the working of an organisation have to be examined, to evolve a modified design for an on-going organisation, in order to ensure their efficiency. Development in information technology requires further dramatic organisational restructuring through organisational National competitiveness will increasingly depend on flexibility requiring fast responses from a government that is enabling rather than providing the directions for change.

This includes details about the levels of supervision, the chian of command, the accountability and transparency in the functioning of an organisation and finally the criteria for evaluation. Organisation building is extremely important in the field of Public Administration. No administrative performance is possible without a suitable organisation."[14]

---

12. Michael Beer, "The Technology of Organisation Development", Marvin D. Dunnette, ed., Handbook of Industrial and Organisational Psychology, Chicago, Rand McNally, 1979, p. 960.
13. Introductory Workshop and Brainstorming Consultation at Colombo, Sri Lanka, 11-12 Jan. 2006, *op. cit.*, p. 31.
14. Following studies carried out by the writer can be studied to understand the practical application of organisational analysis:

According to Dimock and Dimock, "Organisation is the systematic bringing together of interdependent parts to form a unified the whole through which authority, co-ordination and control may be exercised to achieve a given purpose.[15]

According to Mooney, "Organisation is the forum of every human association for the attainment of a common purpose."

Organisational analysis is a technique to ensure the achievement of maximum results with minimum costs, in terms of human and material resources of the organisations. The objective of organisational analysis is to improve pattern of relationships between persons in an organisation and to create harmonious arrangement of work with reference to its main objectives. The need for the design of sound organisational structures for an enterprise and their continual evaluation in terms of suitability through organisational analysis has been recognized as an effective means to promote improvement in corporate performance. Peter F. Drucker has rightly observed: "Good organisation structure does not by itself produce good performance—just as good constitution does not guarantee great Presidents, or good laws a moral society. But a poor organisation structure makes good performance impossible, no matter how good the individuals may be."[16]

6. Incident and Community Participation

Community participation involves members of communities in planning, implementing and monitoring of activities. Thus, community is wholly involved in the programme, rather than being asked to either contribute or to take advantage of the services offered under it. Community participation is the process in which individual, families assume responsibility for their own programme. They come to know their own situation better and are motivated to solve their common problems. This enables them to become agents of their own development, instead of development aid. They, therefore, need to realize that they are not obliged to accept conventional solutions that are not suitable. They have to acquire the capacity to appraise a situation, weigh the various possibilities and estimate what their own contribution can be.

I. Organisation and working of the South-East Asia, Regional Office of WHO, Sterling Publishers, New Delhi, 1977.

II. Organisation and Managerial problems of Apex Co-operative Organisation with special reference to MARKFED, *Cooperative Perspectives*, Vol. 2, No. I, June 1977.

III. Organisation and Management of Co-operative Organisation, *Indian Co-operative Review*, Vol. XIV, No. 2, New Delhi, January, 1977.

IV. Organisation and Administration of Family Planning Field Work: A Case Study of Haryana, PEN, A Magazine of Family Planning Association of India (Haryana Branch) 27 Aug., 1975.

15. Dimock and Dimock: Public Administration, p. 104.

16. Peter F. Drucker: The Practice of Management, Hienemann, London, 1955, p. 225.

7. Incident and Event Planning

Planning is the exercise of intelligence to deal with facts and solutions as they are and find a way to solve problems. Planning is in essence, an organised, conscious and continual attempt to select the best available alternatives to achieve specific goals. Planning is the phase of the total process which leads from the policy statements to the concrete identification of the populations whose needs and demands will be served; the identification of the types of activities that will be performed for these populations with their general attributes, and the specification of the type of instruments that will be required to carry out the activities.

John E. Laing has mentioned the following essentials of planning, kept in mind:

Rational

Much of what passes for planning in executing programmes is is based on unconscious or at best, unexpected thought process of the decision-maker. Such decisions, based on hunches, intuition or past experiences should play an important role in the planning process but only in conjunction with rational consideration of cost benefits and alternatives.

Deliberate

Planning should not involve hurried decision except in special emergencies.

Specific

Whereas policy provides broad guidelines for action, planning should be more specific, breaking each task into its component parts, defining each individual's functions and responsibilities, specifying programmes goals in measurable quantitative terms.

Comprehensive

Planning should cover such diverse components of the programme source allocation, research and evaluation, information and motivation, delivery of services and programme effects.

Systematic

Plan for each component should be both internally consistent and consistent with the plans for the other components.

Continuous

Plans should continuously undergo revision in response changing conditions and to the findings from programme evaluation. If planning for incident operations did not attend to incident operations, this can cause poor use of resources, higher costs and lower effectiveness. Incident action Plan is of great significance for disaster management economically and efficiently.

Critical Appraisal

We have discussed the Incident Command System adopted by Govt. of India through integration in their existing Organisational framework for making disaster management efficient, effective and successful as disaster is vulnerable to development. This is a good attempt to modernize our out-dated disaster management system. However, we have to keep the following facts and suggestions in mind to maintain the system.

I. Training should be Meticulous and Practical

Training connotes that the trainers can influence the performance of the trainees. The influence takes the form of knowledge, attitude and action. The ultimate success of the training depends upon the change in behaviour of the trainees, who in turn can inject efficiency and effectiveness in their services. Action training is aimed at creating a situation in which employees can act optimally. Morton R. Davies rightly mentions the need of Action Training. To quote him, "Action training is designed to achieve explicit, predetermined results which will enhance attainment of an objective of an enterprise in a recognizable, preferably quantifiable way. Action Training is designed to solve a problem, to effect change, to implement a policy or to arrive at 0 observable and predictable results."[17]

One of the key factors in the effort of the government to accomplish its development goals in the area of disaster management is to enhance its administrative capability for development at all levels of administrative hierarchy, which is very much a part of the development process. Such complex problems call for a multi-disciplinary solution to, which concerned people at all levels must apply their technical skills, general knowledge and understanding. The education and training of responsible staff engaged in disaster management are absolutely essential, if worthwhile results are to be obtained. This is true whether they are politicians, administrators, executives, technical people or clerical personnel. But, our experience during the last three decades has demonstrated that the development plans have not been satisfactorily implemented, because of inadequate administrative performance. The reasons for the low level of administrative performance include: organisational defects, lack of coordination, complex and cumbersome administrative and financial procedures, etc. These defects and deficiencies need to be corrected in order to bring about a sharp reduction in the administrative obstacles to disaster management and bridge the gap between aspirations and performance. Simultaneously, the level of competence of public service personnel directly involved in the execution of projects and implementation of development plans can be raised by training them in modern concepts and techniques of disaster administration and management. The following flow chart clearly explains the scientific method of training.

17. Morton R. Davis, Organising for Training, in *I.P.A.*, Jan.-March 1992.

Training should be delivered as close an approximation to the work situation as possible, and that which is intended to achieve the implementation of specified tasks or procedures should be whenever possible, carried out in the work place itself. When training is provided as a framework of action, the overall training process is likely to take the form of a series of projects specifically aimed at implementing new programmes, polices or procedures. One of the major advantages of a project-based training programme is the possibility it affords to identify specific goals and objectives to each element of the programme.

2. Persons identified should be in Continuous use

In India, persons trained on a transferred. As and when, any disaster occupying those positions in the failure through *ad hoc* arrangements.

3. Efficient Organisational Network

For ICS, we need efficient organisational set-up in India, organisational system is like a disaster. The need of the hour is to understand the underlying strengths weaknesses of one's organisation and adopt a strategy, which ensure its continuous growth and progress. Efforts need to be made to capitalize the skills of the fellow members by creating an appropriate environment to stimulate creativity and diffuse leadership. The pursuit for excellence could be imbibed by the rank and file of an orgnaisation, through its core-ideological structure. The structure therefore needs to inspire appropriable innovations and facilitate their execution in such a way that orgnisation is able to sustain its enviable reputation. The role of management, thus, is that of a catalyst, in order to ensure success and survival of an organisation.

4. Planning and Implementation

We in India are good at Planning but implementation which is the real success of planning is not effective. Policy implementation would be more crucial than formulation of policy, as the outcome of policy would be dependent purely on its effective implementation. The modem advancement of information technology has been of a great help to policy-makers, but the art and science of policy implementation has not really progressed. We have formulated excellent education policy, health policy, population policy, industrial policy, but the desired outcome of these policies is nowhere near expectation. Why? Because we are not attending seriously to the meticulous designing of policy implementation contours. An added factor is the human factor upon whose will and determination would depend the outcome of policy implementation. Renis Likert has beautifully brought forth this point. To quote him:

"The performance and output of any enterprise depend entirely upon the quality of the human organisation and its capacity to function as a tightly knit, highly motivated, technically competent entity,, i.e., as a highly effective interaction-influence system. High productivity, high quality products, high earnings, and successful use of research development are not accomplished by impersonal equipment or computers. These goals are achieved by human beings. Successful organisations are those making the best use of competent personnel to perform efficiently all the tasks required by the enterprise."[18]

Richard Elmore has identified four distinct institutional models which describe alternative approaches of implementation process:

1. The "System management model" views implementation as an ordered and goal directed activity;
2. The "bureaucratic process model" views implementation mere as a routine process of continuing direction;
3. The "organisational development model" views implementation as participatory process in which implementers shape policies and claim them as their own; and
4. The "conflicting and bargaining model" views implementation as a conflict and bargaining process. This model is based on the principle of circulatory."[19]

Policy should not remain only on the paper, without yielding any result or subjected to inappropriate implementation. What can be done to ensure that policy implementation is as per the requirements of policy decisions? How can we check this perpetual tendency of neglecting implementation and not bothering about policy issues.

Utilization of Sources

The most serious problem in India is not as much of resource mobilization as that of resource utilization. In the case of Gujarat, there was no dearth of resources yet the desired impact was not produced. Let us discuss the views of some authorities on the subject. In this connection J.L. Iboko has remarked that:

"It is accepted that the inability to manage efficiently or utilize effectively the available and potential resources is the common ill of the all less developed countries. It follows that the successful development demands a sound programme for managerial improvement."[20] It has also been pointed out by an Asian administrator, Y.P. Pant, that it is only after a country is prepared for the possible process of change that international relations or foreign aid would do much to help its onward March.[21]

---

18. Renis Likert, "The Human Organisation: Its Management and Values, New York, Mc-Graw Hill, 1967, International Student Edition, Kogokusha Company, Tokyo, p. 134.
19. Quoted in Q.N. Khan, A Model of Public Policy Implementation Process, in *IJPA*, Jan.-March 1987, p. 354.
20. J.I. Ibokes: Developing the Administration in a Developing Country, *International Review of Administrative Sciences*, Vol. XXVIII, No. 2, 1972, p. 293.
21. Y.P. Pant, Economic Development of Nepal (Allahabad, 1965, p. 24).

Let us understand the nature of these problems which impede and bedevil the effective functioning of the machinery dealing with disaster administration—

(a) Lack of concrete definition of terms, policy and decisions required to mitigate the sufferings of disaster victims and their rehabilitation.
(b) Lack of clear demarcation of authority and responsibilities of personnel engaged in disaster operations resulting in confusion, overlapping and duplication of efforts.
(c) Lack of coordination among the allied agencies and within the units of a department, resulting in duplication and wastage of financial resources.
(d) Lack of reliable, timely and suitable information systems for the formulation, implementation and evaluation of policy.
(e) Widely scattered funding mechanism with little control over costs.
(f) Lack of effective mechanism to involve the employees and beneficiaries in the policy-making and implementation of the rehabilitation programmes of an organisation.
(g) Use of outdated methods and, the financial administration of financial administration.
(h) Lack of interest in improving financial administrative structures and procedures.
(i) Absence of innovative leadership, administrative capability and competence.
(j) Lack of equity in distribution and coverage with respect to the felt need.

Resource mobilization and utilization can be improved to a great extent through improved administrative system especially in the sphere of financial administration. Besides, all the resources must be utilized economically and efficiently and the expenditure on unproductive resources must be curbed. We may conclude by saying that the policy-makers, planners and decision-makers may attend to the following carefully to nurture our resources and to accomplish as much as possible with what is available:

(i) To identify who (action agents) needs how much money (cost) and for what (activities);
(ii) To define criteria for and priority in, allocation of budgetary resources among different activities and different organisations responsible for performance of activities;
(iii) To provide flexibility in budgeting and financing, if necessary beyond bureaucratic control;
(iv) To ensure the timely availability of funds to the programme activities of field level;

(v) To design Management Information System to get timely information on the utilization of resources;

(vi) To arrange statistical analysis to bring out what the performance data truly signify;

(vii) To explore and recommend possibilities of reducing costs with due regards to the maintenance of efficiency and quality;

(viii) To ensure the development of effective linkage among financial, personnel materials and other resources; and

(ix) To ensure the focus on the main objective,, i.e. mitigation of sufferings of disaster victims and their rehabilitation.

5. Effective Utilisation of Resource

The reason for poverty and misery in the developing countries is not essentially the lack of potentialities or resources, human and material but underutilization of these resources. Today, developing countries are not fully utilizing the potential capacity of human beings, owing to inadequate expertise and deficient system of public administration.

ICS has a built in process which allow resource managers at all levels to constantly monitor the status of resources. Resources cost money, therefore, ICS must pay adequate attention to this aspect as there is a danger of corrupt practices.

6. Perfect Management System Essential for ICS

ICS is basically a management system for disasters. Its success requires an efficient and effective management system. ICS has identified important areas of management essential for disaster management but they are independent.

The Incident Command System or ICS broadly refers to a management system to be used for incidents of various kinds and sizes such as earthquakes, floods, cyclones, landslides, etc. or emergencies cuased by train accidents, epidemics. The system provides scope to organize various functions, tasks and staffs within the overall response process while emphasizing greater coordination and communication among different organisations involved. ICS as a system is flexible and adaptable to suit any scale of natural as well as made-made emergency/incidents. It can be useful for routine emergencies such as road and train accidents and for large, complex multi-jurisdictional disasters such as the recent tsunami. In fact, as a management system ICS draws its strengths from its applicability to different wide range of incidents/disasters of varying scales. The main intention in using ICS is to transform the confusion during the early stage of an emergency situation into a we managed response process by providing answers to vital questions such as "who's in charge"? And "What's my job, whom to contact, etc."[22]

---

22. Introduction to Incident Command System, Centre for Disaster Management, LBSNAA, Mussorie, p. 3.

CONCLUSION

ICS is good strategy for disaster management which depends upon good administrative system in the country.

Simple commitment by management is not enough. The improvement process must become as basic and continuous as our concerns. There is no magic approach or solution to be gleaned from either a text-book or a consultant, although either of these can help management discover an effective programme for carrying out its required responsibility. But, the manager remains the key to tapping the most underutilized resource people.[23]

Efficiency programmes comprise both cost reduction (without lower standards) and performances improvement (at no higher, and preferably lower cost). They question whether a task should be done at all, whether it should be done by government directly or by contractors paid by Governments, or done by the private sector.

Since government resources are always under pressure (demand exceeds supply) and expectations exceed what can be afforded), there is an on going requirement to review activities to ensure that resources are used to best effect and that government can demonstrate sound Stewardship. Consequently, the point of entry for programmes to improve efficiency is commonly a requirement to reduce operating costs as part of budgetary restraint.[24]

23. UN: "United Nations Programme in Public Administration", (E/426-ST/TAO/M/38), pp. 11-12.
24. Mohan Kaul, Civil Service Reforms, Learning From Commonwealth Experience, in *IJPA*, July-Sept. 1998, p. 686.

Index